THE PATIENT'S GUIDE

TO MEDICAL TESTS

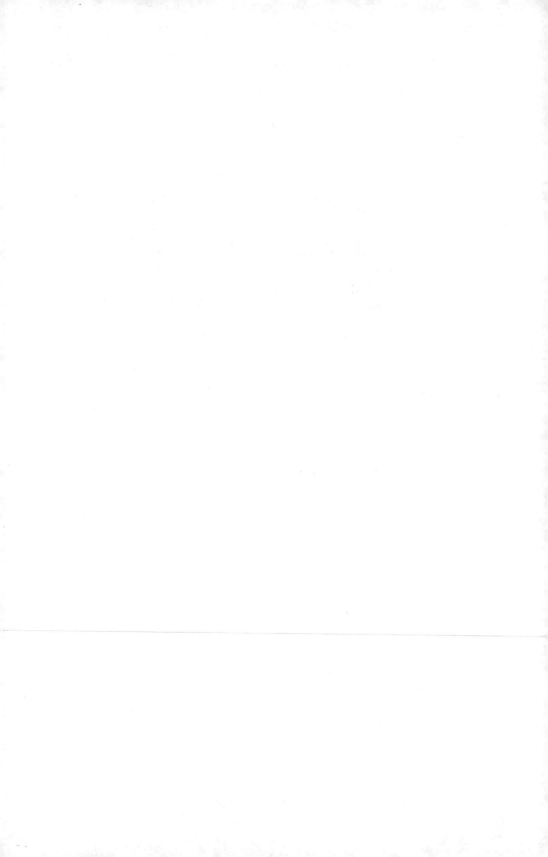

THE PATIENT'S GUIDE
TO MEDICAL TESTS

Everything You Need to Know
About the Tests Your Doctor Prescribes

Joseph C. Segen, M.D.

and

Joseph Stauffer, Ph.D.

Facts On File, Inc.

Facts On File, Inc.
11 Penn Plaza
New York NY 10001

Facts On File books are available at special discounts when purchased in bulk quantities for businesses, associations, institutions or sales promotions. Please call our Special Sales Department in New York at (212) 967-8800 or (800) 322-8755.

Library of Congress Cataloging-in-Publication Data

Segen, J. C.
    The patient's guide to medical tests : everything you need to know about the tests your doctor prescribes / Joseph C. Segen and Joseph Stauffer.
    p.   cm.
    Includes index.
    ISBN 0-8160-3471-0 (hardcover : alk. paper). — ISBN 0-8160-3530-X (pbk. : alk. paper)
    1. Diagnosis — Popular works. 2. Diagnosis, Laboratory — Popular works. 3. Patient education. I. Stauffer, Joseph. II. Title.
    RC71.3S424 1997
    616.07′5—dc21   97-37944

You can find Facts On File on the World Wide Web at
http://www.factsonfile.com

Cover design by Semadar Megged
Text design by Nancy J. Hajeski

Printed in the United States of America

MP NJ 10 9 8 7 6 5 4 3 2 1

This book is printed on acid-free paper

TABLE OF CONTENTS

To our wives, for their patience and tolerance,
and for our children, who give us purpose

Joseph C. Segen, M.D.
&
Joseph Stauffer, Ph.D.

INTRODUCTION

Rapid advances in technology and computers have affected all phases of medical testing. Science has given the medical community a much greater understanding of biological and physiological interactions in the body. Tools developed with this new technology enable the laboratory to provide more accurate, sensitive, and timely results.

High-volume chemistry analyzers can now provide 6,000 or more results an hour. Hematology analyzers can produce accurate determinations of various blood cell types, yielding a complete blood cell count and differentiate between various white blood cells in less than one minute. In microbiology, the aerospace program has led to the development of analyzers that can identify bacteria and determine which antibiotics will be useful in treatment within 24 to 48 hours.

With all this progress, the quality of results has improved tremendously. The most common source of error is specimen mix-up, and this has been minimized through the use of bar codes and positive sample identification procedures that begin from the moment the specimen is obtained. The next step, currently in development, will be the use of robotics for specimen handling; this will further reduce human error in the laboratory.

In the areas of cancer and virology, many new tests have been developed that enhance the diagnosis and monitoring of diseases. New testing methodologies involving analysis of genes are being created; these will yield information on the risk for specific diseases. More sensitive methodologies for detecting viruses are becoming available to the laboratory.

Nuclear magnetic resonance (NMR) and positron magnetic resonance (PMR) procedures are now supplanting X rays in many areas. These new procedures take images of various parts of the body without subjecting patients to radiation. Meanwhile, the interpretation of X-ray images has been made easier by the use of contrast media and image enhancers.

– THE PURPOSE OF A TEST –

Medical tests are used to establish diagnoses, determine the best treatment modality, and monitor treatment. Laboratory tests can yield results that are suggestive of specific diseases but are not reliable when used as the sole indicator of disease. Until 15 to 20 years ago, tests were ordered sequentially to make a diagnosis by a process of elimination. Today the physician is under time constraints and must order batteries of tests, some of which may be unnecessary.

Tests may also be required by employers, schools, or governmental agencies. These tests are generally of the screening type and are used to determine immunity to specific diseases or, in the case of employers, illegal drug use.

– SPECIMEN COLLECTION –

Venous blood represents physiologic conditions throughout the body and is simple to obtain via venipuncture, which is a relatively safe procedure when carried out by a trained phlebotomist. A small needle is inserted into a vein in the arm, and blood is drawn into a tube containing a vacuum. The major risk of this procedure is hematoma at the site used for drawing the sample. Sterile, disposable equipment is used, and the danger of infection to the patient is almost nonexistent. Blood specimens are also obtained from arteries in the thigh when blood gases are ordered. This is generally done in a hospital setting by specialized phlebotomy teams. Capillary blood is used for some microtechniques, usually involving pediatric patients. This is generally done by a phlebotomist pricking a fingertip and drawing the blood drops into a small tube.

Serum is obtained from whole blood by allowing the blood to clot after it is drawn into a specimen container. The resulting clot is centrifuged, and the liquid remaining in the top of the tube is serum. This is the specimen most commonly used for chemistry tests.

Plasma is obtained from whole blood to which anticoagulants have been added. The type of anticoagulant depends on the test requested. The anticoagulated whole blood is centrifuged, and the liquid remaining in the top of the tube is plasma. It is slightly different in composition from serum and cannot always be used as a substitute.

Pleural fluid is found in the lining of the lungs and is increased in various disease states. Pleural fluid is obtained by a procedure called thoracentesis. A needle is inserted into the pleural lining, and fluid is withdrawn. This is generally a hospital-based procedure and carries some risk of pneumothorax (perforation of the lung). There are several chemistry tests run on pleural fluid, but cellular analyses for unusual cells, bacteria, and viruses are the tests most commonly performed on this fluid.

Synovial fluid is also known as joint fluid. It is obtained by inserting a needle into the joint and withdrawing fluid via a syringe. It is usually obtained from swollen joints and is analyzed to determine the cause of the swelling.

Cerebrospinal fluid (CSF) is the fluid found in the spinal cord and throughout the brain. It is obtained by inserting a needle into the spinal column and withdrawing fluid via a syringe, a procedure carried out by a physician. This fluid is usually analyzed when neurological symptoms occur.

Urine specimens are classified as random or 24-hour: Random urine specimens can be obtained at any time by voiding into a clean, dry specimen container. Urine collected over a 24-hour period provides the best specimen for analysis. The first morning's specimen is discarded. All urine voided during the next 24 hours, including the following morning's specimen, is collected in the container provided by the laboratory. For some tests a special preservative is required. This is usually an acid that is placed in the collection container by the laboratory. The container should be clearly marked. Because some of the preservatives are hazardous, special care must be taken when handling these containers.

– WHAT AFFECTS THE RESULTS –

Test results can be affected by a variety of factors. Some of them are due to the manner in which the specimen was obtained and subsequently handled by laboratory personnel. A traumatic phlebotomy, one which causes a hematoma, can affect laboratory tests in several ways. The most common form is seen in hemolysis, a situation in which red blood cells burst and release their contents into the serum. Many tests are adversely affected by hemolysis, and the results cannot be correctly evaluated. Some tests require that the serum or plasma be frozen in order to insure the stability of the substance being analyzed. Failure to freeze the specimen or thawing the specimen in transit will cause false results. Other tests require that the specimen be kept at room temperature because freezing or chilling will cause deterioration of the cellular elements being tested.

Blood, plasma, and serum specimens are drawn into tubes containing various additives. The color of the tube stopper denotes the additive(s) in the tube. Below is a table listing the tube colors and additives.

TUBE CODES

COLOR	ADDITIVE
Light blue	Sodium citrate
Navy blue	No additive (for trace metals)
	Heparin (for trace metals)
Yellow	SPS (for cultures)
FSP (blue)	Thrombin, trypsin inhibitor
Gray	Potassium oxalate, sodium fluoride
Green	Heparin
Lavender	EDTA
Orange	Thrombin
Red	None
Red/gray	Inert barrier material, clot activator
Red/green	Inert barrier material, heparin
Yellow	Acid citrate dextrose (ACD)
Yellow/black	Thrombin

Many tests require that the patient follow a prescribed diet or fast prior to testing. If these restrictions are not strictly observed, test results can be invalid. This is especially true if the patient does not inform the laboratory of failure to follow the prescribed restrictions and the tests are performed as usual.

Aspirin, laxatives, cold pills, cough preparations, sleeping aids, vitamins, nose drops, pain relievers, and stomach antacids can markedly alter a test value. Prescription drugs have an even greater influence on medical testing. The American Association of Clinical Chemists has published a list of over 9,000 adverse effects on laboratory tests caused by drugs alone, and the list continues to grow each year.

A patient's daily routine, including his sleeping habits, can have a direct effect on certain tests, especially hormone evaluations. Many routine blood tests will have different results depending on whether a patient has been lying down or standing up just before blood is taken. Excessive exercise, including running, can produce what seem to be abnormal values even though there is no disease process. If a patient experiences stress or anxiety a few days before a test or at the time the test is performed, the altered mental attitude can produce abnormal test results. Sex, age, height, weight, and body surface area must be taken into account when interpreting the results of a medical test. Many tests have different reference ranges depending on these factors.

– WHERE TESTS ARE PERFORMED –

Clinical laboratory testing is performed in hospitals or commercial laboratories. Testing is closely monitored so that only necessary testing is performed. In order to reduce costs, hospital laboratories generally perform the most routine tests, while less common tests are sent to commercial laboratories. Generally, the larger the hospital, the larger the testing menu. Most physicians, clinics, and hospitals contract with commercial laboratories for services.

– COSTS –

The vast majority of patients do not pay for medical testing directly but have it paid for through health insurance plans. While most people do not question the necessity for medical tests because they rarely see a bill, everyone pays for unnecessary testing through higher premiums. It is, therefore, extremely important to review the invoices that insurance carriers submit.

The major cost involved in medical testing is the cost of equipment and labor. Laboratory analyzers range from $100,000 to $350,000. Most commercial laboratories have several pieces of equipment and must keep them functioning 24 hours a day. The same equipment is available in hospital laboratories. Other specialized testing equipment can cost up to $1 million. Labor is another expense. About six people are involved in handling each specimen from the time it is obtained until the result is available. Behind the scenes there are people involved in billing, client services, and warehousing.

Hospitals and commercial laboratories have become extremely efficient in providing testing services and have been able to keep costs low. In spite of this effort in cost containment, the yearly cost of medical testing in the United States alone is estimated to be $300 billion.

– HOW TO USE THIS BOOK –

The tests in this book are listed in alphabetical order under the name most commonly used by physicians. Because of the large number of tests available, not all tests are listed in this book. We have attempted to list the tests most commonly used by physicians and have surveyed hospitals, commercial labs, and physicians to determine which tests should be included. If there is a particular test not listed in this book, the laboratory or medical facility that performs it will provide you with appropriate literature explaining the test and what procedures should be followed.

Under each listing there is a description of the test, what is required for the performance of the test, the reference range, what abnormal values may signify, and the cost of the test. Any precautions in the evaluation of results and risks to the patient are noted under the comments section. For some tests a full entry (patient preparation, procedure, specimen, reference range, abnormal values, and cost) is not relevant because the test may be new, performed only in major medical centers, or performed only under special circumstances. Many of these tests will instead be discussed briefly in the glossary. Following is a description of the test entry format:

Description: This includes a general description of what the test measures.
Patient preparation: Any instructions for the patient or special procedures involved in performing the test are listed here.
Procedure: The specimen type and particular procedures involved in procuring the specimen are described here.
Reference range: This is the range of values observed for persons free of disease. A value outside of this range does not necessarily mean a disease process is involved. Other test results and physical findings must be evaluated in order to reach a definitive diagnosis.
Abnormal values: The diseases or symptoms that may be associated with abnormal results are listed here. In most cases the ordering physician is using the test to aid in determining the most likely cause of the symptoms.
Cost: The cost of the test is listed as a range. Testing costs vary widely depending on the facility and the locale.
Comments: Any special instructions or precautions are given in this section.

Consumers of medical treatment need to have a basic understanding of the procedures in order to make intelligent choices. This book provides information to help you evaluate your options when seeking medical care.

$$\boxed{A}$$

abdominal tap (belly tap, paracentesis, peritoneal fluid analysis) An invasive procedure in which a very long needle is inserted in the abdominal cavity to obtain fluid for either diagnostic or therapeutic purposes. The abdominal tap is a rapid way for clinicians in a hospital setting to distinguish a "surgical" abdomen (i.e., one requiring surgery) from a "nonsurgical" abdomen. Diagnostic paracentesis is performed to determine the cause of an increase in intraabdominal fluids. This is most commonly due to cirrhosis of the liver but is also caused by carcinoma, inflammation (peritonitis, pancreatitis, ruptured diverticulitis), and abdominal trauma with rupture of organs or blood vessels. One of the more important laboratory values obtained in the analysis of peritoneal fluid is the protein level, which is low in transudates (e.g., ascitic fluid) and high in exudates (e.g., inflammation and malignancy). The abdominal tap provides useful information in about 80% of cases; it may reveal unclotted blood, which indicates that bleeding is occurring within the abdomen; inflammatory cells, which suggests pancreatitis, appendicitis, diverticulitis, or rupture of an organ; or malignant cells, which may be the first indication of cancer.

Patient preparation Before the procedure, patients may be given a tranquilizer.

Procedure The patient lies on his/her back and the abdomen is sterilized with appropriate cleansing solutions. The procedure consists of the insertion of a long, 20- or 18-gauge needle on either side of the navel, from which the physician obtains fluids for chemical analysis and a sample of cells to be examined under the microscope.

Specimen Peritoneal fluid.

Reference range Normally a few mesothelial cells may be seen in the fluid obtained from an abdominal tap.

Abnormal values Fresh blood and inflammatory or malignant cells may be seen as indicated above.

Cost $100–$200.

ACE See *angiotensin-converting enzyme.*

1

acetaminophen (Tylenol®) Acetaminophen is a drug used to relieve pain and reduce fever. It differs from aspirin in that it has little anti-inflammatory activity. Overdose can result in fatal liver failure, and serum levels of acetaminophen are usually requested by the patient's physician when an overdose is suspected.

Patient preparation No preparation is required, other than for drawing blood.

Procedure Acetaminophen is measured by immunoassay procedures, using either fluorescence polarization immunoassay (FPIA) or ELISA.

Specimen Serum, plasma, urine.

Reference rang Up to 25 µg/ml is within the normal therapeutic range.

Abnormal values Toxicity occurs at levels of greater than 50 µg/ml.

Cost $25–$50.

acetone See *urinalysis.*

acetowhite lesion This lesion is a whitish patch on a woman's cervix that is seen by colposcopy when "painted" with Lugol solution (5% acetic acid, vinegar). White (the normal color of the cervix is pink) often indicates changes on the surface of the cervix that pathologists call hyperkeratosis and parakeratosis. These changes may be associated with cancer, precancerous changes known as cervical intraepithelial neoplasia (CIN, also called dysplasia), and infection by the human papillomavirus (HPV), which causes condyloma, a precancerous change.

Patient preparation The preparation is that for a colposcopy.

Procedure The woman lies on her back with her feet in stirrups while the gynecologist examines the cervix with a low-power microscope. The gynecologist coats the cervix with Lugol's solution, which stains the normal tissue a mahogany brown color, leaving the areas of potential disease (e.g., HPV infection, squamous metaplasia, dysplasia, and carcinoma) unstained. Whitish areas that suggest an abnormal lesion are biopsied, and the biopsy is submitted to a pathologist for evaluation.

Specimen Tissue sample, i.e., a biopsy.

Reference range No lesion, or mild inflammation.

Abnormal values HPV infection, metaplasia, dysplasia, and carcinoma.

Cost See *cervical intraepithelial neoplasia, colposcopy, HPV.*

acetylcholine receptor antibodies A family of antibodies that develops in myasthenia gravis, a disease that affects the transmission of nerve impulses. In normal muscle, the chemical acetylcholine is released from nerve endings and binds to the molecules known as receptors, resulting in muscle contraction. In myasthenia gravis, antibodies act against the patient's own acetylcholine receptors. This occurs in up to 95% of patients with myasthenia gravis and prevents the binding of acetylcholine to the receptors, causing muscle weakness.

Patient preparation No preparation is required, other than for drawing blood.

Procedure The antibodies are measured in the serum by a method known as radioimmunoassay.

Specimen Serum. Specimen must be kept at room temperature until analysis.

Reference range Negative, or less than 0.03 nmol/L.

Abnormal values Acetylcholine antibodies are found in myasthenia gravis.

Cost $75–$100.

Comments Failure to maintain the specimen at room temperature will interfere with results. Patients undergoing thymectomy, thoracic duct drainage, immunosuppressive therapy, or plasmapheresis may show reduced levels. Patients with amyotrophic lateral sclerosis may show false-positive results.

acetylcholinesterase See *cholinesterase*.

acetylsalicylic acid See *aspirin*.

acid-fast stain Acid-fast stain is a general term for any number of special stains used to identify *Mycobacterium* species, the most important of which is *M. tuberculosis*, the bacterium that causes tuberculosis. Acid-fastness is related to the composition of the bacterium's outer capsule. While acid-fastness is relatively specific for mycobacteria, it is also seen in some pollens, keratohyaline (a skin protein), lipofuscin (a product of cellular degradation), lead inclusions, and other microorganisms, including *Nocardia*, *Histoplasma*, and other bacteria. There are other, nontuberculous mycobacteria in the environment that stain with the acid-fast technique. In the appropriate setting, however, a positive acid-fast stain is usually regarded as evidence that the person has tuberculosis. Pulmonary tuberculosis is the most serious of the conditions caused by *M. tuberculosis*, which can be diagnosed either on a smear of sputum or on a biopsy of lesions of the lungs that are "suspicious" when the upper respiratory tract is examined by bronchoscopy. Other body sites can be evaluated by aspiration of fluids or by tissue biopsy.

Patient preparation Brush teeth or remove dentures and rinse mouth with water before obtaining a "deep cough" specimen. Saliva from the mouth is of little use. Tuberculosis from other body sites can be evaluated by aspirating fluids or by biopsy of tissues using standard aseptic procedures with local anesthesia.

Procedure Once the specimen is obtained from the patient, it is smeared on a glass slide which is dipped in a number of dyes to determine whether the organism is acid-fast or not. *M. tuberculosis* is slow to grow in culture; identification and determination of sensitivity to antibiotics may take four to six weeks.

Specimen Sputum.

Reference range No acid-fast staining.

Abnormal values Positive staining for acid-fast bacteria indicates the presence of *Mycobacterium* species. This finding must be followed up by a culture to determine the species and its sensitivity to antibiotics. A negative result must also be followed up by a culture since this test is of relatively low sensitivity.

Cost $50–$100.

Comments With the recent increase in tuberculosis and the prevalence of immunosuppressed individuals, particularly those with AIDS, newer techniques have been developed to speed the detection and identification of mycobacteria. The technique of polymerase chain reaction (PCR) may be used to detect early growth of *M. tuberculosis*. PCR shortens the time needed to identify mycobacteria to 24 hours, allowing early administration of antibiotics. A recent phenomenon of considerable concern to public health authorities is the emergence of mycobacteria that are resistant to the antibiotics formerly successful in treating tuberculosis.

acidified serum lysis test   See *Ham test.*

acid infusion test   See *Bernstein test.*

acid mucopolysaccharides   This test is used in the diagnosis of mucopolysaccharidosis, a genetic deficiency in carbohydrate metabolism. An enzyme deficiency causes dermatan sulfate and heparin sulfate to accumulate in tissues. Its most severe form is Hurler's syndrome, also known as gargoylism, which has an early onset and commonly causes death by the age of ten.

Patient preparation No preparation is required, other than for obtaining urine.

Procedure This test is performed on a 24-hour urine specimen that is kept refrigerated and sent to the laboratory immediately after collection. See *timed collection* in Glossary.

Specimen Urine.

Reference range The normal values vary with age and are expressed as milligrams of glucuronic acid per gram of creatinine per 24 hours. At age two, this value is from 8 to 30, by early adolescence, it drops to between 0 and 12.

Abnormal values Values greater than 40 to 50 are suggestive of Hurler's syndrome.

Cost $35–$50 for the screening test.

Comments Improper specimen collection or handling will interfere with interpretation of results. Heparin therapy can cause elevated levels. False-positive levels occur in 5% of urine screening tests for acid mucopolysaccharides.

acid phosphatase   Acid phosphatase is a group of enzymes present in the prostate gland, semen, liver, spleen, red blood cells, bone marrow, and platelets that can be separated and analyzed according to their source. Serum levels of acid phosphatase were formerly measured to diagnose and monitor the progress of prostate cancer. However, an increase in acid phosphatase also occurs in other conditions, thus necessitating newer tests to measure serum levels of PSA (prostatic specific antigen) and a test to measure acid phosphatase of prostatic origin.

Patient preparation Any manipulation of the prostate, such as massage, catheterization, or rectal examination should not be performed within 48 hours of obtaining the specimen.

Procedure The procedure consists of measuring the acid phosphatase in the serum by various laboratory methods.

Specimen Serum. When performed outside the hospital setting, the serum must be separated from the red blood cells and frozen before sending it to the laboratory.

Reference range Less than 3.0 mg/L.

Abnormal values

Increased in: prostatic carcinoma, prostate infarction, Paget's disease, Gaucher's disease, multiple myeloma.

Cost $25–$45.

Comments This test is not specific for prostate cancer and, as previously indicated, has been largely superseded by other tests. Prostate manipulation and hemolysis cause falsely elevated results. Acid phosphatase levels drop abruptly if the specimen is not properly preserved. See *prostate-specific antigen*.

acquired immunodeficiency syndrome (AIDS) This disease has been linked with the human immunodeficiency virus (HIV), which invades specific cells in the immune system. This causes a decline in the body's ability to fight infection, resulting in secondary infections by microorganisms that do not normally cause disease. HIV infection may be present for as long as ten years before the symptoms of AIDS appear. Testing for HIV is strictly regulated by state and federal agencies because of the well-known social impact of HIV positivity. Information about HIV test results are kept confidential and may only be sent to nonphysicians with the written consent of the patient. Currently there are several types of tests used to detect and monitor HIV infection. *Confide* is a new product available through pharmacies. It is a home test; the blood samples are obtained from the finger and placed on a filter paper which is sent to the laboratory via mail. Patient confidentiality is maintained through the use of a 13-digit PIN number attached to the kit. Seven to ten days after mailing the sample, the patient is instructed to call the laboratory and give the assigned PIN number. The results are given to the caller along with the appropriate counseling. Another test, *OraShure,* is available through physicians and uses a sponge to obtain mucosal secretions from the mouth.

Screening tests These tests are known by the acronym ELISA (enzyme-linked immunosorbent assay) and detect antibodies to HIV that may be present in the patient's blood. Screening tests are used by blood banks to detect HIV-infected blood. Transfusion of an HIV-infected unit of blood virtually guarantees that the blood recipient will also become infected with HIV. Screening tests are also used to evaluate a person who may have been infected with HIV. Screening tests generally detect the anti-HIV antibodies approximately four to eight weeks after infection.

Newer tests are being developed to detect the viral antigen, but they are not widely available or approved for clinical use. All screening tests that are positive are then retested by Western blot technique, which, while more reliable than the ELISA procedures, is more costly and difficult to perform.

Monitoring tests These tests monitor the course of AIDS and response to treatment. The p24 ELISA test measures HIV's p24 antigen, which for a time was used to indicate the progression of AIDS. Analysis of the T cell, a type of lymphocyte, is a more comprehensive test that measures the number of T cells in circulation. T cells are a type of white blood cell required for the "cell-mediated" arm of the immune response. The most commonly performed monitoring test for AIDS is the measurement of a subset of T cells, known as CD4 ("helper") T cells, and the ratio of the number of CD4 T cells to another subset of T cells known as CD8 ("suppressor") T cells. CD4 T cells help other cells of the immune system function in an optimal fashion and, in the healthy individual, are more abundant than the CD8 cells. As AIDS progresses, the number of all T cells decreases, especially the CD4 T cells. The number of B cells, the other major type of lymphocyte that is responsible for producing antibodies, usually remains normal throughout the course of AIDS.

New Tests A number of tests are being developed that are more sensitive, allowing earlier detection of HIV infection. Many of these tests are based on polymerase chain reaction (PCR) and are currently used to confirm the presence of HIV. As these tests become easier to perform and more cost efficient, they are likely to become more readily available for monitoring the effectiveness of treatment. These tests are primarily used to determine the number of viruses present in the circulation (viral load).

Patient preparation No preparation is required, other than for drawing blood.

Procedure ELISA is performed on serum. T cell analysis and viral load testing require whole blood specimens which are obtained within 24 hours of testing.

Specimen Serum for ELISA. Heparanized whole blood for T cell and viral load studies, which must be kept at room temperature prior to analysis.

Reference range

ELISA	Negative.
p24	Negative.
PCR	Negative.
T and B cells	Ratio of greater than 1.
CD4 CD8 ratio	Ratio of greater than 1.
CD4 T cells	Greater than 2000.
Western blot	Negative.
HIV RNA Quantitation	Negative.

Abnormal values Positive findings in any of the above tests when confirmed by Western blot are diagnostic of HIV infection.

Cost

ELISA	$25–$50.

p24	$35–$55.
PCR	$100–$150.
T and B cells	$75–$150.
CD4 CD8 ratio	$75–$150.
CD4 T cells	$75–$150.
Western blot	$35–$75.
HIV RNA Quantitation	$200–$300.

Comments False-positive (i.e., reporting a person as positive for HIV who is actually negative) results for HIV testing are extremely unusual given the use of confirmatory tests, particularly the Western blot. False-negative (i.e., reporting a person as negative for HIV who is actually positive) results for HIV can occur during the "window period" interval (i.e., between the time a person is infected with HIV to the time enough anti-HIV antibodies are produced to be detected by the ELISA test).

ACTH   See *adrenocorticotropic hormone.*

activated partial thromboplastin time (aPTT)   The aPTT test is used in preoperative screening for increased bleeding tendencies and to monitor therapy with heparin and oral anticoagulants, drugs used to decrease clot formation. The aPTT test evaluates the time required for the clotting proteins or coagulation factors to form a fibrin clot.
Patient preparation No preparation is required, other than for drawing blood.
Procedure The procedure consists of mixing the patient's plasma with an "activator" and measuring the time required to form a clot.
Specimen Citrated plasma. The sample should be analyzed within two hours of being drawn from the patient, or the plasma should be separated from the red blood cells and frozen.
Reference range A fibrin clot forms 25 to 36 seconds after the addition of the "activator."
Abnormal values
   Increased in: coagulation factor deficiencies (factors V, VIII, IX, X, XI, XII), disseminated intravascular coagulation, Hodgkin's disease, hypofibrinogenemia, leukemia, liver cirrhosis, vitamin K deficiency, von Willebrand's disease, drugs (e.g., heparin, oral anticoagulants, aspirin).
Cost $10–$25.
Comments Sample handling is critical for obtaining correct results. If the venipuncture tube is not properly filled, falsely elevated values in the aPTT test will be obtained.

acute phase reactants (APR)   Acute phase reactants are proteins that rise and fall with acute inflammation. These proteins migrate in specific regions of a slab of gelatin-like material that has been subjected to an electric current. These proteins include α_1-antitrypsin, α_1-acid glycoprotein, amyloid A and P, anti-thrombin III, C-reactive protein, C1-esterase inhibitor, C3 complement, ceruloplasmin, fibrinogen, haptoglobin, orosomucoid, plasminogen, and transferrin. Screening tests for acute phase reaction are nonspecific and include erythrocyte sedimentation rate (ESR), plasma viscosity, and zeta sedimentation rate.

Patient preparation No preparation is required, other than for drawing blood.

Procedure The serum is analyzed by placing it on a special tube and measuring how quickly the red blood cells settle to the bottom, which is known as the erythrocyte sedimentation rate.

Specimen Whole blood.

Reference range The normal ESR is 0 to 20 millimeters/hour.

Abnormal values

Increased in: pregnancy, acute and chronic inflammation, tuberculosis paraproteinemias (e.g., Waldenström's macroglobulinemia), rheumatoid arthritis.

Decreased in: polycythemia, sickle cell anemia, hyperviscosity, low fibrinogen.

Comments The normal range of acute phase reactants increases with age, while the absolute rates of speed at which the blood settles decrease.

adenovirus Any of a family of viruses that cause noninfluenzal acute respiratory disease, pneumonia, epidemic keratoconjunctivitis, acute febrile pharyngitis, and acute hemorrhagic cystitis. The tests for adenovirus either measure antibodies to adenovirus or detect adenovirus antigens by immune (antigen-antibody) reactions. Both types of tests are known as serologic tests because they are performed on the serum. Adenoviruses can also be cultured, but because viral cultures are cumbersome and time-consuming, serologic methods are preferred by many laboratories. Asymptomatic infections (e.g., without flu symptoms) with adenoviruses are common and may make it difficult to interpret the serum levels of the immunoglobulin (antibody) response to infection. As a rule, immunoglobulin M (IgM), a specific antibody, increases when a person is first exposed to a particular microorganism. After the acute infection resolves, an immunoglobulin G (IgG) antibody to the virus is produced, which usually indicates protection against future infections by the causative virus.

Patient preparation For the serologic tests, no preparation is required, other than for drawing blood. There may be some discomfort associated with obtaining specimens from the throat or rectum.

Procedure The serologic procedure consists of measuring the levels of the IgG and IgM antibodies in the serum. To culture a virus, the specimen must be inoculated on one of several cell types, since viruses cannot grow outside of living cells. After a period of several days, the cells are examined by a microscope to detect specific changes caused by adenoviruses.

Specimen Serum for serologic diagnosis. Throat, rectal, and bladder specimens for culturing the virus.

Reference range The normal values for adenovirus antibodies are somewhat patient-specific, as each person differs in his or her ability to produce antibodies. In absence of adenovirus, the culture cells have no changes.

Abnormal values Patients infected with adenovirus usually demonstrate a four-fold increase in titers from the "acute" serum and the "convalescent" serum. Infected cells in culture demonstrate typical changes seen by microscopy.

Cost

    Serology $80–$100.

    Viral culture $110–$150.

ADH See *antidiuretic hormone.*

adrenal antibodies A general term for antibodies that are formed against components of the adrenal gland. These antibodies occur in 40% to 60% of patients with adrenal insufficiency (Addison's disease).

Patient preparation No preparation is required, other than for drawing blood.

Procedure These antibodies are identified by covering a test tissue (e.g., monkey adrenal gland) with the patient's serum. If adrenal antibodies are present, they can be detected by the technique of indirect immunofluorescence.

Specimen Serum.

Reference range None present.

Abnormal values Adrenal antibodies are found in: adrenal insufficiency (Addison's disease), idiopathic hypoparathyroidism.

Cost $75–$115.

adrenocorticotropic hormone (ACTH, corticotropin) ACTH is a hormone secreted by the anterior pituitary gland that signals the adrenal gland to release steroids (cortisol, androgens, and aldosterone), critical to the normal functioning of the body. ACTH levels in the serum vary during the course of the day, peaking in the morning between 6 and 8 a.m. and in the evening between 6 and 11 p.m. ACTH is not routinely measured because it degrades in the plasma and is not required to diagnose routinely encountered clinical conditions. However, in patients with Cushing's syndrome, ACTH measurement is extremely important because ACTH levels help determine where the lesion is located.

Patient preparation The patient's physical activity should be restricted for 10 to 12 hours prior to testing. Medications (particularly corticosteroids) that may interfere with ACTH testing should be withheld for 48 hours if possible. The patient should be placed on a low-carbohydrate diet for two days before testing.

Procedure The serum is analyzed by immunoassay.

Specimen Plasma, frozen within 15 minutes. For suspected adrenal hypofunction, the sample should be obtained from the patient between 6 and 8 a.m. To rule out Cushing's syndrome as a diagnostic consideration, the venipuncture must be performed between 6 and 11 p.m. The sample should be collected in a plastic test tube or a heparinized tube, packed in ice, and sent to the laboratory immediately.

Reference range ACTH levels less than 120 pg/ml.

Abnormal values

Increased in: adrenal insufficiency (Addison's disease), congenital adrenal hyperplasia, Cushing's disease, ectopic ACTH-producing tumors, Nelson's syndrome.

Decreased in: secondary adrenocortical insufficiency, adrenal carcinoma, adenoma.

Cost $50–$75.

Comments Because of ACTH's variability over the course of the day, its diagnostic significance and reliability are limited. Confirmation of increased or decreased ACTH levels may require ACTH suppression or stimulation testing to evaluate changes in the functional activity of the adrenal gland.

aerobic culture   See *bacterial culture.*

AFP   See *alphafetoprotein.*

airway resistance   Airway resistance is the resistance to the flow of air in the upper airways, which is evaluated in pulmonary function tests. Airway resistance is the result of the natural recoil (resiliency) of the upper airway structures (the oral and nasal cavities, larynx, and the nonrespiratory portions of the lungs, including the trachea, bronchi, and bronchioles), through which the air passes on the way to the functional portion of the lungs, the alveoli. Airway resistance testing includes evaluation of airway responsiveness, provocation testing (e.g., bronchial challenge), evaluation of sites of airflow resistance or closures, and characterization of the type of lung disease.

Patient preparation The patient should avoid heavy meals three hours before the test. This is a non-invasive test which measures the pressure of breathing under various conditions.

Procedure Noseclips and a mouthpiece are placed on the patient, who is then seated inside a chamber known as a body plethysmograph. Once the chamber is sealed and the pressure reaches an equilibrium, the patient is told to pant lightly, which reflects the resistance to airflow.

Reference range 0.6–2.8 cm H_2O/liters per second.

Abnormal values

Increased in: asthma, chronic obstructive lung disease, smokers.

Cost $60–$80.

ALA   See *delta-aminolevulinic acid.*

alanine aminotransferase   ALT was formerly called serum glutamine pyruvic transaminase (SGPT), and many physicians continue to use the older name. Alanine aminotransferase is an enzyme found primarily in the liver, with lesser amounts present in the kidneys, heart, and muscles. Under normal conditions, the levels of ALT in the blood are low. When liver damage occurs, ALT is released into the bloodstream, usually before the more obvious clinical findings (e.g., jaundice) of liver damage occur. ALT levels are therefore useful to the physician, because increased ALT is an early indicator of liver damage. The analysis of this enzyme has been automated and is usually included as part of a panel of blood chemistry tests.

Specimen Serum or heparinized plasma.

Reference range

Men	10–32 units/L.
Women	9–24 units/L.
Children	2 times that of adults.

Abnormal values

Increased in: viral or drug-induced hepatitis, infectious mononucleosis, chronic hepatitis, intrahepatic cholestasis, cholecystitis, active cirrhosis acute myocardial infarction.

Cost $10–$20 when performed as a single test.

Comments The measurement of ALT alone has little diagnostic value and must be used in conjunction with other chemistry assays and clinical indicators.

albumin Albumin is the most abundant protein in blood circulation. It is needed to maintain the osmotic pressure within the blood vessels, without which fluids would leak out of the circulation. Albumin provides nutrition to tissues and binds to various molecules, such as hormones, vitamins, drugs, and enzymes, transporting them through the body. Albumin is synthesized in the liver and is extremely sensitive to liver damage. Hypoalbuminemia, the decrease in albumin, may be caused by liver damage, inadequate dietary intake of protein as occurs in malnutrition, and renal disease, in which albumin and other proteins are not retained by the kidneys. Dehydration causes an increase in albumin concentration, known as hyperalbuminemia.

Patient preparation Urine measurements require a 24-hour collection period. See *timed collection*.

Procedure Analysis of albumin is generally done as part of a larger chemistry profile on an automated analyzer.

Specimen Albumin can be measured in many body fluids, including serum, cerebrospinal fluid, and urine. Serum measurements of albumin are usually part of a multichannel chemical analysis of the blood, while albumin in cerebrospinal fluid and urine is measured singly.

Reference range

Serum, male	4.2–5.5 g/dL.
Serum, female	3.7–5.3 g/dl.
Urine	3.9–24.4 mg/24 hrs.
Cerebrospinal fluid	15–45 mg/dL.

Abnormal values
  Increased in: dehydration.
  Decreased in: liver disease, chronic disease, neoplasia, thyroid disease,
     burns, heart failure.
Cost $8–$35 when performed as a single test.
Comments Decreased albumin in serum suggests liver disease. The "liver enzymes" (alanine aminotransferase and aspartate aminotransferase) must be evaluated in conjunction with albumin measurements, to confirm the presence of liver damage. The presence of albumin in urine generally signifies kidney disease.

alcohol The alcohol consumed in alcoholic beverages such as beer, wine, and liquors is ethyl alcohol (ethanol). After ethanol is consumed, it reaches a peak in the blood in about 30 minutes. Approximately three hours are needed to metabolize and eliminate each ounce of ethanol ingested. Blood alcohol measurements are fairly reliable for many hours after an individual ingests the last drink.
  Patient preparation No preparation is required, other than for drawing blood or collecting urine. When blood samples are to be used, the venipuncture site must not be cleaned with alcohol pads because this would contaminate the specimen. The urine collection need not be a timed specimen.
  Procedure Breath measurements are generally carried out by law enforcement officers, often at the site of a traffic violation where alcohol use is suspected. Alcohols are volatile substances; therefore it is important that the specimen container be kept tightly sealed until the time of analysis. Serum and urine ethanol are measured in the laboratory by immunoassay or gas-liquid chromatography; other alcohols are measured by gas-liquid chromatograpy.
  Specimen Ethanol can be measured in the blood, breath, or urine.
  Reference range Negative.
  Abnormal values Greater than 0.05% (50 mg/dL) is considered toxic. Elevated levels of alcohols cause inebriation, liver, and brain damage.
  Cost $25–$75. Higher costs are incurred when the test is used for legal purposes.
  Comments Blood specimens are more accurate than urine when quantitative results are required. Proper specimen handling is extremely important for accurate results.

aldolase Aldolase is an enzyme that converts sugar to energy. Though most prominent in skeletal muscle, it is present in all tissues. Aldolase is elevated in the serum in skeletal muscle disease or injury and is less common in other conditions. It is measured when inflammatory disease of muscle (myopathy) is suspected. The intensity of the increase reflects the severity of the myopathy, and it can be measured serially to monitor the effect of corticosteroid therapy on the course of disease. Aldolase may also be elevated early in the clinical course of patients with muscular dystrophy.

Patient preparation Patient should fast for eight hours prior to the test.

Procedure Aldolase is determined by the conversion of an uncolored substance to a colored substance that is measured by spectrophotometry.

Specimen Serum should be separated and frozen as quickly as possible.

Reference range 3.1–7.5 units/L.

Abnormal values

Increased in: Duchenne's muscular dystrophy, dermatomyositis, polymyositis, trichinosis, metastatic carcinoma, myelocytic leukemia, megaloblastic anemia, hemolytic anemia, tissue death (infarction).

Cost $15–$25.

Comments Because aldolase is relatively nonspecific, it is not commonly requested by clinicians unless they are monitoring muscle diseases.

aldosterone Aldosterone is a hormone of the adrenal gland that helps control the electrolyte balance in the body by regulating the reabsorption of sodium and chloride in exchange for potassium and hydrogen ions in the kidneys. Aldosterone helps maintain blood pressure and blood volume. Secretion of aldosterone is controlled by the renin-angiotensin system which produces an enzyme, angiotensin II, that stimulates the synthesis and secretion of aldosterone. Secretion of aldosterone is also controlled by concentrations of potassium in the circulation. High serum potassium levels elicit secretion of aldosterone, while low concentrations of sodium cause the release of renin which stimulates aldosterone secretion. Aldosterone measurements are used increasingly in the study of hypertension.

Patient preparation The patient should be on a normal salt diet. Diuretics, antihypertensive drugs, oral contraceptives, estrogens, and licorice (which can cause hypertension) should be terminated two to four hours before testing. No recent radionuclide studies (scans) should be performed before drawing the specimen.

Procedure The patient must be at rest and lying down for the first venipuncture. Postural changes are evaluated by drawing another sample while the patient is up and about four hours after the initial specimen is collected. Aldosterone can also be measured in 24-hour urine samples. Measurements are made by RIA methods.

Specimen Serum, plasma, or urine. Specimens should be transported on ice and frozen as soon as possible after being obtained.

Reference range Plasma levels are less than 20 ng/dL in men, 30 ng/dL in non-pregnant women, 100 ng/dL in pregnant women, and 70 ng/dL in children. Urine levels are usually less than 50 µg/24 hours.

Abnormal values

Increased in: adrenocortical adenoma or carcinoma, bilateral adrenal hyperplasia, renovascular hypertension, liver disease, congestive heart failure, cirrhosis, nephrotic syndrome, pregnancy (3rd trimester).

Decreased in: primary hypoaldosteronism, salt losing syndrome, toxemia of pregnancy.

Cost $180–$200.

Comments Failure to observe dietary restrictions or postural procedures interferes with the interpretation of test results. Aldosterone measurements are generally carried out together with potassium, sodium, and renin levels in the evaluation of hypertension and suspected lesions of the adrenal gland.

alkaline phosphatase ("alk phos") Alkaline phosphatase (ALP) is an enzyme normally present in the blood. Various subtypes known as isoenzymes are found in the liver, intestines, and bone cells. ALP is involved in bone calcification, and lipid and metabolite transportation. Conditions that stimulate bone cell activity cause elevated levels of alkaline phosphatase. The liver isoenzyme of ALP is elevated in biliary obstruction. Because an elevated total ALP level can indicate either liver or bone disease, additional studies must be carried out to determine the exact cause of the elevation. Since ALP concentrations rise during active bone formation in growth, infants, children, and adolescents normally have levels up to three times those of adults. Pregnancy can also cause an increase in ALP levels.

Patient preparation No preparation is required.

Procedure Alkaline phosphatase is measured by spectrophotometry.

Specimen Serum.

Reference range Because reference ranges are dependent on the methodology used by the laboratory, these ranges can vary widely. In adult males, the range is 90–250 units/liter; in adult females, 80–200 units/liter.

Abnormal values

Increased in: hepatobiliary disease (e.g., viral hepatitis, severe biliary obstruction, biliary cirrhosis, intrahepatic cholestasis), Paget's disease of bone, osteomalacia, osteogenic sarcoma, bone metastasis, hyperparathyroidism, infectious mononucleosis.

Decreased in: hypophosphatasia, protein deficiency, magnesium deficiency.

Cost $20–$40 when performed as a single test.

Comments Because ALP exists in various tissues, the finding of elevated levels of total ALP must be followed by more specific testing such as ALP isoenzymes. Additional studies of bone or liver chemistries are used to determine the primary cause of elevations. ALP is generally part of a routine chemistry profile.

alkaline phosphatase isoenzymes Alkaline phosphatase is an enzyme with several subtypes known as isoenzymes, which are more common in certain organs. The isoenzymes of greatest clinical significance are those that occur in the liver, bone, intestine, and placenta. The intestinal isoenzyme occurs almost exclusively in individuals with blood group B or O and is markedly elevated eight hours after a fatty meal. The placental isoenzyme first appears in mid to late pregnancy, accounts for half of all alkaline phosphatase during the third trimester, and drops to normal levels after the woman delivers. Another, the Regan isoenzyme, resembles the placental isoenzyme of alkaline phosphatase and is present in some patients with cancer. A number of methods have been developed in the laboratory to separate the isoenzymes according to subtype. The primary use of this test is to determine which type of ALP isoenzyme is predominant when there is an elevation in total alkaline phosphatase.

Patient preparation No preparation is required.

Procedure ALP isoenzymes can be measured by a variety of methods. The older methods involve heating or treating with urea. Currently, electrophoresis or isoelectric focusing are the methods of choice.

Specimen Serum.

Reference range

| Liver | 20–130 units/L. |
| Bone | 20–120 units/L. |

Abnormal values An increase in the bone isoenzymes usually indicates Paget's disease of the bone. Bone isoenzymes are also increased in bone-forming tumors and in pregnancy.

Cost $50–$80.

Comments This test should not be performed if the total alkaline phosphatase levels are within the laboratory's reference (i.e., normal) range, because the results would have little clinical significance. These tests are only semiquantitative and are subject to significant variation. Other laboratory tests and clinical findings should be used in conjunction with alkaline phosphatase isoenzymes when making a diagnosis.

allergy testing See *RAST.*

alpha1-antitrypsin (A1AT) Alpha1-antitrypsin is a protein that inhibits proteolytic enzymes (enzymes that break down proteins). Enzymes that are broken down by A1AT include trypsin, chymotrypsin, elastase, plasmin, thrombin, and others. The normal A1AT serum levels of 2–4 g/L rise nonspecifically during inflammation and are usually increased in acute inflammation, severe infection, and necrosis. The A1AT gene has 25 different forms (e.g., PiMM and PiZZ) which are classified by how they respond to electrophoresis. The PiMM type of A1AT is normal. The most common form seen in A1AT deficiency is designated PiZZ, which is characterized by early-onset emphysema and cholestasis, cirrhosis, hepatic failure, and a markedly increased risk of liver cancer.

Patient preparation The patient should not eat for several hours before drawing the specimen

Procedure A1AT is measured by nephelometry.

Specimen Serum.

Reference range 78–200 mg/dL.

Abnormal values

Increased in: inflammatory disorders, malignancies, hormonal effects, brain infarction, systemic lupus erythematosus, Hashimoto's thyroiditis.

Decreased in: nephrotic syndrome, protein-losing gastroenteropathies, prematurity, acute hepatitis, respiratory distress syndrome, acute pancreatitis, congenital defects, emphysema.

Cost $60–$80.

Comments This test can be a useful indicator in patients at risk for emphysema.

alphafetoprotein Alphafetoprotein (AFP) is a glycoprotein produced by the liver of the fetus. The peak production occurs at 13 weeks of age, after which the production progressively declines. AFP is detected in pregnancy in both the mother's serum and in the amniotic fluid. The AFP levels are greater in twins and in "higher multiple" pregnancies, and its measurement is now a part of routine pregnancy testing. If the fetal neural tube, which develops into the brain and spinal cord, fails to close completely, large quantities of AFP enter the amniotic fluid, resulting in elevated levels in the mother's serum. Neural tube defects associated with increased AFP include spina bifida, anencephaly myelocele, and hydrocephalus. AFP is also elevated in nonneural tube defects, including congenital nephrosis, esophageal atresia, duodenal atresia, and fetal bleeding into the amniotic cavity. AFP levels are usually measured at 13–16 weeks of pregnancy, when the fetal AFP production is highest. Confirmatory tests such as amniocentesis and/or ultrasonography are used to identify neural tube defects when elevated AFP levels are identified. If these tests suggest the presence of significant birth defects, the woman may choose to terminate the pregnancy. After birth, elevated serum AFP levels occur only in conditions of abnormal cell multiplication. Although AFP measurements are not approved by the United States Food and Drug Administration for cancer screening, they are used in practice to detect and monitor therapy of liver cancer (hepatocellular carcinoma) and certain malignant tumors of the gonads (testes and ovaries), retroperitoneum, and mediastinum.

Patient preparation No preparation is required.

Procedure AFP is measured by ELISA, FPIA or chemiluminescent methods.

Specimen Serum or amniotic fluid; when the mother's serum is screened for the presence of AFP, the serum should be drawn between weeks 13–16 of pregnancy.

Reference range

Nonpregnant adults	<30 ng/ml.
Maternal serum (13–16 wks)	<1.0–4.4 ug/dL.
Amniotic fluid (13–16 wks)	0.9–4.1 mg/dL.

Abnormal values

Increased in: liver (hepatocellular) carcinoma, choriocarcinoma, embryonal carcinoma.

Less commonly increased in: pancreatic cancer, stomach cancer, colon cancer, lung cancer.

Cost $60–$90.

Comments When used for monitoring cancer therapy, AFP testing is very reliable. In contrast, the accuracy of only AFP measurements to detect the presence of tube defects is 50%–75%, making it imperative that further tests be performed, including measurements of beta-HCG and estriol (See *triple marker screen*). Multitest formats have dramatically increased the accuracy of predicting the presence of neural tube defects. Because these pregnancy screening methods are based on statistical analysis using maternal age and gestational age to arrive at an assessment of risk, accurate determination of gestational age is extremely important. See *amniocentesis*.

alpha-hydroxybutyric dehydrogenase See *hydroxybutyric dehydrogenase* in Glossary

ALT See *aspartate aminotransferase*.

AMA See *anti-mitochondrial autoantibodies*.

amebiasis An infection by the parasite *Entamoeba histolytica* which causes dysentery that is spread by the fecal-oral route. This is a relatively common cause of diarrhea in homosexual men. Individuals are tested for amebiasis by serology, in which antibodies against the parasite are measured in the serum. Serologic testing is positive in 85% of infected patients. Asymptomatic carriers of *Entamoeba histolytica* have a much lower rate of seropositivity. Microscopic examination of stained stool smears or concentrated stool suspensions are used to document asymptomatic carriers.

Patient preparation No preparation is required.

Procedure Serologic testing is carried out on blood specimens. Stool samples are washed, filtered, and examined by light microscopy to detect amebic cysts and trophozoites.

Specimen Serum or random stool.

Reference range Negative.

Cost

    Serologic Tests $45–$75.

    Stool Exam $25–$50.

Comments See *parasite identification*.

amino acids Amino acids are small molecules that are the building blocks of proteins and peptides. Most of the over 20 amino acids are obtained from dietary intake of proteins, which are broken down in the body and used to synthesize other proteins and enzymes. There are approximately 2000 inherited diseases of metabolism, many of which are caused by specific defects in amino acid metabolism. Most of the diseases that affect amino acid metabolism are extremely rare. In the more common cases, if the metabolic error is diagnosed early enough in the infant's life, it may respond to a special diet.

Patient preparation No preparation is required.

Procedure The diagnostic workup for suspected amino acid disorders is usually performed on newborn infants or young children who have signs of growth or mental retardation or other birth defects. Most states in the United States require that newborns be screened for the presence of one or more of the amino acid disorders. Screening is usually performed on urine, although blood can be used for some tests. The specific tests performed depend on which disease is suspected. The qualitative screen is performed by thin-layer chromatography, which identifies certain amino acids (e.g., methionine, phenylalanine, tyrosine, and others).

Specimen Urine or plasma.

Reference range Each of the 20 amino acids and their metabolites has a different normal value. In the blood, the levels are usually high at birth and lessen with age. In the urine, the opposite is the rule, and the amount excreted in the urine increases with age.

Cost A general screen for the presence of multiple defects in amino acid metabolism costs about $75–$100. Quantitative determinations of the individual amino acid may be as high as $500.

Comments See *hemoglobin*.

ammonia Ammonia is produced in the liver, intestine, and kidneys as the end product of protein metabolism. The liver converts ammonia into urea, which is then excreted by the kidneys. In liver disease, this conversion decreases, resulting in an increase in blood ammonia levels. Repeated measurement of ammonia may be used to follow the clinical progress of hepatic encephalopathy in such conditions as Reye's syndrome.

Patient preparation No preparation is required.

Procedure Ammonia is measured by spectrophotometry.

Specimen Ammonia is measured in whole blood. Because it is volatile, the specimen must be transported to the laboratory on ice and analyzed as quickly as possible.

Reference range 15–49 µg/dL.

Abnormal values

Increased in: hepatic coma, Reye's syndrome, severe congestive heart failure, gastrointestinal hemorrhage, hemolytic disease of the newborn.

Cost $80–$90.

Comments Abnormal blood ammonia levels usually point to the presence of liver disease. Some medications such as diuretics and antibiotics can cause increased ammonia levels.

amniocentesis A procedure in which fluid is obtained from the amniotic cavity by an ultrasound-guided needle (usually at weeks 15–17 of pregnancy) and analyzed for the presence of fetal abnormalities. Accuracy of amniocentesis is reported to be 99.4%. The complication rate of amniocentesis is less than 0.5% above the background pregnancy loss of 2%–3%, and the actual fetal loss is minimal.

Indications for amniocentesis
Maternal age greater than 35.
3+ spontaneous abortions.
Previous history of chromosomally abnormal child.
Metabolic disease.
Neural tube defect.
Patient, father, or family history of chromosomal abnormality.
Possible carrier of X-linked disease.

Defects identified by amniocentesis Cultured amniotic cells can be used for cytogenetic studies, DNA analysis, and enzyme assays. Amniocentesis may not be required in women with increased alphafetoprotein and a normal fetus by ultrasound. See *chorionic villus biopsy*.

Many metabolic diseases (e.g., Tay-Sachs disease) can be diagnosed before birth, as can some physical defects. Chromosome analysis is performed on fetal cells obtained from the amniotic fluid to determine the genetic status of the unborn fetus, and is of use in identifying trisomy 21 (Down's syndrome) and other trisomies. The test is generally performed on pregnant women over age 35, in women with relatives known to have metabolic problems, in women who have previously had children born with Down's syndrome, and in families with a history of chromosome abnormalities.

Patient preparation No preparation is required.

Procedure After locating the exact position of the fetus, usually with ultrasound, the physician places a long, thin needle through the abdomen into the uterus and withdraws the fluid.

Specimen Amniotic fluid.

Reference range No abnormalities identified.

Abnormal values Any elevation, abnormality or defect identified by amniocentesis requires action on the part of the physician.

Cost $700–$900, including chromosome analysis.

Comments There is a slight risk (1%) of needle injury to the fetus, bleeding, and/or infection. Spontaneous abortion occurs in 0.5% and is of unknown cause.

amniotic fluid analysis A general term for a series of tests, obtained by amniocentesis, performed on the amniotic fluid of a woman who is in the second trimester of pregnancy. Amniotic fluid analysis detects the presence of a possible response by the mother's immune system to the fetal red blood cells by measuring bilirubin levels. Analysis of amniotic fluid also detects genetic defects by karyotyping fetal cells and determines fetal maturity, by measuring creatinine, lecithin/sphingomyelin ratio, and surfactant. See *amniocentesis*.

amphetamines See *drug screening*.

amylase Amylase is an enzyme synthesized in the pancreas and salivary glands and secreted into the gastrointestinal tract, which helps digest starch and glycogen in the mouth, stomach, and intestine. The most important use of amylase measurements is in the diagnosis of acute pancreatitis, a condition in which serum and urine levels of amylase peak between four to eight hours after onset of acute pancreatitis, then fall to normal within 48–72 hours. Salivary gland inflammation (parotitis) due to mumps or other causes (e.g., exposure to high-level ionizing radiation) can also release amylase into the circulation. In cases of an elevated serum amylase without clear-cut pancreatitis or parotitis, amylase isoenzymes can be separated and quantified in the laboratory.

Patient preparation Because there are several medications that can affect amylase levels, it is preferable to restrict these medications prior to sampling. Alcohol must also be restricted prior to obtaining specimens, as it may cause false elevations. The ordering physician will instruct the patient whether or not medications can safely be restricted.

Procedure Amylase is measured by spectrophotometric methods.

Specimen Serum, urine.

Reference range Because of the many procedures used to measure amylase levels, the reference ranges vary from laboratory to laboratory. By one method, normal amylase activity is 75–200 units per hour, and by another method 25–125 units per liter.

Abnormal values

Increased in: acute pancreatitis, obstruction of the common bile duct, pancreatic duct, or ampule of Vater, pancreatic injury from perforated peptic ulcer, pancreatic cancer, acute salivary gland disease.
Decreased in: chronic pancreatitis, pancreatic cancer, cirrhosis, hepatitis, toxemia of pregnancy.

Cost $30–$50.

ANA See *antinuclear antibodies.*

anal manometry (balloon manometry for fecal incontinence) This test is a rarely performed procedure that measures the tension in the external and internal anal sphincters, to evaluate constipation or fecal incontinence.

Patient preparation Sedatives may be required by young or anxious patients to alleviate a small amount of discomfort during the procedure. Enemas are usually administered to cleanse the rectum.

Procedure After emptying the bowel with enemas, the patient lies on his/her side. The clinician gently inserts a metal tube to a distance of approximately six inches. A second, thinner tube is inserted through the first, which has a special balloon at its end that is slowly inflated. The pressure response of the inside walls of the rectum to the expanding balloon is measured at baseline and with squeezing.

Specimen The specimen consists of manometric data.

Reference range

Baseline pressure   60 mm Hg.
Squeezing pressure   200 mm Hg.

Abnormal values Low baseline pressures indicate failure of the internal anal

muscles. Low squeezing pressures indicate failure of the external anal muscles. High baseline pressures are typically seen in Hirschsprung's disease, which most commonly affects children.
Cost $500–$750.

androstenedione Androstenedione is a steroid produced by the adrenal cortex and the gonads which is converted to estrone by enzymes in the liver and in fat cells. Estrone is an estrogen (a "female" hormone) with very low biological activity; it is the major estrogen in children and postmenopausal women. An increased production of estrone may induce premature sexual development in children and renewed hormonal activity in the ovaries of postmenopausal women. It is increased in obese females and may interfere with the menstrual cycle. In men, overproduction of androstenedione can cause feminizing signs (e.g., loss of body hair, change of fat contour).
Patient preparation No preparation is required, other than for drawing blood.
Procedure Androstenedione is measured by radioimmunoassay methods.
Specimen Serum.
Reference range
  Females
    Premenopausal   0.6–3 ng/ml.
    Postmenopausal   0.3–8 ng/ml.
  Males   0.9–1.7 ng/ml.
Abnormal values
  Increased in: Cushing's syndrome, ovarian, testicular, or adrenocortical
    tumors.
  Decreased in: hypogonadism.
Cost $190–$210.

anemia panel A group of laboratory measurements that are cost-efficient, sensitive, and specific for evaluating a patient with anemia. An anemia panel includes the CBC (complete blood count) with indices and reticulocyte counts. If the red blood cells seen in the anemia are small (microcytic) and have reduced amounts of hemoglobin (hypochromic), the panel should measure iron levels, iron-binding capacity, and levels and percent saturation of ferritin, all of which would confirm the presence or absence of iron-deficiency anemia. If the red blood cells seen in the anemia are markedly enlarged (macrocytic), then vitamin B_{12} and folate levels are measured, as macrocytic anemia is often due to a deficiency of vitamin B_{12} and folic acid. See *organ panel* in Glossary.

angiography Angiography is an invasive procedure that allows the physician to see defects in the wall of the arteries or veins. Angiography can also be used to evaluate the blood flow through the heart and its valves (coronary catherization), lungs (pulmonary angiography), and brain (cerebral arteriography). Angiography is usually carried out when initial, noninvasive procedures are insufficient in revealing the cause of a suspected vascular defect.

Patient preparation No preparation is required.

Procedure This procedure is normally carried out in a hospital setting. A hollow, flexible tube (catheter) is inserted into an artery or vein near the organ being studied. A radio-opaque dye is injected through the catheter to make the vessels being studied visible by X ray.

Reference range No alterations in the flow of blood.

Abnormal values Any alteration in the flow of blood through valves or vessels is abnormal; these alterations include reduced flow due to narrowing (also known as stenosis) or reversed flow (known as regurgitation) through the vessels. Depending on the phase of the study, angiography allows examination of arterial (early phase) or venous (late phase) blood flow.

Cost $4000–$6000.

Comments This is an invasive procedure requiring anesthesia and skilled physicians that is often performed in a hospital setting.

angiotensin-converting enzyme (ACE)   Angiotensin-converting enzyme is found in high concentrations in pulmonary capillaries and in lesser amounts in blood vessels and kidneys. It is a key component in the renin-angiotensin system, which regulates arterial blood pressure by converting angiotensin I to angiotensin II, a powerful vasoconstrictor. Although ACE plays a role in regulating blood pressure, there is no correlation between ACE levels and blood pressure. Measurement of ACE is primarily used in the differential diagnosis of sarcoidosis.

Patient preparation Patient should fast for 12 hours before having the specimen drawn.

Procedure ACE is measured spectrophotometrically.

Specimen Serum or heparanized plasma. Specimen should be sent to the laboratory as quickly as possible or frozen until analysis.

Reference range 18–67 U/L.

Abnormal values

Increased in: sarcoidosis, Gaucher's disease, leprosy.

Decreased in: corticosteroid therapy for sarcoidosis.

Cost $75–$85.

Comments ACE measurement is used to confirm clinical findings in the diagnosis of sarcoidosis. Once the diagnosis has been established, ACE levels may be used to monitor treatment response.

anion gap   The anion gap is a mathematical approximation of the difference in the body between the unmeasured negative ions (anions), which include phosphate, sulfates, proteins, and organic acids, and the unmeasured positive ions (cations), which include calcium and magnesium. This gap reflects the state of serum electrolytes and helps distinguish among the types of electrolyte imbalances without resorting to the more expensive and time-consuming measurement of each serum electrolyte. The anion gap is calculated as the difference between the sum of the measured anions or negative ions (chloride and bicarbonate) and that of the measured cations or positive ions (sodium and potassium), a value that is usually 8–16 milliequivalents per liter. The calculation is based on a simple principle that the total concentrations of positive and negative ions are normally equal and thus maintain electrical neutrality in serum. Sodium and potassium account for more than 90% of circulating positive ions, while chloride and bicarbonate together account for 85% of the counterbalancing negative ions. The difference between the measured positive and negative ions corresponds to those negative ions that are not routinely measured. The anion gap allows the physician to evaluate metabolic defects in the form of metabolic acidosis, diabetic ketoacidosis, and lactic acidosis, as well as to monitor renal function and intravenous hyperalimentation. The urinary anion gap is calculated as sodium plus potassium minus chloride, which is a crude index of the levels of urinary ammonium, and is used to evaluate hyperchloremic metabolic acidosis.

Patient preparation No preparation is required.

Procedure The sum of the chloride and bicarbonate in mEq/L obtained on a chemistry panel are subtracted from the sum of sodium and potassium in mEq/L.

Specimen Serum or heparinized plasma.

Reference range 8–14 mEq/L.

Abnormal values

  Increased in: renal failure, ketoacidosis caused by malnutrition in diabetes mellitus or alcohol abuse, lactic acidosis, overdose (e.g., salicylates, methanol, ethylene glycol, paraldehyde).

  Decreased in: hypermagnesemia, multiple myeloma, Waldenström's macroglobinemia.

Cost $10–$20

Comments There are many factors that can cause a falsely increased or decreased anion gap. Further investigation and diagnostic tests are usually necessary to determine the specific cause of metabolic acidosis.

anoscopy See *proctoscopy.*

antibiotic sensitivity and identification A test performed in the microbiology laboratory after a disease-causing bacteria has been identified by culture. In many laboratories this is an automated procedure.

Patient preparation None required, other than for drawing blood or obtaining urine or sputum.

Procedure After being cultured on an agar plate, the bacterium is recultured on an agar plate that contains paper disks impregnated with many different antibiotics in concentrations similar to the concentrations attained in the body. The most common susceptibility test in the clinical laboratory is the diffusion test, in which the bacterium of interest is grown to confluence (i.e., a "lawn") on a culture plate, and paper disks impregnated with specific amounts of various antibiotics are placed on the culture plate. The amount of growth inhibition (i.e., the diameter of nongrowth) around the paper disk is measured. Lack of growth around the paper disks implies bacterial sensitivity to the corresponding antibiotic(s). The laboratory then generates a list of antibiotics to which the bacterium is sensitive or resistant. This list is used to guide the physician as to which antibiotic is most likely to be effective in treating a particular infection.

Specimen Blood, urine, sputum.

Reference range Sensitivity to an antibiotic is determined by the diameter of the inhibition of growth surrounding a 6 millimeter paper disk impregnated with any number of antibiotics.

Abnormal values The smaller the diameter of inhibited growth around the paper disk, the more resistant the bacterium is to the antibiotic in the paper disk.

Cost $15–30, in addition to the cost of the culture.

antibody   See *immunoglobulins.*

antibody screen and identification of red cell antigens   One of the most critical tests performed in the laboratory is the screening of blood intended for transfusion for the presence of red blood cell antigens and antibodies to those antigens. Certain groups of red blood cell antigens (in particular the Rh and ABO blood groups) are associated with extremely brisk and potentially fatal hemolytic reactions if the recipient's blood has antibodies to the red blood cell antigens being transfused. Few tests performed in the laboratory have a greater impact on a patient than antibody screening; thus it requires more attention to detail because there is a genuine risk for serious complications and/or death. "Type and screens" (T&S) are carried out as part of a person's preadmission testing before surgery. T&S are also used to detect anti-Rho(D) or other anti-Rh antibodies in the blood of an Rh-negative woman who is pregnant with an Rh-positive fetus, which will determine the need for Rho(D) immune globulin (RhoGam) administration.

Patient preparation No preparation is required.

Procedure This type of testing is carried out by visually observing whether or not a reaction occurs when various antigenic components are exposed to the patient's red blood cells. There is little automation available at this time; however, several companies are preparing instrumentation for FDA approval.

Specimen Whole blood drawn in a red-top tube, *not* a serum separator tube, as the red blood cells themselves are being evaluated.

Reference range No abnormal antibodies detected.

Abnormal values A positive T&S indicates the presence of antibodies to red blood cell antigen(s) and demostrates probable incompatibility between the blood donor and recipient. A positive T&S may also occur in acquired hemolytic anemia. Positivity in pregnancy indicates antibodies to Rh factor from either a previous pregnancy with an Rh-positive fetus or a prior transfusion with incompatible blood, which is exceedingly rare.

Cost $35–$55.

anticardiolipin antibodies (cardiolipin antibodies)   Cardiolipins are a part of many phospholipid membranes. Antibodies against cardiolipin (ACA) are found in systemic lupus erythematosus (where they are also known as lupus anticoagulants) and related connective tissue diseases and may be found in normal individuals. Anticardiolipin antibodies (ACA) include immunoglobulins (IgM, IgG, and IgA types) and are associated with various clinical and laboratory abnormalities, including thrombocytopenia, false-positive RPR test (for syphilis), and prolonged activated partial thromboplastin time. IgG ACAs are more influenced by disease activity than are IgM ACAs.

Patient preparation No preparation is required.

Procedure Anticardiolipins are measured using ELISA methods.

Specimen Serum collected in a red-top tube.

Reference range None detected.

Abnormal values Anticardiolipins antibodies may be present in: recurrent thromboses, lupus-like syndromes, false-positive RPR (for syphilis), recurrent fetal loss.

Cost
IgM	$75–$90.
IgG	$75–$90.
IgA	$75–$90.

Comments The most commonly ordered ACA tests are for IgG and IgM. Measurement of IgA type ACA is not believed to be clinically useful.

antidiuretic hormone (vasopressin, ADH)   ADH is a small peptide secreted by the posterior pituitary gland. ADH increases the water reabsorption in the kidneys in response to increased osmolality (relative water deficiency with increased sodium and solutes). When the osmolality falls in the presence of excess water, the secretion of ADH falls, allowing an increased excretion of water to maintain the balance of fluids.

Patient preparation Restrictions in diet, medications, and activity are required prior to obtaining the specimen.

Procedure ADH is measured by radioimmunoassay (RIA).

Specimen Serum. After obtaining a blood sample, the serum must be separated from the clot immediately.

Reference range 1–3 picograms per milliliter

Abnormal values

Increased in: acute porphyria, Addison's disease, bronchogenic carcinoma, hypothyroidism, cirrhosis, infectious hepatitis, severe hemorrhage, circulatory shock.

Decreased in: diabetes insipidus, viral infection, metastatic disease, sarcoidosis, tuberculosis, histiocytosis X (Hand-Schuller-Christian disease), syphilis, head trauma.

Cost $100.

Comments Measurement of ADH is used in the differential diagnosis of diabetes insipidus and syndrome of inappropriate antidiuretic hormone secretion (SIADH).

anti-DNase B (ADB test)   Infections with streptococci evoke the production of various antibodies, e.g., anti-DNase B and antistreptolysin O (ASO). The ADB test can detect antibodies to both pharyngeal and skin streptococcal infections and may be superior to the ASO test for diagnosing acute poststreptococcal glomerulonephritis.
Patient preparation No preparation is required.
Procedure Latex or hemagglutination techniques are used to determine the presence of ADB.
Specimen Serum.
Reference range A titer of less than 1:640.
Abnormal values A titer of greater than 1:1280 is considered significant and indicates presence of group A streptococci.
Cost $100–$120.
Comments ASO continues to be the most common test ordered to identify streptococcal infections. The ADB test is used as a second-line test when there is suspicion that the ASO test is falsely negative. See *antistreptolysin O test.*

anti-double-stranded-DNA antibodies (anti-ds DNA antibodies)   An autoantibody (an anti-"self" antibody) that is directed against DNA and is commonly present in systemic lupus erythematosus. Anti-ds-DNA antibodies are usually measured as part of a battery of antibodies in a workup of a patient known to have antinuclear antibodies. High levels of anti-ds DNA antibodies are associated with glomerulonephritis, one of the complications of lupus erythematosus, which is associated with increased risk of death.
Patient preparation No preparation is required.
Procedure The most common method in use today is indirect fluorescent antibody identification (IFA). ELISA methods, which are much less subjective, are becoming available.
Specimen Serum.
Reference range None detected.
Abnormal values Elevated levels of anti-ds-DNA antibodies are found in most cases of lupus erythematosus.
Cost $70–$90.
Comments Anti-ds DNA antibodies testing is more specific than the older, often subjective interpretation of fluorescent staining patterns. See *anti-single-stranded-DNA antibodies.*

antiendomysial antibodies   Endomysin is a specific portion of muscle fibers. Antiendomysial antibodies have been associated with allergies to wheat and hypersensitivity to gluten, the major protein found in wheat.
Patient preparation No preparation is required.

Procedure Antiendomysial antibodies are measured by ELISA techniques.
Specimen Serum.
Reference range No antibodies detected.
Abnormal values Antiendomysial antibodies may be present in: dermatitis herpetiformis, gluten-sensitive enteropathy (celiac disease), nontropical sprue.
Cost $110–$130.

antigen capture assay A laboratory test used to detect low levels of an antigen in the serum. In this assay, a solid surface (e.g., a bead) is coated with purified and concentrated antibody to an antigen of interest. A body fluid which is presumed to contain the antigen is washed over the solid surface, and the antigen, if present, is "captured." This is followed by a step in which a second antibody with an attached marker (e.g., an enzyme) is washed over the solid surface. If the antigen of interest is present in the fluid, the enzyme will cause a reaction (e.g., a colored dye reaction), allowing the detection of the captured antigen. The antigen capture assay was used briefly to detect HIV but proved far less sensitive than the polymerase chain reaction. See *polymerase chain reaction.*

antigliadin antibodies Gliadins are a class of proteins found in the gluten of wheat and rye grains. In genetically susceptible individuals, certain gliadins may evoke the production of immunoglobulin A (IgA) and G (IgG) antibodies, resulting in a malabsorption syndrome known as celiac disease or celiac enteropathy.
Patient preparation No preparation is required.
Procedure Antigliadin antibodies are measured by ELISA techniques.
Specimen Serum.
Reference range None detected.
Abnormal values Each laboratory that performs this reference test establishes its own normal and abnormal values.
Comments IgG is more sensitive than IgA, but IgA is more specific when evaluating celiac disease.
Cost $150–$170.

antiglobulin test See *direct antiglobulin test, indirect antiglobulin test.*

antiglomerular basement membrane antibodies Anti-GBM antibodies are usually found in a disease that affects the lungs and kidneys known as Goodpasture syndrome. Anti-GBM antibodies may be useful in monitoring treatment of Goodpasture syndrome and may be measured together with anti-neutrophil cytoplasmic antibodies (ANCA) in the rare disease known as Wegener's granulomatosis which, like Goodpasture syndrome, affects the lungs and kidneys.
Patient preparation Specimen is obtained via surgical procedures carried out in a hospital setting.

Procedure Biopsy specimens obtained via surgery or serum are treated with special immunological stains and read by a pathologist.
Specimen Serum or tissue from the lungs or kidneys that must be transported frozen in liquid nitrogen.
Reference range None detected.
Abnormal values IgG antiglomerular basement membrane antibodies are present in the serum or in renal biopsies of patients with Goodpasture's syndrome.
Cost $145–$175.

antihistone antibodies Histones are proteins of unknown function that interact with DNA. Antibodies to histones are found in nearly all patients with symptomatic drug (e.g., procainamide)-induced lupus erythematosus.
Patient preparation No preparation is required.
Procedure Antihistone antibodies are measured by ELISA techniques.
Specimen Serum.
Reference range None detected.
Abnormal values Antihistone antibodies are used to differentiate procainamide-induced lupus erythematosus from the autoimmune form of systemic lupus erythematosus.
Cost $70–$90.

anti-islet cell antibodies See *antipancreatic islet cell antibodies* in Glossary.

anti-Jo1 antibody The Jo-1 antigen corresponds to the neural enzyme. Anti-Jo1 antibodies are found in patients with muscle inflammation (myositis) and interstitial lung disease and are more common in certain connective tissue diseases. The anti-Jo1 antibody is more commonly seen in a condition known as polymyositis than in dermatomyositis and may be associated with interstitial lung disease. It is virtually absent in normal subjects or those with other rheumatic diseases.
Patient preparation No preparation is required.
Procedure Anti-Jo1 antibodies are measured by ELISA techniques.
Specimen Serum.
Reference range None detected.
Abnormal values Anti-Jo1 antibodies may be present in myositis and interstitial lung disease (e.g., cryptogenic fibrosing alveolitis or pulmonary interstitial fibrosis).
Cost $75–$95.
Comments Most laboratories use the ANA (antinuclear antibody) test to screen for autoantibodies, although a negative ANA test does not exclude the presence of Jo-1 antibodies.

antimicrobial susceptibility test See *antibiotic sensitivity and identification*.

antimicrosomal antibodies Antimicrosomal antibodies are those that are antineutrophil cytoplasmic antibody ■ 29

directed against components of the thyroid gland. Of all the tests for antithyroid antibodies, those for antimicrosomal antibodies are the most useful. Antimicrosomal antibodies are often present in thyroid disease, in higher concentrations than antithyroglobulin antibodies, especially in younger patients. See *antithyroglobulin antibodies, antithyroid antibodies.*

Patient preparation No preparation is required.

Procedure Antimicrosomal antibodies are measured by ELISA techniques.

Specimen Serum.

Reference range None detected.

Abnormal values

Increased in: Hashimoto's thyroiditis (nearly 100% positive), Grave's disease (80%), hypothyroidism, atrophic thyroiditis, elderly individuals

Cost $65–$85.

Comments The antibodies can be measured using a number of different techniques including complement fixation, fluorescent antibody detection on unfixed tissue, radioimmunoassay (RIA), and tanned red blood cell agglutination.

antimitochondrial antibodies A family of antibodies that reacts with various antigens in mitochondria. Mitochondria are small organelles present in all cells and are particularly abundant in the renal tubules, gastric mucosa, and other organs in which the cells expend large amounts of energy. One of the mitochondrial antigens evokes the production of a specific antimitochondrial antibody that is present in 90%–95% of patients with primary biliary cirrhosis, some of whom also have a disease known as scleroderma. The antibody is directed against a lipoprotein present on the mitochondrial membrane.

Patient preparation No preparation is required.

Procedure Antimicrochondrial antibodies are measured by IFA or ELISA techniques.

Specimen Serum.

Reference range The titer of antimitochondrial antibodies is usually less than or equal to 20.

Abnormal values

Increased in: primary biliary cirrhosis, chronic active hepatitis, drug-induced hepatitis, cirrhosis of the liver of unknown etiology, autoimmune diseases.

Cost $65–$85.

Comments The presence of antimitochondrial antibodies is not diagnostic for primary biliary cirrhosis; clinical evaluation is needed.

antineutrophil cytoplasmic antibody (ANCA, anticytoplasmic antibody) ANCA antibodies are autoantibodies with varied specificities against myeloid-specific lysosomal enzymes. ANCA are most common in certain forms of systemic vasculitis (e.g., necrotizing vasculitis, active Wegener's granulomatosis [84%–100% are positive], and polyarteritis nodosa) as well as unexplained renal failure. There are two major patterns of ANCA:

1. Cytoplasmic ANCA, which is most commonly positive in Wegener's granulomatosis. See *antiglomerular basement membrane antibodies.*
2. Perinuclear ANCA is specific for myeloperoxidase and is most commonly positive in idiopathic crescentic glomerulonephritis.

Patient preparation No preparation is required.
Procedure ANCA antibodies are measured by ELISA techniques.
Specimen Serum. The specimen must be separated from clotted blood and frozen as quickly as possible.
Reference range None detected.
Abnormal values

Increased in: Wegener's granulomatosis, polyarteritis nodosa, necrotizing vasculitis, Churg-Strauss syndrome, inflammatory bowel disease, drug-induced lupus erythematosus, systemic lupus erythematosus, rheumatoid arthritis.

Cost $150–$180.
Comments ANCA antibodies are quantified by indirect fluorescent microscopy and may be increased in inflammation of the lungs and kidneys, in crescentic glomerulonephritis, and in HIV infection. This is a technically demanding procedure, with both false-positive and false-negative results. A negative result does not exclude Wegener's granulomatosus.

antinuclear antibodies (ANA)   A group of circulating antibodies, commonly seen in connective tissue diseases, that are directed against various antigens in the nucleus, including histones, double- and single-stranded DNA, and ribonucleoprotein. ANAs, like all other autoantibodies, appear when the body's immune system perceives "self" antigens as foreign. Although the antibodies are not themselves harmful, they sometimes form antigen-antibody complexes that cause tissue damage.
Patient preparation No preparation is required.
Procedure ANAs are detected by fluorescent microscopy.
Specimen Serum.
Reference range A titer of less than 180 is negative.
Abnormal values
NUCLEAR STAINING PATTERNS

Homogenous and peripheral	SLE, MCTD, RA, PSS, SS
Speckled	SLE, MCTD, SS, PSS, RA
Nucleolar	PSS, SS
Centromere	CREST syndrome

CYTOPLASMIC STAINING PATTERNS

| Mitochondrial | Primary biliary cirrhosis |
| Smooth muscle | Chronic active hepatitis |

Abbreviations

| MCTD | Mixed connective tissue disease |
| PSS | Progressive systemic sclerosis, scleroderma |

RA	Rheumatoid arthritis
SS	Sjögren's syndrome
SLE	Systemic lupus erythematosus

Cost $45–$75.

Comments The primary purpose of this test is to screen for systemic lupus erythematosus. Positive results may be obtained in normal healthy individuals. The false-positive rate increases with age, as autoantibodies are more common in older individuals.

antiparietal cell antibody (parietal cell antibodies)   Parietal cells are present in the mucosa of the stomach and are involved in acid production. Parietal cell antibodies classically occur in patients with pernicious anemia (50%–100%, who may also have antithyroid antibodies) and in severe atrophic gastritis. Despite the frequency with which this antibody is seen in pernicious anemia, it is nonetheless a nonspecific antibody which is also found in 20%–30% of patients with various autoimmune disorders; it is also found in 2% of the normal population and increases with age—16% of asymptomatic individuals older than 60 years have antiparietal cell antibodies.

Patient preparation No preparation is required.

Procedure These antibodies are identified by the indirect immunofluorescence technique performed on nonhuman cells grown in culture.

Specimen Serum.

Reference range None detected.

Abnormal values Antiparietal cell antibodies are present in: pernicious anemia, atrophic gastritis, chronic gastritis.

Cost $60–$80.

antiphospholipid antibody syndrome   The antiphospholipid antibody syndrome is a clinical condition characterized by the presence of circulating antiphospholipid antibodies (APA), in particular against cardiolipin, which overlap with the so-called lupus anticoagulants. Antiphospholipid antibodies are identified in patients with systemic lupus erythematosus and are associated with thromboembolism, the formation of clots within blood vessels. This condition is classically associated with

1. HABITUAL ABORTION, with midpregnancy fetal loss ("wastage") due to clotting within placental vessels, myocardial infarction due to coronary thrombosis, pulmonary hypertension, and occasionally kidney infarction. These findings often occur in a background of systemic lupus erythematosus.

2. NEUROLOGIC DYSFUNCTION, e.g., cerebrovascular accidents, chorea, epilepsy, Guillain-Barré syndrome, migraines, multiple sclerosis-like disease, myelopathy, and strokes.

These antibodies are thought to cause disease by acting on platelet membranes or on vessel walls. High titers of IgG anticardiolipin antibodies are reported to be relatively specific for the antiphospholipid syndrome. In absence of previous spontaneous fetal loss, the presence of these antibodies is not necessarily a risk factor for fetal loss. These antibodies are known to cross-react with DNA, explaining the false-positive tests for syphilis, which is commonly seen in patients with systemic lupus erythematosus.

Patient preparation No preparation is required other than for drawing blood.

Procedure Antiphospholipid antibodies are measured by ELISA.

Specimen Serum.

Reference range

IgG	Less than 15 GPL units.
IgM	Less than 5 MPL units.

Abnormal values

Low positive	IgG	16–40 GPL units.
	IgM	6–20 MPL units.
Moderate positive	IgG	41–80 GPL units.
	IgM	21–40 MPL units.
High positive	IgG	Greater than 80 GPL units.
	IgM	Greater than 40 MPL units.

Cost $100–$200.

Comments Antiphospholipid and anticardiolipin antibodies are often associated with, but are not identical to, the lupus antibodies (i.e., an elevated ACA titer may not always coexist with positive lupus antibodies). Synonyms include circulating lupus anticoagulant syndrome, anticardiolipin antibody syndrome, lupus anticoagulant-antiphospholipid antibody syndrome.

antiplatelet antibody test   This test is used to detect auto- or alloantibodies directed against platelet antigens in cases of thrombocytopenia or patients who appear refractory (i.e., do not respond) to platelet transfusions.

Patient preparation No preparation is required.

Procedure Platelet antibodies are measured by several methods, including ELISA, complement fixation, and immunofluorescence.

Specimen Plasma. The plasma must be separated from red blood cells and frozen in a plastic vial for transportation to the laboratory. An alternative method is to collect the specimen in acid citrate dextrose (ACD) tubes.

Reference range Each laboratory establishes its own normal range.

Abnormal values These antibodies are found in immune thrombocytopenia.

Cost $130–$160.

Comments This very difficult and costly test is not widely available.

anti-PRP antibody   A serotype-specific antibody against the bacterial polyribosylribitol phosphate, which confers protection against invasive *Haemophilus influenzae* infection. Anti-PRP antibody may be induced by vaccination with the *H. influenzae* type b polysaccharide vaccine or other types of vaccines and may be measured in children and in people with AIDS.

Patient preparation No preparation is required.

Procedure Anti-PRP antibodies are measured by ELISA.

Specimen Serum.

Reference range Anti-PRP antibodies are present in those protected against *Haemophilus influenzae.*

Abnormal values Anti-PRP antibodies are absent in those susceptible to *Haemophilus influenzae.*

Cost $100–$200.

antireticulin antibodies The presence of antibodies to reticulin is a non-specific finding that has been described in untreated celiac disease and dermatitis herpetiformis and can be used to monitor compliance with a gluten-free diet.

Patient preparation No special preparation is required.

Procedure Antireticulin antibodies are measured by ELISA techniques.

Specimen Serum.

Reference range None detected.

Abnormal values Each laboratory establishes its own normal and abnormal values.

Cost $90–$110.

antiribosomal antibodies Ribosomal antibodies are found in 5%–12% of patients with systemic lupus erythematosus and rarely in other rheumatic diseases. This test is used in conjunction with antinuclear antibody testing (ANA) and extractable nuclear antigen (ENA) to diagnose rheumatic diseases. See *antinuclear antibodies, extractable nuclear antigens.*

antiscleroderma antibodies Scleroderma antibodies (Scl-70) are found in approximately 30% of patients with diffuse scleroderma.

Patient preparation No special preparation is required.

Procedure Antiscleroderma antibodies are measured by IFA or ELISA techniques.

Specimen Serum.

Reference range None detected.

Abnormal values Antiscleroderma antibodies are detected in diffuse scleroderma.

Cost $90–$100.

anti-single-stranded-DNA antibodies (anti-ss DNA antibodies) This anti-DNA autoantibody, like its anti-double-stranded "cousin," occurs in so-called connective tissue (or collagen vascular) diseases, the prototypic form being systemic lupus erythematosus. It is used in the same context as the test for anti-double-stranded DNA antibodies.

Patient preparation No preparation is required.

Procedure Anti-single-stranded DNA antibodies are measured by IFA techniques.

Specimen Serum.

Reference range None detected.
Abnormal values Elevated levels may be found in lupus erythematosus.
Cost $90–$100.
Comments The test for anti-single-stranded DNA antibodies is thought to be less useful than that for anti-double-stranded DNA antibodies.

anti-smooth muscle antibodies A group of antibodies that have been identified in a number of liver diseases, including chronic viral (formerly known as chronic active) hepatitis and primary biliary cirrhosis, as well as infectious mononucleosis and asthma. These antibodies do not cause liver damage, and thus have been described as a "passenger" phenomenon.
Patient preparation No special preparation is required.
Procedure Smooth muscle antibodies are measured by indirect immunofluorescence.
Specimen Serum.
Reference range Titers of less than 1:40.
Abnormal values Titers of 1:80 to 1:320 are seen in chronic active hepatitis. Smooth muscle antibodies are also present in primary biliary cirrhosis, infectious mononucleosis, asthma, and in tumors.
Cost $100–$150.

antisperm antibodies Although sperm antibodies occur in infertility, their presence has not been associated with a specific type of infertility. Sperm antibodies may be found in the circulation, either free or as immune complexes, in seminal fluid and/or attached to the sperm surface.
Patient preparation No special preparation is required.
Procedure Antisperm antibodies are measured by IFA or ELISA.
Specimen Serum, semen.
Reference range None detected.
Abnormal values Presence of antisperm antibodies may be associated with infertility.
Cost $120–$140.
Comments The serum test can be negative in spite of the presence of antibodies on the sperm surface; therefore, antibodies must be measured in both serum and semen.

antistreptolysin O test (ASO) The antistreptolysin O test is a serologic test that monitors group A β-hemolytic streptococcal infection (strep throat) and acute streptococcal glomerulonephritis. High titers usually occur only after prolonged or recurrent infections and identify patients at risk for nonepidemic pharyngitis. Serial titers provide a more reliable diagnosis than a single titer.
Patient preparation No preparation is required.
Procedure ASO is measured by latex agglutination or hemagglutination procedures.
Specimen Serum.

Reference range

Adults, preschool children	Less than 85 Todd units.
School-age children	Less than 170 Todd units.

Abnormal values

Low-level increase	Uncomplicated streptococcal infection
Increase to 250 Todd units	Inactive rheumatic fever
Greater than 500 Todd units	Acute rheumatic fever
	Acute poststreptococcal glomerulonephritis

Cost $30–$50.

Comments Even healthy persons have some detectable ASO titer from previous minor streptococcal infections. Patients with streptococcal skin infections rarely have abnormal ASO titers. A more recent test, anti-DNase B (ADB), can detect both pharyngeal and skin infections, making it superior to ASO. Antibiotic or corticosteroid therapy may suppress the ASO response.

antitetanus toxoid antibodies   Measurement of antibodies to tetanus toxoid is used to assess the status of tetanus immunity. IgM antibodies are increased following acute exposure and IgG antibodies are present in individuals who have adequate serum levels of antitetanus antibodies.

Patient preparation No special preparation is required.

Procedure Antitetanus toxoid antibodies are measured by ELISA.

Specimen Serum.

Reference range Antitetanus antibodies are present in immunized individuals.

Abnormal values Antitetanus antibodies are absent in individuals susceptible to tetanus.

Comments Most people have been immunized to tetanus. The assay is of no use in managing acute clinical tetanus. This test should be used if there is a question as to the immune status of a patient.

antithrombin III   Antithrombin III (AT-III) is a serine protease inhibitor formed in the liver that can be decreased in liver disease (due to decreased production) and disseminated intravascular coagulation (due to "consumption"). AT-III preferentially binds thrombin as well as some other enzymes (known as serine proteases) in the coagulation cascade and neutralizes their activity, an action that slows or stops the clotting of blood. Heparin anticoagulant activity hinges on the activation of AT-III, and AT-III-deficient individuals derive no benefit from heparin therapy.

Patient preparation No special preparation is required.

Procedure Two procedures can be used. The most common is the functional assay which actually measures the activity of AT-III using chromogenic substrates. The more sensitive test is the total assay which uses ELISA or radioimmunoassay (RIA) to measure AT-III.

Specimen Citrated plasma that has been frozen.

Reference range 17–25 mg/dL.

Abnormal values
   Increased in: acute hepatitis, following renal transplant, inflammation, menstruation, vitamin K deficiency.
   Decreased in: congenital deficiency, liver transplant, disseminated intravascular coagulopathy, nephrotic syndrome, cirrhosis, carcinoma, mid-menstrual cycle, chronic liver failure, other liver diseases.
Cost $35–$50.
Comments A decrease in AT-III may predispose patients to thrombosis and failure to respond to heparin therapy.

antithyroglobulin antibodies   Thyroglobulin is the major protein produced by the thyroid gland and is the primary carrier molecule for the thyroid hormones thyroxine (T_4) and T_3. Antithyroglobulin antibodies are found in autoimmune diseases of the thyroid and are usually measured as part of the diagnostic workup for hypothyroidism.
   Patient preparation No preparation is required.
   Procedure Antithyroglobulin antibodies are measured by IFA and ELISA.
   Specimen Serum.
   Reference range None detected.
   Abnormal values Antithyroglobulin antibodies are present in: Hashimoto's thyroiditis (circa 85% positive), Graves' disease (30%), hypothyroidism, atrophic thyroiditis, elderly individuals.
   Cost $65–$85.
   Comments Because antithyroid antibodies occur in other autoimmune diseases, further tests (e.g., assays for antimicrosomal antibodies) are needed to reach a definitive diagnosis. See *antimicrosomal antibodies, antithyroid antibodies.*

antithyroid antibodies (thyroid antibodies)   Any of a number of antibodies directed against "self" antigens which may be either cellular components (e.g., antimicrosomal antibodies) or proteins (e.g., thyroglobulin) of thyroid origin that are often present in autoimmune diseases. Antimicrosomal and antithyroglobulin antibodies are the most commonly measured. These antibodies damage the thyroid and are found in patients with autoimmune diseases of the thyroid and other organs.
   Patient preparation No special preparation is required.
   Procedure These antibodies are measured by ELISA or IFA.
   Specimen Serum.
   Reference range Titers of less than 1:32 (antithyroglobulin) and less than 1:100 (antimicrosomal) are classified as negative.
   Abnormal values
   Increased in: chronic thyroiditis (40%–70%), Graves' disease (thyrotoxicosis), Hashimoto's thyroiditis, hypothyroidism, pernicious anemia, rheumatoid arthritis, systemic lupus erythematosus.
   Cost $75–$100. See *antimicrosomal antibodies, antithyroglobulin antibodies.*

apexcardiography Apexcardiography is a technique that graphically records the movements of the chest wall caused by the beating heart. It is used to evaluate left ventricular function, myocardial infarction, aneurysms, ischemia, and pericarditis. The apexcardiogram provides ancillary (extra) information and is used in conjunction with electrocardiography, phonocardiography, and carotid or jugular vein pulse tracings.

Patient preparation No preparation is required.

Procedure A transducer is placed on the patient's chest that converts the mechanical force of the moving chest wall into electrical energy. This energy is then converted into waves known as apexcardiograms.

Reference range No abnormalities in amplitude (size) or appearance of waves.

Abnormal values Absent or abnormal waves may be present in atrial fibrillation, mitral and aortic valve stenosis, systemic hypertension, hypertrophic cardiomyopathy, ventricular aneurysm, ischemia, infarction, and in coronary artery disease.

Cost $150–$200.

apolipoproteins A family of molecules (including Apo A-I, Apo A-II, and Apo B) that corresponds to the protein portion of lipoproteins. Some reports in medical literature link coronary artery disease to decreased Apo A-I, Apo A-II, and HDL-cholesterol and/or increased Apo B, total cholesterol, triglycerides, and LDL-cholesterol. Apo A and Apo B may be measured in conjuncution with cholesterol and triglycerides to determine risk of coronary heart disease.

Patient preparation Patient must fast for 12–24 hours prior to the test.

Procedure Apolipoproteins are measured by nephelometry or turbidimetry.

Specimen Serum.

Reference range

	Apo A	Apo B
Males	66–151 mg/dL	49–123 mg/dL
Females	75–170 mg/dL	26–119 mg/dL

Abnormal values

	Apo A	Apo B
Males	Less than 60 mg/dL	Less than 45 mg/dL
	Greater than 160 mg/dL	Greater than 130 mg/dL
Females	Less than 70 mg/dL	Less than 20 mg/dL
	Greater than 175 mg/dL	Greater than 125 mg/dL

Cost $100–$150.

Comments There is much controversy over the utility of Apo A and Apo B measurements as a means of determining the risk for coronary artery disease and atherosclerosis. Some experts believe more data is needed to determine their value.

aPTT Activated partial thromboplastin time. See *partial thromboplastin time.*

arterial blood gas Blood gas determinations are used to assess pulmonary function, acid-base level of the blood, and to monitor respiratory therapy.

Patient preparation No preparation is required. This test is normally done in a hospital setting because its primary use is in monitoring patients in pulmonary distress.

Procedure Blood gases are measured manometrically using specialized instruments.

Specimen Whole blood obtained from an artery. Because the analytes (e.g., oxygen and carbon dioxide) are not stable, the test cannot be performed outside of a hospital setting; the specimen must be rushed to the laboratory on ice and the test performed immediately.

Reference range

pO_2	75–100 mm Hg.
pCO_2	35–45 mm Hg.
pH	7.35–7.42.
O_2Ct	15%–23%.
O_2sat	94%–100%.
HCO_3	22–26 mEq/L.

Abnormal values Respiratory defects, decreased O_2, acidosis, defects in pH and bicarbonate.

Cost $50–$100.

Comments Outpatient clinical laboratories normally do not perform these tests. See the following entries in the Glossary: *metabolic acidosis, metabolic alkalosis, respiratory acidosis, respiratory alkalosis.*

arterial blood oximetry A clinical test that quantifies carboxyhemoglobin and methemoglobin and calculates the content of oxygen bound to hemoglobin. Arterial blood oximetry is conducted on patients with anemia or polycythemia for evaluation of altered hemoglobins and oxygen content of the blood and to correlate the findings of arterial blood gas analysis.

Patient preparation No preparation is required, other than for drawing blood from an arterial source.

Procedure This is a manometric test which utilizes specialized instrumentation.

Specimen Blood obtained from an artery. Because the analyte, carbon monoxide, is not stable, the test cannot be performed outside of a hospital setting; the specimen must be rushed to the laboratory on ice and the test performed immediately.

Reference range	Carboxyhemoglobin	Less than 1.5%.
Abnormal values	Heavy smokers	Up to 5% or more.
Cost $50–$100.		

arterial catheterization (arterial cannulation) The insertion of an indwelling catheter in order to monitor a particular parameter in the peripheral blood in "real time." Arterial catheterization is used to monitor a hemodynamically unstable patient who may be hypo– or hypertensive and currently being treated with vasopressor or vasodilator agents; to sample blood on a regular basis to assess blood gases (oxygen, carbon dioxide) in a patient receiving mechanical ventilation; and to determine cardiac output.

Cost Arterial catheterization is usually performed in a hospital setting and is rarely a separately billed procedure.

arterial study See *arteriography*.

arteriography (arterial study) A general term for the visualization of the arteries by injection of a radiocontrast material into an area of clinical concern and/or stenosis. Arteriograms are performed on arteries that are severely affected by atherosclerosis which, if untreated, may lead to infarction (death of tissue) of a limb or organ, long-term disability, or in the extreme case, death. Arteriograms are commonly performed on the carotid arteries (which are a major conduit of blood to the brain), the coronary arteries (heart), and femoral arteries (legs), each of which may respond to surgical or medical (i.e., nonsurgical) therapy if the artery is severely occluded.

Patient preparation Informed consent is required. The patient must be on a clear liquid diet before the procedure. Baseline chemistries (BUN, creatine platelets, partial thromboplastin time, and prothrombin time) are necessary.

Procedure A local anesthetic is injected at the site of insertion of the angiographic catheter. The catheter is inserted and a radiologic device—the fluoroscope—is used to guide the catheter to the artery being evaluated. An opaque (contrast) material is injected into the artery.

Reference range No blockages, atherosclerosis, or strictures of the vessels are identified.

Abnormal values Atherosclerosis and vascular spasms cause local or diffuse narrowing of the arteries.

Cost $250–$800.

arthritis panel A standard panel of laboratory tests used to evaluate possible causes of arthritis and used for Medicare or Medicaid reimbursement. The panel must include a fluorescent antibody screen for antinuclear antibodies, quantification of rheumatoid factor and uric acid, and nonautomated erythrocyte sedimentation rate. See *synovial fluid analysis*.

arthrography A procedure in which air or radiocontrast medium is injected into various joints (e.g., shoulder, wrist, knee, ankle) to allow visualization of the articular space. Arthrography has waned in popularity as improvements in instruments and greater understanding of the anatomy and derangements of the joint have made arthroscopy the preferred method for diagnosing joint disease.

Patient preparation Informed consent is required. The patient should not vigorously exercise the joint being examined for 24 hours before the procedure.

Procedure Local anesthesia is injected adjacent to the joint being examined. A 22-gauge needle is used to aspirate fluid for bacterial and chemical analysis. The same needle is used to inject the radiocontrast material and air into the joint space under fluoroscopic guidance. Computed tomography images and standard X-ray films are obtained from the joint.

Specimen Fluid for bacterial and chemical analysis; film and CT scans from the joint.

Reference range No abnormalities are identified.

Abnormal values Increase in fluid in joints; defects or alterations in the cartilage and/or meniscus may require treatment.

Cost $200–$400.

arthroscopy A procedure in which an endoscope is inserted into a joint (e.g., shoulder, wrist, knee, ankle) to directly examine an articular space of interest. Arthroscopy has become one of the most commonly performed procedures in medicine in general and orthopedics in particular. It can be used to diagnose diseases of the meniscus, synovium, and extrasynovial tissues and, if necessary, to obtain biopsies. It is also used to treat some of the diseases diagnosed during the procedure.

Patient preparation This procedure requires preoperative preparation such as sterilization of the field. In addition, either local, spinal, or general anesthesia is required.

Procedure Depending on the joint to be examined, small incisions are made through which the endoscope is inserted into the joint. The endoscope is then used to visualize the joint, obtain specimens, or trim torn cartilage.

Abnormal values
Baker's cyst, chondromalacia, chondromatosis, fractures, osteochondral disruption and fractures, osteochondritis dissecans, rheumatic disease, synovial defects, tears of the capsule, ligaments.

Cost $750–$1000.

Comments Since this is a surgical procedure, there is generally some minor discomfort. See *synovial fluid analysis.*

ascorbic acid Ascorbic acid, more commonly known as vitamin C, is a cofactor for protocollagen; it promotes the conversion of tropocollagen to collagen. Vitamin C deficiency is known as scurvy.

Patient preparation The patient should not eat after midnight before the specimen is obtained.

Procedure Ascorbic acid is measured by high-performance liquid chromotography.

Specimen Serum, preferably collected in a green-top tube. White blood cells or urine may also be used.

Reference range
Serum   0.6–2.0 mg/dL.
White blood cells   20–50 mg/10^8 white blood cells.

Abnormal values
Decreased in: scurvy, malabsorption, alcoholism, pregnancy, hyperthyroidism, renal failure.

Cost $100–$150.

aspartate aminotransferase (AST, GOT, glutamate oxaloacetate transaminase) Aspartate aminotransferase is an enzyme found primarily in the liver and heart. It is released into the bloodstream in hepatic, myocardial, renal and cerebral infarction, and in hepatic and skeletal muscle disease.

Patient preparation No preparation is required.

Procedure AST is measured spectrophometrically. AST assays are automated and usually included as part of standard panels of blood chemistry tests.

Specimen Serum or heparinized plasma.

Reference range

Newborn	25–75 U/L.
Infant	15–60 U/L.
Adult	8–20 U/L.
Elderly adult	10–25 U/L.

Abnormal values

Increased in: severe hepatitis, liver cell necrosis, necrosis or trauma of heart muscle, necrosis, or trauma of skeletal muscle

Cost $10–$20 when performed as a single test.

aspiration biopsy (fine needle aspiration biopsy) The removal of minute tissue fragments by a needle and syringe under suction to prepare a smear for cytological examination or to make a cell block.

Patient preparation Informed consent is required. A sedative may be necessary for anxious patients.

Procedure A local anesthetic is injected near the biopsy site (e.g., breast, thyroid). A 22-gauge needle is attached to a syringe, and cells and tissue are aspirated using suction. A smear is made of the cells and/or a cell block is produced, which are examined by a pathologist or cytopathologist.

Specimen Smear of cells, cell block.

Reference range Normal cells and/or tissue.

Abnormal values Inflammatory cells, malignant cells, or microorganisms may be present.

Cost $100–$250.

aspiration cytology A formal term for diagnostic cells and other material from internal organs (e.g., breast, liver, lymph node, prostate, salivary gland, thyroid) and other relatively inaccessible sites which are obtained by fine needle aspiration. See *exfoliative cytology.*

aspirin (acetylsalicylic acid) A widely used analgesic that is also used to "thin" the blood in patients at risk for coronary artery disease. The various forms of aspirin (e.g., salicylic acid) have similar effects of relieving pain, reducing fever, and diminishing inflammation. Aspirin induces a prolonged functional defect in platelets by permanently inactivating prostaglandin synthase, which converts arachidonate to prostaglandin H_2; this effect is detected clinically as a prolonged bleeding time. Aspirin is an over-the-counter medication which can have serious side effects when abused. Children who take aspirin for upper respiratory infection of viral etiology are at risk for Reye's syndrome (acute hepatic fatty degeneration and encephalopathy), even at low doses. Due to the risk of Reye's syndrome, the American Academy of Pediatrics has recommended that no child receive aspirin if he/she has had chickenpox or influenza; most pediatricians have stopped prescribing aspirin for any fever in children. Moreover, aspirin can cause bleeding in susceptible patients. Salicylate overdose can be a very serious medical situation and laboratory measurements are usually ordered when an overdose is suspected.

Patient preparation No preparation is required.

Procedure Acetylsalicylic acid is measured spectrophotometrically.

Specimen Serum.

Reference range 2–20 mg/dL.

Abnormal values Greater than 30 mg/dL.

Cost $25–$50.

Comments Aspirin use during pregnancy was formerly thought to increase the incidence of congenital cardiac malformations. Early testing methods were inconsistent due to interfering substances. Newer methodologies using immunoassays are much more reliable.

audiometric test See *hearing function test.*

autohemolysis test A test that measures the amount of hemolysis (destruction of red blood cells) that occurs spontaneously during 24 hours. The test is used to detect hereditary spherocytosis, a rare type of anemia, and separate it from other forms of hemolytic anemia.

Patient preparation No preparation is required.

Procedure Defibrinated blood is incubated with differing concentrations of salt for 24 hours at 37° C (body temperature). The results are compared with those of identical blood that has glucose or ATP added before incubation.

Specimen Blood.

Reference range 50% hemolysis of normal red blood cells occurs at 0.4%–0.5% saline solutions.

Abnormal values

Increased in: hereditary spherocytosis, osmotic fragility.

Decreased in: thalassemia.

Cost $150–$300.

Babesia microti *Babesia* is an intraerythrocytic parasite that can cause symptoms resembling those of malaria. Immunocompromised persons and the elderly are at the greatest risk, although immunocompetent persons can also develop the disease, known as babesiosis. Infections are detected by serological tests and by microscopic examination of peripheral blood smears.

Patient preparation No preparation is required.

Procedure The serum is analyzed by ELISA techniques. A thick smear of blood is stained and examined by light microscopy.

Specimen Serum is used for the serological tests. Whole blood collected in EDTA is used for microscopic evaluation.

Reference range Titers of less than 1:8 for serologic examination by ELISA techniques. No organisms detected by light microscopy.

Abnormal values Titers of greater than or equal to 1:16 by ELISA techniques. Organisms detected on smear of blood.

Cost Serologic tests $75–$100.
Microscopic evaluation $50–$75.

Comments Babesia microti infection has been found to occur simultaneously with Lyme disease.

bacterial culture Microbiology cultures can be separated into two distinct types: aerobic (the most common type of culture) and anaerobic. Aerobic bacteria grow in the presence of oxygen and are the most common causes of infection. Anaerobic bacteria grow in the absence of oxygen or under conditions of reduced oxygen. Anaerobic bacteria are commonly present in wounds, and thus wound cultures are performed under both aerobic and anerobic conditions.

Patient preparation No preparation is required except for drawing blood and obtaining urine and other specimens (e.g., from the throat and lungs).

Procedure A specimen obtained from a patient with a suspected anaerobic infection requires special handling because oxygen (i.e., open air) is toxic to these bacteria and may be responsible for a culture-negative result.

Once the specimen arrives in the microbiology laboratory, it is processed under conditions of reduced oxygen and any bacteria identified are recultured to determine the bacteria's sensitivity to antibiotics.

Specimen Blood, urine, sputum, and material from wounds is collected into a low-oxygen transportation material and sent quickly to the laboratory.

Reference range No bacteria are cultured after a period of two to five days.

Abnormal values Bacteria are identified in one or more of the cultures.

Cost $50–$100.

bactericidal activity testing See *antibiotic sensitivity and identification, susceptibility test.*

BAER See *brainstem auditory evoked response.*

balloon angioplasty A general term for an invasive cardiology procedure in which a catheter with an inflatable balloon is "snaked" to a previously identified (by angiography) zone of arterial stenosis or occlusion; once in place, the balloon is inflated, expanding the lumen of the occluded vessel. Balloon angioplasty is used for coronary and carotid arteries and for other vessels. See *percutaneous transluminal coronary angioplasty.*

band test See *lupus band test* in Glossary.

barium enema (lower GI series) A radiographic procedure for examining the large intestine in which barium sulfate (a substance that blocks the passage of X rays), either alone (single contrast) or with air (double contrast), is instilled by enema until the large bowel is filled. Any regional or zonal defects in the appearance of the column of barium may indicate disease in the form of inflammation, polyps, or tumors; in contrast, visible pouches of barium can indicate diverticuli. A barium enema is a critical component of a diagnostic workup in patients with histories of altered bowel habits, lower abdominal pain, or the passage of blood, mucus, or pus in the stool. If these changes are of acute and/or recent onset and accompanied by weight loss, malignancy becomes a primary consideration; definitive diagnosis requires proctoscopy or sigmoidoscopy, accompanied by a biopsy.

Patient preparation The following may be ordered:
1. Low-residue diet for one to three days.
2. Only clear liquids the day before the test.
3. As much water or clear liquids as possible for 12–24 hours before the test.
4. Laxatives the afternoon prior to the test.
5. Suppository and/or enemas in the evening or early morning of test.
6. Light breakfast of toast and black coffee or clear tea the morning of test.
7. Patient must be instructed as to the importance of retaining the barium enema.

Procedure
1. Patient is placed in supine position and initial X rays are taken.
2. Patient is then placed in Sims position, and a well-lubricated rectal tube is inserted through the anus.
3. Barium is then administered slowly, and the filling process is followed fluoroscopically as the patient assumes varied positions.
4. Spot films are taken during the flow of barium.
5. The rectal tube is withdrawn, after which the patient evacuates as much barium as possible.
6. After evacuation, an additional film is taken.

Specimen The diagnostic "specimen" consists of X rays of the large intestine.

Reference range Uniform filling and passage of barium through the colon.

Abnormal values Carcinoma, diverticulitis, chronic ulcerative colitis, granulomatous colitis, polyps, intussusception, gastroenteritis, stenosis, irritable colon, vascular injury, some cases of acute appendicitis.

Cost $300–$500.

Comments If a complete GI series is to be performed, this test should be done before the barium swallow because residual barium may interfere. Several conditions are contraindications for this test, including tachycardia, severe ulcerative colitis, toxic megacolon, or suspected perforation of the large intestine.

barium swallow (upper GI series)   A technique in which a radiocontrast "milkshake" of barium sulfate is swallowed to detect benign or malignant lesions of the pharynx, esophagus, stomach and small intestine and to visualize the integrity of the swallowing mechanism. The progress of the barium is followed radiographically to detect filling defects (places where the normal outline of barium should be seen but is not). Barium swallow is used to detect foreign bodies, strictures, tumors, Barrett's esophagus, fistulas, and reflux. Definitive diagnosis of lesions of the region requires endoscopic biopsy.

Patient preparation Foods, fluids, and antacids should be restricted after midnight the night before the test. The patient should be aware that the term "milkshake" refers to the barium preparation's consistency and not its rather unpleasant taste.

Procedure
1. Patient is placed in an upright position behind a fluoroscope, and the heart, lungs, and abdomen are examined.
2. Patient takes one swallow of the barium mixture, and the pharyngeal action is recorded by cineradiography.
3. Patient takes several swallows of the barium mixture, and the passage of barium is examined fluoroscopically; spot films of the esophageal region are taken.
4. Patient is placed in other positions and instructed to swallow barium. Additional fluoroscopic observation and spot films are taken.

5. The cardia and fundus of the patient's stomach are also observed.

Specimen The diagnostic "specimen" consists of X rays of the esophagus and stomach.

Reference range No abnormalities in filling noted.

Abnormal values Hiatus hernia, esophageal diverticula, esophageal varices, esophageal strictures, tumors, polyps, ulcers, pharyngeal muscular disorders, esophageal spasms, achalasia.

Cost $100–$500.

Comments If this test is part of a GI series, the barium enema must be done first. Stools will be chalky and light-colored for 24–72 hours after test. Barium may cause obstruction or fecal impaction, and the physician should be notified if barium is not expelled in two to three days. Synonyms include barium esophagram, esophagram, and esophagogram.

Barr body (sex chromatin) A condensed clump of chromatin which corresponds to an inactivated X chromosome. The number of Barr bodies per cell is one less than the number of X chromosomes.

Patient preparation In adults, the mouth should be rinsed before obtaining a specimen. In children, the specimen should be collected between feedings.

Procedure The buccal (inner cheek) mucosa is scraped twice, once to clean debris and a second time with a clean tongue depressor to obtain surface epithelial cells. The material from the second scraping is spread on a glass slide. The slide is fixed in alcohol and examined by fluorescence microscopy.

Specimen Scrapings from buccal mucosa, or in some women, from the vaginal wall.

Reference range

Males	No Barr bodies are seen.
Females	One Barr body is seen.

Abnormal values

Males	One or more Barr bodies are seen.
Females	Two or more Barr bodies are seen.

Cost $75–$125.

barrier tube See *Corvac tube* in Glossary.

basal acid output (BAO) A measure of the amount of hydrogen ions (H^+) produced by the resting stomach (i.e., not been stimulated by sight, smells, or thoughts which would cause production of acid). Basal acid output serves to measure the completeness of vagotomy used in patients with gastrectomy.

Patient preparation Discontinue all anticholinergics, antidepressants, and tranquilizers 24 to 48 hours before testing. No food or liquids after midnight the night before the procedure. No antacids, cimetidine, alcohol, tobacco, propranolol, or ranitidine.

Procedure The stomach is intubated, and the gastric content is aspirated to determine basal acid output.

Specimen Gastric juice.
Reference range 0–10 mmol of H^+/hour
Abnormal values
   Increased in: gastric cancer, hypothyroidism (myxedema),
   megaloblastic (pernicious) anemia, rheumatoid arthritis, Zollinger-
   Ellison syndrome.
Cost $75–$125.

"belly" tap   See *abdominal tap.*

Bence-Jones protein   Bence-Jones proteins are abnormal, light-chain immunoglobulins derived from the clonal expansions of lymphocytes. They are found in the urine of patients with multiple myeloma (a cancer of the bone marrow) and Waldenström's macroglobulinemia.
   Patient preparation No preparation is required.
   Procedure The old procedure was a manual precipitation of protein with sulfosalycilic acid and observation of the precipitate after boiling the solution. The current method is immunofixation electrophoresis, which is much more specific and sensitive.
   Specimen Urine.
   Reference range None detected.
   Abnormal values Bence-Jones proteins are often present in Waldenström's macroglobulinemia (most patients) and multiple myeloma (50%–80%).
   Cost $45–$65.
   Comments False-positive results can occur in connective tissue disease, renal insufficiency, and some malignancies. Immunofixation electrophoresis is the preferred method for detecting Bence-Jones proteins; heat treatment methods have fallen into disuse.

Bernstein test (esophageal acid perfusion, acid infusion test)   A clinical test to determine if a patient's heartburn symptoms are related to reflux by exposing the esophagus to acid. The Bernstein test is especially useful when endoscopic examination and distal esophageal biopsy results are negative.
   Patient preparation The patient should not eat or drink eight hours before the procedure. Antacids and H_2 blockers (e.g., ranitidine, cimetidine) must be discontinued before the test.
   Procedure A nasogastric tube is inserted into the esophagus, and low concentrations (0.1 normal) of hydrochloric acid are instilled on the esophageal mucosa. The patient is told to describe any symptons, such as burning pains, during the test. The test is ended after 30 minutes, after which the mucosa is washed with saline solution.
   Specimen The "specimen" consists of symptoms described by the patient during the procedure.
   Reference range No symptoms reported by the patient during the acid perfusion or saline perfusion.

Abnormal values Typical heartburn is described by the patient during acid, but not during saline perfusion.
Cost $300–$600.

beta-carotene See *carotene.*

beta-2-microglobulin Beta-2-microglobulin is an amino acid cell membrane-associated protein that is nonspecifically increased in inflammation, renal disease, AIDS, and in some malignancies. Because the urinary levels of beta-2-microglobulin are affected by kidney disease, it is reported to be useful in diabetics to monitor renal involvement.
Patient preparation No preparation is required.
Procedure Beta-2-microglobulin is measured by nephelometric or ELISA techniques.
Specimen Serum, urine (24-hour specimen).
Reference range
   Serum   Less than 2mg/ml.
   Urine   Less than 120 mg/24 hrs.
Abnormal values
   Serum increased in: inflammation, chronic lymphocytic leukemia, glomerular disease.
   Serum decreased in: renal tubular disease.
   Urine increased in: renal tubular disease.
   Urine decreased in: glomerular disease.
Cost $20–$40.

bicarbonate Bicarbonate is the most important buffer compound in the blood. A buffer maintains the pH (acid-base balance) of the blood at a proper level, slightly on the acid side of a neutral pH of 7.0. Bicarbonate is easily regulated by the kidney, which excretes it in excess and retains it when needed.
Patient preparation No preparation is required.
Procedure Bicarbonate is measured spectrophotometrically. It is generally part of a larger profile including electrolytes and glucose.
Specimen Serum.
Reference range 24–26 mEq/L.
Abnormal values
   Increased in: ingestion of excessive amounts of antacids, diuretics, steroids.
   Decreased in: diarrhea, liver disease, renal disease, chemical poisoning.
Cost $10–$15.
Comments Bicarbonate levels are not used to diagnose a specific disease but to measure the degree of metabolic pH imbalance, which is of greatest use in acute situations. It is also used to monitor the response to rehydration or administration of electrolytes. In the past, bicarbonate levels were determined as part of the general health screen, a practice that has been largely

discontinued given the relative instability of bicarbonate when transported. Bicarbonate levels are useful if appropriate precautions are taken during transportation, and the length of time between obtaining the specimen and analysis can be minimized. See *arterial blood gas.*

bilirubin Bilirubin is a metabolized product of hemoglobin when red blood cells break down at the end of their usual lifespan of four months. Bilirubin becomes part of the bile fluid that is transported from the liver to the gallbladder to the intestines, most of which is normally eliminated by the bowels. Excessive production or decreased excretion of bilirubin increases the minute amounts normally present in the blood, and its unique color, when increased, causes a yellowing (jaundice) of the skin and the whites of the eyes. Bilirubin that has not been metabolized in the liver is attached to albumin in the blood; in this state it is called indirect bilirubin. After hepatic metabolism, the bilirubin is no longer bound to proteins and is called direct bilirubin. The sum of direct and indirect bilirubin is called total bilirubin. Total bilirubin is usually measured as part of a routine chemistry profile and in liver profiles. If the total bilirubin is elevated, the laboratory will measure the direct bilirubin (reflex diagnostic testing). In the laboratory, total and direct bilirubin can be easily measured, while indirect bilirubin is calculated from the difference.

Patient preparation No preparation is required.

Procedure Bilirubin is measured spectrophotometrically on automated analyzers.

Specimen Serum, urine, amniotic fluid. Because bilirubin breaks down when exposed to light, specimens should be protected from exposure to strong ultraviolet light.

Reference range

TOTAL BILIRUBIN

Umbilical cord	Less than 2.0 mg/dL
0–1 days	Less than 6.0 mg/dL
1–2 days	Less than 8.0 mg/dL
3–5 days	Less than 12 mg/dL
Beyond day 5	Less than 0.2–1.0 mg/dL

DIRECT BILIRUBIN
0.0–0.2 mg/dL

URINE
Negative

AMNIOTIC FLUID

| 28 weeks | Less than 0.075 mg/dL |
| 40 weeks | Less than 0.025 mg/dL |

Abnormal values

Total bilirubin increased in: hepatic damage, hemolytic anemia, certain congenital enzyme deficiencies.

Direct bilirubin decreased in: biliary obstruction.

Direct and indirect bilirubin increased in: chronic hemolysis, biliary obstruction with hepatic damage.

Cost $10–$15.

Comments Bilirubin in newborns is normally high. If the levels go above 20 mg/dL, exchange transfusion must be considered in order to avoid permanent damage in the form of kernicterus, the accumulation of bilirubin in the brain. Bilirubin can be found in the urine in certain diseases. Total bilirubin is increased with liver cirrhosis. Some drugs (e.g., Thorazine, hormones, antibiotics) can increase direct bilirubin.

biophysical profile   Measurement of five fetal activities that usually identify a fetus at risk for potentially poor outcome. Except for the nonstress test, the other parameters may be measured simultaneously by dynamic ultrasound imaging. Fetal breathing movement, non-stress test, fetal muscle tone, fetal movement, and amniotic fluid volume are the five fetal activities measured.

Cost $500.

biopsy   A term referring to both the surgical procedure in which a small piece of tissue is removed from a patient and the tissue itself. The changes in the biopsy are interpreted by a pathologist, who renders a diagnosis based on relatively standard morphologic criteria. Biopsies are used to diagnose a disease; determine the extent of the disease (e.g., metastasis in cancer); and determine the adequacy of surgical removal (e.g., tumors).

Patient preparation Informed consent is required. Mild sedatives may be required in anxious patients.

Procedure Many biopsies are performed in an ambulatory (outpatient) setting, require no hospitalization, and can be obtained by direct visualization or during endoscopic procedures of the gastrointestinal tract and elsewhere. When a suspicious lesion is detected, a small pincer is inserted, and a small portion is removed for microscopic evaluation. A relatively recent development is the fine needle aspiration biopsy (FNA). In this procedure, the physician inserts a fine needle into the suspicious area and withdraws a small sample. The needle is guided by fluoroscopy and can reach most internal organs with little risk to the patient. In the usual sequence, the tissue is fixed, processed in various solvents, embedded in paraffin, stained, and examined by light microscopy; less commonly, other techniques (e.g., immunofluorescence and electron microscopy) may be required to establish a diagnosis.

Specimen Tissue from various body sites.

Reference range No abnormalities are seen by microscopy.

Abnormal values Inflammation, tumors and malignancies, infections, and other lesions may be seen in biopsied material.

Cost The fees hinge on the procedure being performed, taking into account the difficulty in obtaining the tissue. They usually cost several hundred dollars.

Comments While most biopsies can be readily evaluated by an experienced pathologist, there are cases in which the tissue is sent to expert consultants for further evaluation and diagnosis. See *aspiration biopsy, biochemical biopsy* in Glossary, *breast biopsy, chorionic villus biopsy, endobronchial biopsy, excisional biopsy, needle biopsy, nerve biopsy, punch biopsy, wedge resection*.

blastogenesis assay   See *mitogenic assay*.

bleeding time   Bleeding time (i.e., the time required for bleeding to stop) depends on the number and functional capacity of the platelets as well as the elasticity of the blood vessel wall and is a crude measure of the effectiveness of a person's responses to vascular injury. The bleeding time test is part of the routine preoperative evaluation and is also performed on patients with a history of bleeding disorders. Bleeding time was commonly ordered in the past, but with the advent of specific coagulation tests and accurate platelet measurements, it is used only in specific circumstances.

Patient preparation No preparation is required.

Procedure The most common method is the template method.

1. A blood pressure cuff is wrapped around the upper arm and inflated to 40 mmHg.
2. An area of the forearm free of superficial veins is cleansed and dried.
3. A template is applied to the forearm and a spring-loaded blade is used to make two incisions, 1 mm deep and 5 mm long.
4. A stopwatch is started.
5. Taking care not to touch the cuts, drops of blood are gently blotted every 30 seconds until the bleeding of both cuts stops. The bleeding time is the average of the two.

Reference range 2–8 minutes.

Abnormal values 10–15 minutes.

   Increased in: Hodgkin's disease, acute leukemia, disseminated intravascular coagulation, hemolytic disease of the newborn, severe hepatic disease, coagulation factor deficiencies—factors I, II, V, VII, VIII, IX, and XI.

Cost $15–$25.

Comments The bleeding time test is not recommended for patients with low platelet counts. The incisions are very small and do not cause significant pain. Falsely elevated bleeding times can be due to several drugs, including aspirin.

blood gas analysis   See *arterial blood gas*.

blood urea nitrogen   See *BUN*.

blot (blotting)   A technique used in molecular biology in which a nitrocellulose or nylon membrane bearing a molecule of interest (e.g., DNA, RNA, or protein) is transferred to the membrane from an electrophoretic gel by either osmosis or vacuum. After transferring the molecule of interest, the membrane is bathed in a solution that contains a mirror-image molecule of the one that is already on the membrane, producing a hybridization blot. See *Northern blot* in Glossary, *Southern blot* in Glossary, *Western blot*.

bone biopsy A biopsy of bone that is obtained in the context of suspected skeletal or rheumatic disease. If an infection is suspected, the biopsy should be obtained under sterile conditions so that a portion of the material can be submitted for culture. Biopsies of bone and/or synovial membrane may confirm or exclude the presence of degenerative bone disease (e.g., osteoarthritis). See *bone marrow aspiration and biopsy*.

bone densitometry The measurement of a bone's mass or density to determine its strength or density, which is reduced in patients with osteoporosis (bone loss).
Patient preparation No preparation is required.
Procedure All of the current methods (single-photon absorptiometry, dual-energy photon absorptiometry, dual-energy X-ray absorptiometry, computed tomography) of bone densitometry are based on a tissue's absorption of photons derived from either a radionuclide or an X-ray tube, the latter of which has an increased accuracy and shorter scan time. Bone densitometry objectively assesses the risk of suffering fractures by quantifying bone loss. Other methods of evaluating osteopenia include "eyeballing" a plain film of a bone; this requires a bone loss of at least 30% before osteoporosis can be diagnosed with certainty. The "feel" of the bone when it is drilled by a surgeon at the time of joint replacement is an even cruder method of evaluating osteopenia.
Specimen A film of bone.
Reference range Normal bone density.
Abnormal values
  Bone density is decreased in: estrogen deficiency, osteopenia, long-term glucocorticoid therapy, primary asymptomatic hyperparathyroidism.
Cost $100–$250.

bone/joint panel A group of laboratory tests that have been determined to be most cost effective, sensitive, and specific in evaluating a patient with bone and joint complaints; the bone/joint panel includes measurement of uric acid, calcium, phosphorous, alkaline phosphatase, total protein, and albumin. See *organ panel* in Glossary.

bone marrow aspiration and biopsy Bone marrow is the soft tissue found in the medulla of long bones and the interstitium of cancellous bone and is the site where red blood cells, white blood cells, and platelets are produced. A bone marrow aspiration and biopsy is obtained when there is a marked and/or chronic decrease in red blood cells (i.e., anemia), white blood cells (leukopenia), platelets (thrombocytopenia), or all three hematopoietic cell lines (known as aplastic anemia). The procedure is also indicated in the presence of increased white blood cells (as occurs in leukemias and lymphomas), red blood cells (polycythemia vera), and platelets (myelodysplastic syndromes).

Patient preparation Informed consent is required. Mild sedatives may be required for anxious patients.

Procedure The four common sites for this procedure are the posterosuperior iliac spine, the sternum, the spinous process of the vertebrum, and the tibia. After preparing the skin over the biopsy site and applying local anesthetic, the needle is inserted. For an aspiration analysis, a fluid specimen in which marrow is suspended is removed. For a biopsy specimen, a core of marrow cells is removed. After the marrow is removed, the fluid portion is spread on glass slides for staining. Tissues removed are placed in a fixative and prepared for examination by a pathologist. These procedures are generally used to diagnose leukemia, certain anemias, lymphoma, myelofibrosis, and multiple myeloma and to follow the effectiveness of therapy for these diseases.

Specimen Fluid and tissue.

Reference range No abnormalities are present. The white blood cells, red blood cells, and platelets are present in normal amounts and proportions.

Abnormal values
Decreased in: anemia, pancytopenia, chemotherapy, drug toxicity.
Increased in: leukemia (increased white blood cells), polycythemia vera (increased red blood cells), idiopathic thrombocytopenic purpura (increased platelets).

Cost $150–$350.

Comments These procedures are associated with deep, aching pain.

bone scan (bone scintigraphy) A method in which a radioactive compound (^{99m}Tc IDA) is administered; its distribution in the body is analyzed by a scintillation camera for increased or decreased uptake of the radioactive compound in the bone, which is a sensitive indicator of infection or malignancy.

Patient preparation All blood that is to be analyzed by RIA (radioimmunoassay) must be drawn before performing the scan.

Procedure A radioisotope 99m-technetium is injected and the resulting image of the entire skeleton is recorded two to three hours later with a gamma camera.

Specimen Scintillation scans.

Reference range A low level of diffuse uptake is present in all bones.

Abnormal values Focal increased or decreased uptake may be seen in primary or metastatic cancer, infection, arthritis, metabolic disease, trauma, avascular necrosis of bone, and in joint prosthesis (artificial joint).

Cost $625–$800.

Borrelia burgdorferi See *Lyme disease.*

brain scan A term used in nuclear medicine as a synonym for brain scintigraphy and in radiology for a CT scan of the brain.

brain scintigraphy A procedure in which a dose of a radioisotope is administered intravenously and its distribution monitored with a gamma camera. Brain scintigraphy provides information on the adequacy of blood flow to the cerebral cortex and detects abnormalities in the brain before they can be detected by CT or MR scans. Brain scintigraphy is used in the evaluation of strokes, transient ischemic attacks, seizure activity, and organic brain disease; it can also be used to diagnose tumors and psychiatric abnormalities. When it is performed in conjunction with the technique known as single-photon emission tomography, it is regarded by some experts as being of considerable diagnostic utility.

brainstem auditory evoked response (BAER) A clinical method for evaluating hearing, using clicking sounds and recording the responses (auditory evoked potentials) with electroencephalogram electrodes placed on the scalp. BAER is an objective means of establishing the diagnosis and localization of early lesions of the auditory system.
Patient preparation No preparation is required. The hair should be washed before the procedure.
Procedure Electrodes are attached to the scalp. The patient is exposed to clicking sounds that cause responses on the electroencephalograph. The shape and timing of these responses indicate the location of the auditory system and the brain.
Specimen Graphic recordings from the electroencephalograph.
Reference range No abnormalities in timing and shape of brain waves.
Abnormal values BAER is abnormal in: acoustic neuroma, intrinsic brain stem lesions, including multiple sclerosis, infarction, gliomas, and degenerative disease (e.g., Charcot-Marie-Tooth disease, olivopontocerebellar degeneration, Wilson's disease), increased intracranial pressure, brain death.
Cost $200–$450.

breast biopsy A general term for a sampling of breast tissue with a lesion (lump) identified by physical examination or mammography.
Patient preparation Informed consent is required. A mild sedative may be required in anxious patients.
Procedure A 14- to 18-gauge needle is inserted into a breast mass. The amount of tissue obtained in a breast biopsy can be miniscule, as is typical in a "skinny needle" biopsy in which the core of tissue measures one millimeter or less in diameter, to relatively substantial, measuring one or more centimeters in diameter. In general, pathologists who interpret breast biopsies prefer larger biopsies because the sampling error is lessened, and there is more background tissue (stroma), which provides a useful architectural boundary. All tissues are stained and examined by a pathologist. As a general rule (with many exceptions), breast biopsies in younger women are more commonly benign and include fibroadenomas and fibrocystic disease; in older women, clinically identified lumps are more often malignant.

Specimen The specimens obtained depend on the type of procedure. For a breast aspiration, cells and small tissue fragments are spread on slides, and a cell block may be produced. For biopsies using larger gauge needles, tissue fragments are placed in formalin. "Open" breast biopsies are relatively large and are performed in the hospital.
Reference range No abnormalities are seen by microscopy.
Abnormal values Benign lesions (e.g., fibrocystic disease, inflammation), benign tumors (fibroadenoma), and malignant tumors (cancer).
Cost $150–$350.

breast (cancer) markers Any of a number of antigens variably present in breast tissue that may be of use in differentiating between benign or malignant lesions of the breast, or in identifying the breast as the site of origin in tumor metastases; breast markers include estrogen receptor, progesterone receptor, zinc-α_2-glycoprotein, GCDFP-15 (gross cystic disease fluid protein 15), casein, α-lactalbumin, lactoferrin, B73.2, TAG-12, MAM-6, MCA b-12, and MMTV-related antigens.

bronchial brushings (brush biopsy) A procedure in which cells from the mucosa of the upper airways (trachea, bronchi, bronchioles) are obtained for cytologic evaluation under direct bronchoscopic visualization of suspicious mucosal lesions. A soft, nylon brush is advanced through the bronchoscope and gently brushed over the lesion(s) of interest, thereby obtaining cells that are analyzed by a cytopathologist. Bronchial brushings are primarily used to establish a diagnosis of malignancy and have a high degree of accuracy, comparing favorably with the biopsy in confirming the presence of malignancy. If used in conjunction with a protected brush catheter, the relatively uncontaminated material can be cultured for various organisms in the face of suspected pneumonia. See *bronchial washings*.

bronchial challenge testing (bronchial provocation testing, mecholyl challenge, methacholine provocation test) A test administered to an individual after a battery of tests establishes a baseline of the functional status of his/her lungs; the individual inhales methacholine, a histaminic agent that reduces the values of pulmonary function tests in patients with asthma. Methacholine has no effect on patients with decreased pulmonary function due to causes such as heart failure, sinus infections, or intrathoracic tumors. Cold air can be administered as another form of bronchial inhalation challenge with similar responses in asthmatic patients. See *pulmonary function test*. The bronchial challenge is used to identify and determine the severity of nonspecific bronchial hypersensitivity and to evaluate the efficacy of drugs used to treat bronchospasm.

bronchial inhalation challenge See *bronchial challenge testing*.

bronchial provocation testing See *bronchial challenge testing*.

bronchial washings (bronchoalveolar lavage)   A procedure in which 3–5 ml of isotonic saline is instilled through a bronchoscope, and fluid (usually 1–2 ml is recovered) containing cells, microorganisms, or other material from the upper airways (trachea, bronchi, bronchioles) is aspirated into a trap. The material is centrifuged, stained, and examined by light microscopy if an infection is suspected. The diagnostic yield from bronchial washings is less than that of bronchial brushings but is of particular use in obtaining cytologic specimens that are beyond (i.e., too far down in the lungs) the visual reach of the bronchoscope. A definitive diagnosis of malignancy can be established from bronchoscopically visible lesions in approximately 75% of patients with bronchial washings, in contrast to over 90% yield with bronchial brushings. For the deeper tumors that are beyond reach by bronchoscopy and by extension the bronchial brush, washings have a 50% diagnostic yield in contrast to none with the bronchial brush. See *bronchial brushings, bronchoscopy.*

bronchoalveolar lavage   See *bronchial washings.*

bronchoscopy (fiberoptic bronchoscopy)   The use of a flexible device to directly examine the upper airways, vocal cords, and the tracheobronchial tree to the fourth to sixth division. Bronchoscopy is used to evaluate suspected malignancy or infections, hemoptysis (coughing up of blood), persistent coughing, and occasionally to remove foreign bodies in the upper airways. Bronchoscopy should not be performed unless absolutely necessary in patients with asthma, severe hypoxia, unstable angina pectoris, or recent myocardial infarction. The bronchoscope has a halogen or xenon light source, a 2–2.5 mm channel that allows the obtention of diagnostic material in the form of biopsies, brushings, and washings, as well as the instillation of medicine and mechanical components that allow it to be easily guided through the tracheobronchial tree. See *bronchial brushings, bronchial washings.*

Patient preparation The patient is given a mild anesthetic to ease the passage of the bronchoscope through the airway.

Procedure A flexible tube equipped with fiber optic cables is inserted through the mouth and down the airway to the lungs. The physician can observe the bronchi and obtain biopsies or washings.

Reference range No abnormalities, lesions, erosions, or discolorations are seen.

Abnormal values Infection (e.g., *Premocystis carinii*, tuberculosis), inflammation, interstitial lung disease, sarcoidosis, benign tumors, and cancer.

Cost $1000–$1500.

BUN (blood urea nitrogen)   Urea nitrogen is one of the waste products of protein metabolism and is excreted through the kidneys. Measurement of urea nitrogen reflects the ratio between urea production and clearance. Increased urea nitrogen may be due to increased production or decreased excretion. Although the expression "BUN" is commonly used, most laboratories use serum and occasionally plasma or urine but never whole blood. BUN is normally measured in conjunction with creatinine as an indicator of kidney function.

Patient preparation No preparation is required. If urine measurements are to be carried out, see instructions for 24-hour urine collection.

Procedure Usually a spectrophotometric analysis is used on automated equipment. Conductometric measurements are also used on some analyzers.

Specimen Serum, plasma, or urine. Lithium, heparin, and EDTA may be used as anticoagulants.

Reference range

Birth to 1 year	4–16 mg/dL.
1 to 40 years	5–20 mg/dL.

Over 40, there is a gradual increase.

Abnormal values

Increased in: chronic glomerulonephritis, pyelonephritis, other chronic renal disease, acute renal failure, urinary tract obstruction.

Decreased in: pregnancy, decreased protein intake, severe liver damage.

Cost $15–$25 as a single test. Usually performed as part of a larger profile.

CA 15-3 (cancer antigen 15-3)   A group of mucin-like 300–450 kD glyco-proteins that are increased in approximately one-third of all patients with breast cancer. 5% with stage I to 95% with stage IV have serum levels of greater than 25 U/ml, which correlates with tumor bulk. As with most cancer antigen assays, the utility of this assay is the postoperative monitoring of patients.   This is NOT a screening test for breast cancer, although most patients with combined local and systemic disease have elevated levels.

Patient preparation No preparation is required.
Procedure CA 15-3 is measured using RIA methodology.
Specimen Serum.
Reference range Less than 25–30 U/ml.
Abnormal values
    Increased in: widespread breast cancer, benign breast disease.
Cost $45–75. This test is not currently approved by the FDA.
Comments Individuals who have developed antibodies to mouse immunoglobulins may exhibit falsely elevated results. Because 2% of normal healthy subjects and 9% of those with benign breast disease have serum levels of greater than 30 U/ml, CA 15-3 is not used as a screening test.

CA 19-9 (cancer antigen 19-9)   A tumor-associated carbohydrate antigen that is an epitope located on the Lewis A blood group antigen. Serum levels of greater than 37 U/ml are found in 72%–100% of patients with pancreatic carcinoma (97% of those with levels above 1000 U/ml), in $\frac{2}{3}$ of those with hepatocellular carcinoma, over $\frac{1}{2}$ of those with gastric carcinoma, and $\frac{1}{5}$ of those with colorectal carcinoma. Although the monoclonal antibody to CA 19-9 cannot be used to screen for pancreatic cancer, it can be used to detect postsurgical recurrence and to differentiate between benign and malignant disease of the pancreas.

Patient preparation No preparation is required.
Procedure CA 19-9 is measured by RIA methodologies.
Specimen Serum.
Reference range Less than 37 U/ml.

Abnormal values

Increased in: pancreatic cancer, gastrointestinal cancers, head and
neck tumors

Cost $45–$75. This test is currently not approved by the FDA and therefore may not be reimbursed by Medicare, Medicaid, and most insurance
companies.

Comments False positives have been seen in hepatic cirrhosis and may be
seen in individuals who have antibodies against mouse immunoglobulins.
Individuals who are Lewis (a-b-) phenotype (blood group) cannot synthesize CA 19-9 and therefore may be false negative. Because 0.6% of
healthy blood donors and 18% of those with benign pancreatic disease
have serum levels of greater than 37 U/ml, CA 19-9 is not used as a
screening test.

CA 125 (cancer antigen-125)   A cell surface glycoprotein first identified in
mucinous ovarian carcinomas that is also expressed on adenocarcinomas of
the uterine cervix, endometrium, gastrointestinal tract, and breast. CA 125
is expressed on the cell membrane of normal ovarian tissue and 80% of nonmucinous (usually serous type) epithelial ovarian cancers and can be measured in the serum, where rising levels indicate a poor prognosis. CA 125
may also be found in nongynecologic cancers, liver disease, acute pancreatitis, renal failure, lymphoma, and occasionally in normal females. Because of
the high false-positive rate, CA 125 cannot be used as a screening test. It is
used primarily to monitor disease progression in nonmucinous common
epithelial neoplasms of the ovary. Baseline levels should be obtained prior to
surgery and initiation of therapy.

Patient preparation No preparation is required.

Procedure CA 125 is measured using RIA methodology. There are automated chemiluminescent procedures currently undergoing the FDA
approval process.

Specimen Serum.

Reference range Less than 35 U/ml.

Abnormal values

Increased in: cancers of the cervix, endometrium, and ovary.

Cost $45–$75. The RIA version of this test has been approved by the FDA
and is reimbursable when used for monitoring purposes.

Comments False-positive results are seen in patients who have antibodies
against mouse immunoglobulins.

CA 549 (cancer antigen 549)   A cancer marker that is normally present in
breast, colon, and kidney tissue and increased in breast cancer.

Patient preparation No preparation is required.

Procedure CA 549 is measured by RIA methodologies.

Specimen Serum.

Reference range None established.

Comments This tumor antigen is not readily available and is primarily used in a research setting. There has not been sufficient data to determine its effectiveness as a diagnostic tool.

calcitonin Calcitonin is a polypeptide hormone produced by the C or parafollicular cells in the thyroid gland, the release of which is stimulated by rising serum calcium levels. Calcitonin is a parathyroid hormone (PTH) antagonist that lowers serum calcium levels by inhibiting bone resorption and increasing excretion of calcium by the kidneys. Calcitonin is also produced by several neoplasms, particularly medullary carcinoma of the thyroid. Increased serum levels of calcitonin are characteristic of this tumor, which may in turn be associated with other tumors of the endocrine system; calcitonin levels in the serum may be used to monitor therapy.

Patient preparation Patient should fast overnight prior to the test.
Procedure Calcitonin is measured by RIA methodology.
Specimen Serum or plasma. The blood specimen should be collected into a chilled tube, separated in a refrigerated centrifuge, placed into a plastic tube, and frozen.
Reference range Less than 19 pg/ml.
Abnormal values
   Increased in: medullary carcinoma of the thyroid, oat cell carcinoma of the lung, breast carcinoma.
Cost $45–$75.
Comments In some patients with medullary carcinoma of the thyroid, baseline calcitonin levels may be normal; the diagnosis of this tumor requires a calcitonin stimulation test with pentagastrin. Occasionally, falsely elevated calcitonin levels are encountered. These may be caused by antibodies present in the test kits, as some patients have calcitonin that lacks immunoreactivity, thus causing incorrect results. CEA measurements may be used as an adjunct to calcitonin levels.

calcitonin stimulation test In patients with normal levels of calcitonin but suspected medullary carcinoma, this test can be used to confirm the diagnosis.
Patient preparation Patient should fast overnight prior to the test.
Procedure A baseline specimen is taken just prior to the infusion. Calcium is then infused (15 mg/kg) for four hours. Samples are taken at three and four hours postinfusion.
Specimen Serial serum specimens drawn in EDTA tubes prior to infusion and at 90 seconds, 5 minutes, and 10 minutes after infusion.
Reference range
   Males   Less than 265 pg/mL.
   Females   Less than 120 pg/mL.
Abnormal values A rapidly rising calcitonin level indicates medullary carcinoma.
Cost $75–$100.
Comments There is now a second test available. Pentagastrin (0.5 mcg/kg)

is infused over a period of 5–10 seconds. A blood specimen is obtained immediately prior to pentagastrin infusion, at 90 seconds, 5 minutes, and 10 minutes after infusion.

calcium (serum) The body contains large amounts of calcium, predominantly in the bones and teeth. In addition to being the most critical component of bone, calcium is also needed to maintain many metabolic processes in the body such as muscle contraction, transmission of neural impulses, the clotting of blood, and inhibition of cell destruction. A daily intake of about 400 mg is required to fulfill the body's needs for calcium. Serum calcium levels are controlled by a balance between parathyroid hormone (PTH, produced by the parathyroid glands) and calcitonin (produced by the C or parafollicular cells of the thyroid). PTH increases serum calcium levels by increasing bone resorption and mobilizing calcium, and it indirectly increases gastrointestinal absorption of calcium by increasing the production of vitamin D. PTH also increases phosphate excretion in the urine. Calcitonin decreases serum calcium and phosphate levels by inhibiting bone resorption.

Patient preparation No preparation is required.

Procedure Calcium is measured spectrophotometrically on automated chemistry instruments.

Specimen Serum or plasma. EDTA cannot be used as the anticoagulant for plasma measurements.

Reference range

Infant to 1 month	7.0–11.5 mg/dL.
1 month to 1 year	8.6–11.2 mg/dL.
Older than 1 year	8.2–10.2 mg/dL.

Abnormal values

Increased in: hyperparathyroidism, parathyroid tumors, Paget's disease of bone, multiple myeloma, metastatic carcinoma, multiple fractures, prolonged immobilization, renal disease, adrenal insufficiency, excessive calcium ingestion, excessive use of antacids.

Decreased in: hypoparathyroidism, malabsorption, Cushing's syndrome, renal failure, acute pancreatitis, peritonitis.

Cost $10–$15. Calcium levels are usually measured as part of a chemistry profile.

Comments Acute hyper- or hypocalcemia can be life threatening. Close monitoring and rapid therapy is crucial. Excess ingestion of vitamin D and other agents can cause falsely elevated levels. Chronic abuse of laxatives, excessive transfusions, and various drugs can suppress calcium levels.

calcium (urine) Measurement of calcium levels in the urine and serum levels are used to diagnose and monitor disorders of calcium metabolism. Urinary calcium levels reflect the intake, rates of intestinal absorption, bone resorption and renal loss. This test is also used in stone evaluation and followup.

Patient preparation For stone evaluation the patient should continue a normal diet for at least three days prior to the test.

Procedure Calcium is measured spectrophotometrically on an automated chemistry instrument.

Specimen A 24-hour urine collection is required.

Reference range 100–250 mg/24 hours.

Abnormal values

Increased in: hyperparathyroidism, Paget's disease of bone, renal disease, carcinoma.

Decreased in: renal osteodystrophy, rickets, hypoparathyroidsm, pre-eclampsia.

Cost $15–$35.

Comments Certain drugs such as thiazide diuretics and oral contraceptives cause decreased levels.

caloric test A test of vestibular function in which the ear canal is irrigated with cold and hot water. This test often identifies an impairment or loss of thermally induced nystagmus on the involved side.

Patient preparation No specific preparation is required. Sedatives and motion sickness medication should be discontinued.

Procedure The patient's head is tilted forward 30° from horizontal, bringing the horizontal semicircular canal into a vertical plane, which allows the greatest sensitivity for thermal stimulation. Each canal is irrigated separately for 30 seconds, first at 7°C below, then 7°C above body temperature, separated by 5 minutes.

Specimen Clinical findings.

Reference range

Cold water	Rotary nystagmus (involuntary rapid eye movements) away from irrigated ear.
Hot water	Nystagmus toward the irrigated eye.

Abnormal values

Caloric tests are altered in: acoustic neuroma, inflammation, infarction, or tumors of the brain stem or cerebellum, vestibular or cochlear inflammation or tumors.

Cost $500–$750.

Campylobacter pylori See *Helicobacter pylori*.

cancer antigen 15-3 See *CA 15-3*.

cancer antigen 19-9 See *CA 19-9*.

cancer antigen 125 See *CA 125*.

cancer screen Any measurable clinical or laboratory parameter that can be used to detect early malignancy. Although these tests are relatively nonspecific, they are highly sensitive and detect the majority of subjects who are "abnormal" for the parameter being measured. The most common cancer screens are those that detect occult blood in the stool as a screen for colon cancer and mammography for identifying microcalcifications and geographic densities which are common radiologic findings in breast cancer. Cancer screens must be viewed in the context of a cost-benefit ratio and are not available for many of the more common malignancies such as lung cancer (which theoretically could be detected by annual chest films, although this has not been recommended).

carbon dioxide content   The blood picks up oxygen (O_2), and as it passes through the lungs releases carbon dioxide (CO_2) which with water are the end products of oxygen metabolism. Some of the CO_2 in the blood is changed to bicarbonate and is excreted in the kidneys. Measurement of CO_2 is generally part of what is called "blood gas measurement" and is used to evaluate the ease with which gases are exchanged through the lungs and to determine the factors affecting the acid-base balance (pH) of the blood.

Patient preparation No preparation is required.

Procedure CO_2 is measured manometrically using specialized equipment.

Specimen Either venous or arterial blood which is collected in a special sealed syringe to avoid any contact with air.

Reference range

Infancy to 2 years	18–28 mmol/L.
2 years and older (venous)	22–26 mmol/L.
2 years and older (arterial)	22–29 mmol/L.

Abnormal values

Decreased in: respiratory alkalosis, hyperventilation, metabolic acidosis.

Increased in: severe vomiting, continuous gastric drainage, hypoventilation, e.g., emphysema, pneumonia.

Cost $50–$70 as part of a blood gas determination.

Comments This procedure is normally carried out in a hospital setting. Obtaining arterial blood requires a specially trained phlebotomist.

carboxyhemoglobin   Carbon monoxide (CO) irreversibly binds to hemoglobin in blood to form carboxyhemoglobin (COHb). COHb is a natural metabolic product of hemoglobin breakdown and is normally present in the blood in minimal amounts. Increased COHb occurs in individuals who have been exposed to carbon monoxide, which can be quantified to determine the intensity of exposure to CO. The increased turnover of hemoglobin in the newborn in combination with the decreased efficiency of the infant's respiratory system may lead to higher levels of carboxyhemoglobin.

Patient preparation No preparation is required.

Procedure CO is measured manometrically using a specialized instrument called an oximeter.

Specimen Whole blood. The specimen should be obtained prior to the patient beginning oxygen therapy.

Reference range

Newborns	10%–12%
Nonsmokers	Less than 2%
Smokers	
1–2 packs/day	4%–5%
More than 2 packs/day	8%–10%

Cost $40–$60.

Comments The primary use of this test is to determine exposure to carbon monoxide, which may originate from fires, vehicular exhaust garage exposure, and so forth. Carboxyhemoglobin determination is of little use in screening for tobacco use because of its rapid excretion.

carcinoembryonic antigen (CEA) A glycoprotein present in the circulation in nanogram amounts first described as a relatively specific finding in occult primary adenocarcinomas; it is increased in up to 30% of colorectal, lung, liver, pancreas, breast, head and neck, bladder, cervix, prostate, and medullary thyroid carcinomas. CEA is also less commonly increased in lymphoproliferative disorders, (e.g., lymphomas, leukemias), malignant melanoma, and in heavy smokers. Although increased CEA is not a reliable cancer screen, it is useful for monitoring recurrent colon cancer; some experts believe that a 35% increase of CEA above a patient's postresective surgery baseline levels is reason for a "second look" operation to rule out metastases. CEA is increased in 60%–90% of metastatic lung cancer. CEA is normally found in the fetal and embryonic gut, in smokers, or in inflammatory bowel disease. Any gain in overall survival by CEA monitoring is small, and possibly less than 1% of patients survive after resection of liver metastasis. In HIV-infected patients with *Pneumocystis carinii* pneumonia, an increase in CEA (8.8 vs. 2.7 ng/ml in normals) is associated with a poor short-term prognosis and a mortality rate of ± 80% if CEA is greater than 20 ng/ml. If CEA is elevated before colon surgery, it is a poor prognostic sign and may identify patients at increased risk of cancer recurrence. This test is not used as a screening test and its primary use is monitoring the patient for cancer recurrence after surgery or chemotherapy.

Patient preparation No preparation is required.

Procedure CEA is measured by radioimmunoassay, enzyme immunoassay, and chemiluminescence.

Specimen Serum and plasma. When monitoring a patient's CEA levels it is important to use the same specimen type each time.

Reference range

Adult (nonsmoker)	Less than 2.5 ng/ml.
Adult (smoker)	Less than 5 ng/ml.

Abnormal values

Malignant: colorectal cancer, breast cancer, giant cell carcinomas of thyroid, pancreatic cancer, ovarian cancer.

Nonmalignant: Smokers, inflammation, inflammatory bowel disease pancreatitis, hypothyroidism, cirrhosis.

Cost $45–$75.

Comments CEA is NOT a screening test for cancer and early cancers may be negative for CEA. The CEA levels may be normal even in patients with advanced malignancy. Because there are several manufacturers supplying kits for CEA measurement, it is critical that the same kit manufacturer be used each time a specimen is submitted to a laboratory, as variations in methods may give slightly different results. If the physician changes laboratories or the laboratory changes to a new manufacturer, several specimens must be run utilizing both kits in order to establish a new baseline. This is crucial because many surgeons will perform a subsequent surgery (exploratory) if there is a noticeable rise in CEA levels. Changes in methodology must be ruled out as a cause of the elevation when evaluating the data.

cardiac catheterization   A procedure in which a long catheter is inserted through a peripheral blood vessel, usually a vein of the leg (femoral vein) or arm (antecubital vein), passed through the inferior vena cava, and under fluoroscopic guidance, placed in the region(s) of interest. Cardiac catheterization can be used to;

1. Evaluate heart valves and detect stenosis and regurgitation.
2. Determine regional blood pressure and detect pulmonary hypertension.
3. Obtain blood samples to evaluate oxygenation of blood.
4. Inject dye and evaluate heart function in "real time" (cardiac angiography) and assess the patency of the coronary arteries (coronary angiography).

Right-sided cardiac catheterization is used to evaluate tricuspid and pulmonary valve function and to measure pressures of and take blood samples from the right atrium, ventricle, and pulmonary artery. Left-sided cardiac catheterization is used to evaluate mitral and aortic valve function and evaluate the coronary arteries. Some cardiologists believe cardiac catheterization may be replaced by the noninvasive technique Doppler echocardiology.

Patient preparation A small incision is made in the upper interior thigh to allow access to the vein. Minimal discomfort is experienced.

Procedure The catheter is snaked through the opening made to the heart where dye can be injected, samples can be obtained, or occlusion can be reduced. The progress of the catheter is followed via radiologic imaging.

Abnormal values

Right side: pulmonary hypertension, pulmonary valve stenosis, tricuspid valve stenosis, atrial and ventricular septal defects.

Left side: aortic valve regurgitation, coronary artery disease (stenosis or occlusion), mitral valve stenosis or regurgitation, ventricular hypertrophy or aneurysm.

Cost $3000–$4000.

Comments Complications of the procedure include cardiac arrhythmias, embolism (cerebral, pulmonary), myocardial infarction, and pericardial tamponade.

cardiac enzymes   A group of three enzymes formerly used to monitor suspected myocardial infarction (muscle death that occurs in a heart attack). Cardiac enzymes include creatine phosphokinase (CPK), aspartate aminotransferase (AST, formerly GOT-glutamate-oxaloacetate transaminase), and lactate dehydrogenase (LDH). Following myocardial infarction, these three enzymes rise and fall in the same order over a period of a week. This "first generation" of serum tests that indicate the presence of damage to the myocardium (heart muscle) have been abandoned in favor of newer, more specific cardiac markers. See *cardiac marker, creatine phosphokinase isoenzymes, flipped pattern* in Glossary, *troponin* in Glossary.

cardiac output   See *angiography.*

cardiopulmonary sleep study   See *polysomnography.*

carotene   (beta-carotene)   Beta-carotene is among the retinoid compounds found in fresh fruits and vegetables which is categorized as a fat-soluble provitamin, metabolized to vitamin A. The test is relatively insensitive in the face of low levels of carotene and results vary among laboratories. It is used to confirm the diagnosis of carotenoderma (carotene deposits in the skin) and to screen for the presence of fat malabsorption as occurs in steatorrhea, the malabsorption of fat.
   Patient preparation Patient must fast for 12 hours prior to obtaining the specimen.
   Procedure Carotene is measured spectrophotometrically.
   Specimen Serum. Specimen must be protected from light.
   Reference range 50–250 μg/dL, which varies according to diet and laboratory.
   Cost $40–$60.
   Comments The use of this test is controversial because of its low sensitivity and interlaboratory variability.

CAT scan   See *computed tomography.*

catecholamines   Catecholamines are a group of substances secreted by the adrenal medulla. They include epinephrine (adrenaline), norepinephrine noradrenaline (which is also produced by the sympathetic nerve endings), and dopamine. Catecholamines are measured in the blood and urine of patients with hypertension to exclude the possibility of pheochromocytoma, a relatively uncommon but eminently treatable tumor of the adrenal medulla that characteristically causes hypertension.
   Patient preparation It is extremely important that the patient avoid stress and strenuous exercise prior to obtaining the specimens, because these may cause a spurious increase of the catecholamines.
   Procedure Catecholamines are currently measured by a combination of column chromatography and spectrophotometry. Newer methods have incor-

porated high-pressure (or performance) liquid chromatography to allow analysis of all catecholamines simultaneously. HPLC is becoming more available and will supplant more manual methods in the near future.

Specimen Plasma, urine. Two plasma specimens are generally taken: one when the patient is standing and the other when the patient has been recumbent for at least 30 minutes. It is recommended that an indwelling catheter be used because the act of venipuncture can cause elevated levels.

Reference range

Lying down	Epinephrine	Less than 110 pg/ml.
(supine)	Norepinephrine	70–750 pg/ml.
	Dopamine	Less than 130 pg/ml.
Standing	Epinephrine	Less than 1140 pg/ml.
	Norpinephrine	200–1700 pg/ml.
	Dopamine	Less than 130 mg/ml.
Urine	Epinephrine	Less than 12 ug/ml.
	Norepinephrine	15–80 ug/ml.
	Dopamine	35–400 ug/24 hours.

Abnormal values

Increased in: pheochromocytoma, neuroblastoma, paragangliomas, multiple endocrine neoplasia syndrome.

Cost $50–$75.

Comments Catecholamines are measured in the workup of palpitation, severe headache, and diaphoresis. Urine is the preferred specimen if a tumor is suspected in the presence of hypertension. Metanephrines, HVA (homovanillic acid), and VMA (vanillylmandelic acid) are urinary metabolites of catecholamines used to confirm diagnosis.

cathepsin D Cathepsins are a group of lysosomal proteinases or endopeptidases that function optimally at an acidic pH. Cathepsin D is an experimental tumor marker which has shown promise in determining breast cancer prognosis; it has been found to be increased in hormone-dependent breast carcinoma, the serum levels of which are predictive of early recurrence and death in node-negative cases. High levels of cathepsin D are associated with an increased risk of 2.6 for recurrence and a relative risk of 3.9 for death in breast cancer. The test is not currently available outside a research setting. See *metastasis* in Glossary.

CBC See *complete blood count.*

CEA See *carcinoembryonic antigen.*

ceruloplasmin Ceruloplasmin is an α-globulin that is produced in the liver and serves as the carrier protein for copper (each molecule contains eight copper ions). Ceruloplasmin has ferroxidase and polyamine oxidase activity and is thus thought to be involved with iron metabolism.

Patient preparation No preparation is required.

Procedure Ceruloplasmin is measured by nephelometric or turbidimetric methods.

Specimen Serum.

Reference range 20–40 mg/dL. Adult levels are reached 3–6 months after birth.

Abnormal values

Increased in: tumors, inflammation, liver disease, rheumatoid arthritis, systemic lupus erythematosus, pregnancy, oral contraceptives.

Decreased in: Menkes' "kinky hair" syndrome, hepatitis, cirrhosis.

Absent in: Wilson's disease.

Cost $35–$65.

Comments Excessive use of zinc may block intestinal absorption of copper and is associated with low ceruloplasmin levels.

cervical biopsy   A biopsy of the uterine cervix that is usually performed several days to weeks after a pap smear reveals cellular changes, in particular epithelial cell abnormalities warranting further evaluation. See *Bethesda system* in Glossary, *cervical intraepithelial neoplasia, colposcopy, pap smear.*

Patient preparation Informed consent is required.

Procedure Cervical biopsies are performed using either Tischler or Kevorkian-Younge biopsy forceps which "chomp" out a piece of cervical tissue believed to contain the lesion causing the changes found on the pap smear. The tissue is placed in formalin, processed in paraffin, cut into thin sections, stained, and interpreted by a pathologist.

Specimen Cervical tissue.

Reference range No abnormalities are seen.

Abnormal values HPV (human papilloma virus) changes, CIN I–III (cervical intraepithelial neoplasia), and cervical cancer may be seen.

Cost $75–$150.

Comments Complications of the cervical biopsy include discomfort and occasional bleeding. In the United States, the findings in pap smears are interpreted based on the Bethesda System, which divides the cellular changes seen in pap smears into benign cellular changes with or without infection and epithelial cell abnormalities (which can be either squamous cell or glandular cell abnormalities). Because benign cellular changes are normal, they represent a clean bill of health. If the pap smear was adequate, the patient requires no further diagnostic evaluation except for the usual annual follow-up. On the other hand, epithelial cell abnormalities range from atypical cells with reactive changes to premalignant (low-grade squamous intraepithelial lesion, high-grade squamous intraepithelial lesion) and frankly malignant (carcinoma in situ, squamous cell carcinoma) changes. All epithelial cell abnormalities require further evaluation (e.g., a cervical biopsy and/or colposcopy).

cervical intraepithelial neoplasia (CIN)   A premalignant state arising in uterine cervical epithelium and confined to this tissue. CIN represents a continuum of histologic changes ranging from well-differentiated CIN 1 (mild dysplasia) to severe dysplasia/carcinoma in situ (CIN 3). The higher grade the lesion the greater the tendency to progress to invasive epidermoid carcinoma. CIN typically arises in a background of infection with the human papillomavirus, which has a number of subtypes: HPV 6 and 11 are associated with benign condylomas; HPV types 16 and 18 occur in CIN 3; types 31, 33, 35, 52, and 56 may appear in lower-grade CIN; 78% of women who are positive for HPV, especially HPV 16 and 18, develop CIN 2–3. See *carcinoma in situ* in Glossary, *intraepithelial neoplasia* in Glossary.

chemistry profile (routine chemistry profile)   A battery of tests performed on serum measuring the substances in the blood that may be obtained in common diseases. Often included in a profile are albumin, BUN (with nitrogen), calcium, cholesterol, creatinine, glucose, alkaline phosphatase, lactate dehydrogenase phosphorus, ALA, AST, and electrolytes.

Patient preparation An 8–12 hour fast is preferred before obtaining the specimen.

Specimen Serum in red-top tube.

	REFERENCE RANGE	ABNORMAL VALUES
Albumin	3.2–4.5 g/dL	<3.0 g/dL
Alanine aminotransferase		
(ALT, GPT)	8–45 U/L	50 U/L
Alkaline phosphatase	35–100 U/L	125 U/L
Asparate aminotransferase		
(AST, GOT)	8–45 U/L	100 U/L
Bicarbonate (HCO$_3$)	21–28 mmol/L	<20 mmol/L >30 mmol/L
BUN	5–20 mg/dL	>25 mg/dL
Calcium	8–10 mg/dL	<7 mg/dL >11.5 mg/dL
Chloride	97–107 mmol/L	<90 mmol/L >112 mmol/L
Cholesterol	150–200 mg/dL	240 mg/dL
Creatinine	<1.2 mg/dL	1.5 mg/dL
Glucose	70–125 mg/dL	<60 mg/dL >140 mg/dL
Lactate dehydrogenase	<200 U/L	>250 U/L
Phosphorus	2.5–4.5 mg/dL	<1.5 mg/dL
Potassium	3.5–5.0 mmol/L	<2.5 mmol/L >7.0 mmol/L
Protein (total)	6–8 g/dL	<4.5 g/dL >9 g/dL
Sodium	135–145 mmol/L	<125 mmol/L >155 mmol/L
Uric acid	2.5–7.0 mg/dL	7.0 mg/dL

Cost $25–$60.

Chlamydia   Three species of chlamydia (*C. trachomatis, C. pneumoniae,* and *C. psittaci)* are pathogenic for humans. These bacteria are very common worldwide and are transmitted by sexual contact or through exudates. Chlamydia is a major cause of blindness. Because many chlamydial infections are asymptomatic, it is common practice to screen all pregnant women as part of their prenatal workup. *C. psittaci* is an important cause of infection in animals, especially birds, which in turn can transmit it to humans, causing severe respiratory infection. *C. pneumoniae* (also known as *C. psittaci* TWAR) is a frequent cause of upper respiratory infection and mild lower respiratory infection in adolescents and young adults. *C. trachomatis* causes nonspecific urethritis; it is the only chlamydia that can be routinely cultured. Laboratory diagnosis of *C. psittaci* and *C. pneumoniae* are made on the basis of serologic evaluation. Newer tests have been developed for *C. trachomatis* that have multiple serovarieties, allowing easier screening and more rapid diagnosis. These tests include direct fluorescence antibody (DFA), ELISA, DNA probe, and polymerase chain reaction (PCR) which is the newest method and is not yet widely available. Because PCR can be used on urine specimens, it may lead to more widespread screening of males.

Patient preparation No preparation is required.

Procedure There are many modalities currently utilized to detect infection by chlamydia. The modality used is generally related to cost; DFA and ELISA methods are the least sensitive but also cost the least. DNA probe and PCR methods have only recently been FDA approved. The reagent kits for the latter two methods are only available from two sources, GenProbe and Roche Diagnostics. When there is more competition and more widespread use, the prices will decrease significantly.

Specimen Vaginal or urethral swab for DFA, ELISA, and DNA probe. Urine, vaginal, or urethral swab for PCR. Ocular swab for culture.

Reference range Negative.

Abnormal values Presence of chlamydia antigens.

Cost $35–$55.

chloride Chloride is the major negative electrolyte (anion) in the extracellular fluid and interacts with sodium to maintain the osmotic pressure of blood, thereby regulating blood volume and arterial pressure. Chloride can be measured in many body fluids, and its concentration in sweat is used as an indicator of cystic fibrosis.

Patient preparation No preparation is required.

Procedure Chloride is currently measured electronically using ion selective electrodes on automated chemistry instruments. Older spectrophotometric methods employing mercuric thiocyanate created disposal problems and have been discontinued.

Specimen Serum/plasma, 24-hour urine, CSF, sweat.

Reference range

Serum/Plasma	95–110 mmol/L.
Urine	110–250 mmol/24 hours.
Sweat	5–40 mmol/L.

Abnormal values

Serum/Plasma	Less than 90 mmol/L.
	Greater than 115 mmol/L.

Urine	Less than 20 mmol/L.
Sweat	Greater than 60 mmol/L.

Cost $15–$25 as a single test. Usually chloride is measured in a general chemistry or renal profile and in conjunction with pH and electrolytes to determine the metabolic baseline.

cholangiography   A test performed by a radiologist that consists of a fluoroscopic examination of the biliary ducts after injection of iodinated radio-contrast material. Cholangiography is used primarily to determine the cause and location of biliary obstruction after the region was visualized by computed tomography (CT) or with ultrasonography. Cholangiography gives the most detailed view of the obstruction. Because of the invasive nature and potential risk of serious side effects, this procedure is used only when necessary.

Patient preparation This procedure is generally performed in a hospital setting. Local or general anesthesia is used because this can be a painful procedure.

Procedure The patient is placed in a supine position, and a needle is placed in the liver under the guidance of fluoroscopy. When bile can be aspirated from the duct, contrast medium is injected. Films are taken at various intervals for further study.

Specimen X rays.

Reference range No anatomic defects, obstruction, or dilatation are seen.

Abnormal values Obstructive jaundice, cholelithiasis, biliary tract carcinoma, carcinoma of the pancreas, carcinoma of the papilla of Vater.

Cost $250–$350.

Comments Transient pain is associated with the placement of the needle and injection of the contrast medium. The patient must rest for six hours after the procedure. The patient must be assessed for hypersensitivity to the contrast medium. Uncorrected coagulopathy is a contraindication to the performance of the test.

cholecystography (gallbladder series)   A radiographic procedure for studying the gallbladder and biliary tract. An ingested contrast medium concentrates in the gallbladder, making it visible under X-ray evaluation. The procedure is also carried out after a fatty meal to evaluate the emptying of the contrast medium from the gallbladder. The results can indicate suspected gallbladder disease in the form of inflammation (cholecystitis), gallstones (cholelithiasis), or colicky upper right quadrant pain.

Patient preparation The patient is given contrast medium (six tablets of iopanoic acid) two to three hours after the evening meal. Water and food are then restricted until the radiographic films are taken the next day.

Procedure X-ray and fluoroscopic studies are carried out 12–14 hours after ingestion of the contrast medium.

Specimen X rays.

Reference range No anatomic defects, obstruction, or dilatation are seen.

Abnormal values Gallstones (cholelithiasis), cholecystitis, cholesterol polyps, benign and malignant tumors.

Cost $250–$400.

Comments This method has waned in popularity and provides little information that cannot be obtained by gallbladder ultrasonography. Contraindications are severe renal or hepatic disease and hypersensitivity to the contrast medium.

cholesterol Cholesterol is a normal structural component in cell membranes and plasma lipoproteins that is absorbed from the diet and synthesized in the liver. It is a precursor of steroid hormones and bile acids. A diet high in saturated fat raises cholesterol levels and a low-saturated-fat diet tends to lower them. Because increased cholesterol has been associated with atherosclerosis, coronary artery disease, and an increased risk of death due to heart attacks, (total) cholesterol is commonly measured and included in most routine chemistry panels. Cholesterol is transported through the circulation by carrier proteins. Cholesterol that circulates attached to high-density lipoprotein (HDL-cholesterol) is metabolized in an optimal fashion and is known as "good" cholesterol. Cholesterol that circulates attached to low-density lipoprotein (LDL-cholesterol) and to very low-density lipoprotein (VLDL) is known as "bad" cholesterol. When the total cholesterol is elevated (usually above 200 mg/dL), it is common practice to measure the levels of HDL-cholesterol and LDL-cholesterol.

Patient preparation For optimal results, the patient should fast for 12 hours prior to the test.

Procedure Cholesterol is measured spectrophotometrically using automated chemistry instruments.

Specimen Serum.

Reference range

Less than 200 mg/dL	Low risk of cardiovascular disease.
200–240 mg/dL	Intermediate risk.
Greater than 240 mg/dL	Therapy needed.

Abnormal values

Increased in: hypercholesterolemia, nephrotic syndrome, hypothyroidism, biliary cirrhosis.

Decreased in: malnutrition, hyperthyroidism.

Cost $10–$30 when used as an initial screening. It is generally part of a routine chemistry panel.

Comments Although many studies have shown a relationship between cholesterol levels and risk of coronary artery disease, there is some controversy as to cause and effect.

cholinesterase There are two forms of cholinesterase, one is synthesized in red blood cells and the other (pseudocholinesterase) in the serum/plasma of the liver. Both forms are used to determine the extent of organophosphate (pesticide) exposure. The serum/plasma form (i.e., pseudocholinesterase) is more useful in detecting acute toxicity while the red blood cell form better reflects chronic exposure. Some persons have a genetic variant that acts more slowly on substrates than the normal enzyme and experience prolonged apnea after anesthesia with suxamethonium-type muscle relaxants. These abnormal enzymes can be detected by a screening procedure prior to undergoing anesthesia.

Patient preparation No preparation is required.

Procedure Cholinesterase is measured spectrophotometrically on automated chemistry analyzers.

Specimen Heparinized whole blood.

Reference range The levels are not well established and are laboratory dependent.

Abnormal values
Increased in: hemolysis.
Decreased in: organophosphate pesticide poisoning, carbamate exposure, atypical variant of cholinesterase.

Cost $50–$75.

Comments Red blood cell cholinesterase is not normally present in amniotic fluid but when found in conjunction with increased alphafetoprotein levels suggests the presence of an open neural tube defect in the fetus.

chorionic villus biopsy A method for early (first trimester) prenatal diagnosis of fetal chromosomal abnormalities and other disease; placental tissue is obtained at 9–11 weeks (vs. the 16th week for amniotic fluid analysis) from the developing placenta by ultrasound-guided, transcervical catheter aspiration biopsy. The tissue obtained is from the chorion frondosum, the layer from which the chorionic villi develop.

Patient preparation Informed consent is required. The patient should void before the procedure.

Procedure There are two approaches for chorionic villus biopsy: the transcervical and the transabdominal. The transabdominal carries a lower risk of infection, uses a needle that can be aimed with more accuracy (versus a plastic catheter used in the transcervical approach), and has a lower rate of spontaneous fetal loss. Once the biopsy is obtained it is submitted to a reference laboratory for chromosome analysis.

Specimen Tissue that is maintained in a "living" state, placed in a transport medium.

Reference range No biochemical, chromosome, or DNA abnormalities.

Abnormal values Defects include increased or decreased number of chromosomes and increased alphafetoprotein.

Cost $300–$700.

Comments The diagnostic yield of chorionic villus biopsy is 97.8%; the yield of amniocentesis performed at 16 gestational weeks is 99.4%. The chorionic villus biopsy has a slightly higher rate of fetal wastage. Chorionic villus biopsy may be associated with an increase in defects of the extremities and/or digits. See *amniocentesis, biophysical profile.*

chromium An essential mineral present in trace amounts in the body; it is present in various enzymes and potentiates the action of insulin. Chromium deficiency is rare and characterized by weight loss, glucose intolerance, insulin resistance, decreased respiratory quotients, and peripheral neuropathy. Chromium is present in a wide range of foods from brewer's yeast to skim milk. Toxic levels result from industrial exposure to chromium-laden fumes and dusts in electroplating, manufacture of steel, dyes, and chemicals, leather tanning, and photography. The clinical findings of acute chromium poisoning include allergic reactions, conjunctivitis, dermatitis, and edema. Chronic exposure is associated with gastrointestinal symptoms, hepatitis, and an increased incidence of lung cancer.

Patient preparation The patient should fast for 12 hours prior to the drawing of the specimen.

Procedure Chromium levels are determined by atomic absorption spectrophotometry.

Specimen Whole blood, serum, urine. For serum collection, a special trace-element blood collection tube is required. For urine collection, a 24-hour specimen must be collected in a plastic, metal-free container supplied by the laboratory.

Reference range

Serum	0.05–0.15 ng/mL.
Urine	Less than 1ng/24 hours.

Abnormal values

Chromium deficiency	Less than 0.01 ng/mL.
Chromium intoxication	Greater than 10.0 ng/mL.

Cost $75–$100.

chromogenic (enzyme) substrate test Any of a number of biochemical tests used in microbiology to detect the presence of an enzyme, such as β-lactamase. In this test a specific biochemical reagent is incorporated into the bacterial culture medium, which upon hydrolysis changes color, confirming the presence of the enzyme of interest.

chromosome analysis (karyotyping) A laboratory procedure in which cells of fetal origin (obtained either in the first trimester by chorionic villus biopsy or later in pregnancy by amniocentesis) are grown in a tissue culture medium to detect major chromosomal defects. There are several techniques used in chromosome analysis. Karyotyping is the oldest and most commonly performed method and allows visual detection of defects in chromosome structure; the defects are then classified according to type (e.g., breakage or loss of chromosomes, duplication, inversion). While karyotyping continues to be the gold standard for chromosome analysis, it is slow, labor-intensive, expensive, and thus likely to be replaced by newer techniques such as polymerase chain reaction (PCR) and fluorescent in situ hybridization (FISH). Chromosome analysis is indicated for congenital anomalies with mental or growth retardation, infertility, in cryptorchidic testes, ambiguous genitalia, repeated neonatal death, advanced maternal age, and in analysis of neoplasia. See *DNA hybridization, polymerase chain reaction.*

Patient preparation For serum, fluid, and buccal smear specimens, no special preparation is required. For the bone marrow specimen, local anesthetic is used at the puncture site.

Procedure The lymphocytes are separated from the other cells by differential centrifugation. They are then exposed to hypotonic solutions to disrupt the cellular membranes. The chromosomes are then harvested by differential ultracentrifugation and analyzed by microscopy.

Specimen Blood, bone marrow, amniotic fluid, buccal smear.

Reference range No chromosome defects are identified.

Abnormal values Various leukemias, Turner syndrome, Klinefelter's syndrome, genetic defects.

Cost $300–$900.

Comments Newer, more specific methods are being developed rapidly. These methods will not only allow the detection of an abnormality that is the cause of a specific genetic syndrome but will also detect genes that may put an individual at risk for various cancers (breast, colon) or other diseases. This area of laboratory medicine is known as molecular biology.

CIN See *cervical intraepithelial neoplasia.*

CIS See *carcinoma in situ* in Glossary.

CK-MB See *creatine phosphokinase.*

clonidine suppression test A test used to identify pheochromocytoma, a tumor of the adrenal gland.

Patient preparation The patient should not eat anything for four hours before the test. Certain foods (e.g., bananas and walnuts) and drugs (Aldomet, epinephrine, levodopa, methenamine mandelate) should not be ingested before the test.

Procedure Blood is collected to measure baseline production of catecholamines. 0.3 mg of clonidine is administered by mouth. After three hours, blood is collected a second time to measure (by RIA) any changes in the concentrations of catecholamines.

Specimen Plasma.

Reference range
Epinephrine	Less than 88 pg/mL.
Norepinephrine	100–550 pg/mL.
Dopamine	Less than 140 pg/mL.

Abnormal values
Epinephrine	Greater than 90 pg/mL.
Norepinephrine	Greater than 550 pg/mL.
Dopamine	Greater than 150 pg/mL.

Cost $125–$200.

Clostridium difficile   This bacterium is the major cause of antibiotic-associated enterocolitis. It can be detected on culture, but a positive culture is not significant because asymptomatic individuals can have a positive culture. There are laboratory tests that can detect the toxins released by this bacterium and are usually analyzed in specimens from symptomatic patients.

Patient preparation No preparation is required.

Procedure Clostridium difficile toxins are extracted from the stool specimens and measured by ELISA methodology.

Specimen Stool or proctoscopic specimen.

Reference range Negative.

Abnormal values Antibiotic-associated pseudomembranous colitis.

Cost $35–$50.

CMV   See *cytomegalovirus.*

coagulation panel   A group of assays designed to efficiently identify a probable cause of hemorrhage in a patient who is bleeding. The assays include prothrombin time, activated partial thromboplastic time, platelet count, and bleeding time.

Comments Patients who have bleeding tendencies are usually referred to a hematologist experienced in coagulopathies. This field is rapidly expanding and the tests, especially for the more difficult cases, are carried out in only a few reference laboratories which are usually in university-associated hospitals.

coagulation studies   Coagulation is the process by which blood clots. The coagulation system generates thrombin, an enzyme that acts on soluble fibrinogen to produce insoluble fibrin. Fibrin is the end product of coagulation and the last step in a highly complex series of protein reactions known as the coagulation cascade. The coagulation factors are identified by Roman numerals (e.g., factor V, factor VIII) or descriptive names (e.g., fibrinogen, von Willebrand factor). Almost all of these coagulation factors are present in circulating blood in an inactive form. There are many tests used to measure various abnormalities involved in the coagulation process. Some tests are commonly performed as part of a routine workup and include prothrombin time (PT), activated partial thrombin time (aPTT), and platelet count. Other coagulation tests are rarely performed (e.g., bleeding time) or esoteric (e.g., platelet studies, specific factor analysis) and only performed when specific coagulation defects are being evaluated.

cocaine   A powder derived from the plant *Erythoxylon coca* that evokes intense physical and psychological addiction. Cocaine causes many undesired effects on the heart (e.g., arrhythmias in the form of ventricular tachycardia and fibrillation, myocarditis, and myocardial infarction), as well as sudden death, convulsions, hyperpyrexia, cerebral vasculitis, loss of sense of smell, decreased oxygen diffusing capacity, spontaneous pneumomediastinum, and eating disorders such as bulimia and anorexia.

Urine and serum may be screened for benzoylecgonine, cocaine's major metabolite, by enzyme-labelled competitive immunoassay and confirmed for legal purposes by the gold standard method, gas chromatography-mass spectrometry. See *drug screening, EMIT* in Glossary.

coccidioidomycosis   An infection by airborne arthroconidia of the soil fungus *Coccidioides immitis,* which is endemic to the southwestern United States and the western hemisphere. The mycelial form is easily cultured on artificial media and is highly infectious but cannot be definitively identified; serological testing reveals transient increase of IgM antibodies in 75%.
Patient preparation No preparation is required.
Procedure Serological testing is carried out using ELISA methodology or complement fixation.
Specimen Serum.
Reference range Titers of less than 1:8 are negative.
Abnormal values Titers of greater than 1:16 are positive.
Cost $50–$75.

cold agglutinin   Cold agglutinins are autoantibodies that agglutinate red blood cells at very low temperatures. They are detectable at low levels in normal patients, increase after certain infections, and are of no significance if they are non-hemolytic (i.e., do not cause hemolysis of red blood cells). Cold agglutinins are used to aid in the diagnosis of primary atypical pneumonia and certain hemolytic anemias. Cold agglutinins that are detected at $20°C$ can interfere with antibody screening in blood bank testing and can cause pain, thrombosis, and hemolysis.
Patient preparation No preparation is required.
Procedure The serum is incubated at cold temperatures $(10°C)$ and observed for the formation of precipitate which disappears upon warming.
Specimen Serum.
Reference range Negative.
Abnormal values Cold agglutinins are present in mycoplasma pneumonia and hemolytic anemias.
Cost $20–$30.

colonoscopy   The visual examination of the large intestine with a flexible fiberoptic endoscope.
Patient preparation The patient must maintain a clear liquid diet for 48 hours prior to the test, after which the large intestine is cleansed with laxatives until the return is clear. The procedure is generally safe but somewhat uncomfortable.
Procedure A water-soluble lubricant is applied to the patient's anus and the tip of the colonoscope. The colonoscope is then inserted and guided through the colon. Air is passed through the colonoscope to distend the

bowel and provide better visualization. The endoscope is equipped with a lens to allow the physician to view and photograph the lining of the bowel, known as the mucosa. If a suspicious lesion is observed, a biopsy is obtained through a channel in the endoscope.

Specimen Any abnormalities may be photographed and/or biopsied.

Reference range The normal colonic mucosa is a pale reddish pink.

Abnormal values Bleeding, diverticulosis, polyps, stricture, tumor (benign or malignant), inflammatory bowel disease (e.g., ulcerative colitis, Crohn's disease).

Cost $700–$1000.

Comments There is some risk of intestinal perforation.

colposcopy A technique in which a colposcope is used to evaluate and/or biopsy lesions of the uterine cervix and upper vagina, the presence of which had been previously identified by a pap smear.

Patient preparation No preparation is required.

Procedure The woman lies on the examination table with her feet in stirrups. The gynecologist looks through a colposcope and examines the vaginal wall and uterine cervix. The colposcopist may coat the area of interest with an iodinated liquid (e.g., Lugol's solution), highlighting the suspicious areas in gray-white on a mahogany brown background.

Specimen The gynecologist may photograph and/or biopsy suspicious areas.

Reference range No abnormalities are seen.

Abnormal values Gray-white patches often correspond to hyperkeratosis and parakeratosis, histological lesions that are associated with premalignant and malignant lesions. See *cervical biopsy.*

Cost $150–$350.

combined anterior pituitary test (CAP test) A dynamic test of pituitary function that may be performed in an ambulatory care (i.e., outpatient) setting.

Patient preparation Hormonal therapy (cortisosteroids, contraceptives, thyroid hormones) should be documented and, if possible, discontinued.

Procedure Four hypothalamic releasing hormones (RH, corticotropin-RH growth hormone-RH, luteinizing hormone-RH, and thyrotropin-RH) are administered sequentially over a space of 20 seconds. Serum levels of the target hormones (adrenocorticotropic hormone [ACTH], growth hormone [GH], follicle-stimulating hormone [FSH], luteinizing hormone [LH], thyroid-stimulating hormone [TSH], and prolactin) are drawn and measured at -30, 0, 30, 60, 90, and 120 minutes. Hormones are measured by RIA or ELISA.

Specimen Serum.

Reference range

ACTH	25–100 pg/mL
GH	0.4–10 ng/mL
FSH	
Males	4–25 mU/mL

Females, premenopause	4–30 mU/mL
Females, postmenopause	40–250 mU/mL
Females, midcycle	10–90 mU/mL
LH	
Males	6–23 mU/mL
Females, premenopause	3–40 mU/mL
Females, postmenopause	30–200 mU/mL
Females, midcycle	75–150 mU/mL
TSH	
Males	2.0–7.5 µU/mL
Females	2.0–17.0 µU/mL

Abnormal values

ACTH	Less than 20, greater than 125 pg/mL
GH	Less than 0.2, greater than 12.5 ng/mL
FSH	
Males	Less than 2, greater than 30 mU/mL
Females, premenopause	Less than 2, greater than 50 mU/mL
Females, postmenopause	Less than 20, greater than 400 mU/mL
Females, midcycle	Less than 4, greater than 125 mU/mL
LH	
Males	Less than 2, greater than 40 mU/mL
Females, premenopause	Less than 1.5, greater than 60 mU/mL
Females, postmenopause	Less than 15, greater than 300 mU/mL
Females, midcycle	Less than 40, greater than 250 mU/mL
TSH	
Males	Less than 1, greater than 10 µU/mL
Females	Less than 1, greater than 25 µU/mL

Cost $200–$400.

complement Complement is a group of more than 25 proteins present in the serum that mediate the nonspecific inflammatory response to various antigens through a complex sequence of enzymatic cleavages. The cleavages result in the activation of one of two molecular pathways: the classic pathway (which responds to antigen-antibody complexes) and the alternative (or properdin) pathway (which responds to fungi and bacteria, in addition to antigen-antibody complexes). Either pathway leads to a common pathway of molecular activation, and in the final stage, lysis of a cell membrane occurs. Complement results in a number of biologically active products which are implicated in numerous diseases with an immunologic basis. Complement proteins are designated as C1 through C9. Not all complements are routinely measured in the laboratory.

Patient preparation No preparation is required.
Procedure Complements are measured using ELISA methodology.
Specimen Serum.
Reference range
Total complement   40–100 units

C1q	70 µg/ml
C1r	34 µg/ml
C1s	31 µg/ml
C2	25 µg/ml
C3	1600 µg/ml
C4	600 µg/ml
C5	85 µg/ml
C6	75 µg/ml
C7	55 µg/ml
C8	55 µg/ml
C9	60 µg/ml
Factor B	200 µg/ml
Factor D	1 µg/ml

Abnormal values
Deficiencies in:

C1r	Systemic lupus erythematosus (SLE), renal disease, repeated infections
C1s	Systemic lupus erythematosus
C4	Systemic lupus erythematosus
C2	Systemic lupus erythematosus, vasculitis, membrano-proliferative glomerulonephritis, dermatomyositis
C3	Repeated infections
C5	Systemic lupus erythematosus, gonococcal infection
C6	Relapsing meningococcal meningitis, gonococcal infection
C7	Raynaud's disease, chronic renal disease, gonococcal infection
C8	Systemic lupus erythematosus, gonococcal infection

Cost $45–$100, depending on the test.

Comments In general, the initial screen measures the total complement, C3 and C4, which encompass all three complement pathways and is found useful in evaluating rheumatic disorders such as lupus erythematosus, arteritis, and arthritis.

complement fixation test An assay of broad clinical application which depends on the ability of serum complement to interact with antigen-antibody (Ag-Ab) complexes. In the first stage of the test, complement is incubated with a solution that may contain the antigen and antibody of interest. If Ag-Ab complexes are formed, they interact with the complement, and the complement is consumed ("fixed"); in the second stage, sensitized sheep red (EA) cells are added to the milieu and incubated at 37°C for one hour. If the serum contained the antibody of interest, the complement was previously consumed ("fixed") and not available to lyse the EA cells; therefore, the absence of lysis indicates a positive test. Complement fixation can be used to detect Ag-Ab complexes, soluble and particulate Ags, Abs, bacteria, fungi, and gamma globulins.

complete blood count Most commonly known as CBC, the complete blood count is one of the most commonly ordered tests and involves the measurement of the cellular components of blood and hemoglobin by highly automated instruments. The CBC measures hematocrit, hemoglobin, the volume of each red blood cell (MCV), hemoglobin per red blood cell (MCH), number of red blood cells, white blood cells, and platelets; a differential count enumerates lymphocytes, monocytes, eosinophils, basophils, and neutrophils. If the automated differential is abnormal, a manual differential is performed to verify the results. The manual differential is labor intensive and involves the preparation of a microscope slide and visually counting the cellular components under a microscope.

Patient preparation No preparation is required.

Procedure The current generation of automated instruments are specialized flow cytometers which measure cell size, DNA content, and hemoglobin to determine the quantity of each cell type. Some of the parameters such as hematocrit, MCV, and MCHC are calculated from the measured results.

Specimen Whole blood with EDTA anticoagulant, which may be obtained by venipuncture, fingerstick, or heel stick.

Reference range (adult)

RBCs	
Male	$4.5–6.2 \times 10^6/mm^3$
Female	$4.2–5.4 \times 10^6/mm^3$
MCV	84–99 fL/cell
MCH	26–32 pg/cell
MCHC	30%–36%
Hematocrit	
Male	42%–54%
Female	38%–46%
Hemoglobin	
Male	14–18 g/dL
Female	12–16 g/dL
WBCs	$4,100–10,900/mm^3$
Neutrophils	48%–77%
Lymphocytes	16%–43%
Monocytes	0.6%–9.6%
Eosinophils	0.3%–7%
Basophils	0.3%–2%
Platelets	$140–400,000/mm^3$

Abnormal values	DECREASED IN	INCREASED IN
WBC	Viral infection	Bacterial infection, leukemia
Hematocrit	Anemia	Polycythemia
	Hemodilution	Hemoconcentration due to blood loss
Hemoglobin	Anemia	Hemoconcentration due to
	Hemorrhage	polycythemia or dehydration
	Fluid retention	
RBCs	Anemia	Polycythemia

Abnormal values (cont.)	DECREASED IN	INCREASED IN
RBCs	Fluid overload	Dehydration, Hemorrhage
MCV	Iron deficiency Anemia	Macrocytic anemia Thalassemia
	Vitamin B_{12} or folate deficiency Reticulocytosis Genetic DNA disorder	
MCH	Microcytic anemia	Macrocytic anemia
MCHC	Iron deficiency anemia	Spherocytosis

NEUTROPHILS

Increased in: infections, myocardial infarction, metabolic diseases stress, inflammation.

Decreased by: radiation or cytotoxic drugs, infections, hypersplenism hepatic disease, collagen vascular disease, folic acid or vitamin B_{12} deficiency.

EOSINOPHILS

Increased in: allergy, parasitic infections, skin disorders, neoplastic diseases, collagen vascular disease.

Decreased in: stress, Cushing's syndrome.

BASOPHILS

Increased in: chronic myelocytic leukemia, polycythemia vera, Hodgkin's disease, certain anemias.

Decreased in: hyperthyroidism, ovulation, pregnancy, stress.

LYMPHOCYTES

Increased in: infections, lymphocytic leukemia, certain immune diseases, ulcerative colitis.

Decreased in: chronic debilitating illness, immunodeficiency.

MONOCYTES

Increased in: infections, collagen vascular disease, carcinomas, monocytic leukemia, lymphomas.

Cost $25–$50.

Comments The CBC is a general screen and can indicate various disease processes. It is used as a first test and is followed by more comprehensive testing if indicated. See *platelet count, red blood cell count.*

computed tomography (CT imaging, CT scanning)   A procedure in which a three-dimensional image is constructed from a series of two-dimensional radiologic "slices" of a particular region of the body. Like conventional radiology, the images are obtained based on the simple principle that different tissue densities (designated fat, water, air, and muscle) will have a different appearance on the film. In contrast to conventional radiology, CT scanning results in a thousand-fold increase in the sharpness of images of a body region and can often pinpoint lesions measuring less than 2 mm in greatest dimension. The indications for CT scanning and MRIs overlap considerably and both have proven effective in detecting lesions from virtually any body region. Computed tomography has revolutionized the field of radiology and with its sister technologies, magnetic resonance imaging (MRI) and ultrasonography, has increased the yields and accuracy of noninvasive methods used in diagnostic medicine. See *MRI, ultrasonography.*

cone biopsy See *conization.*

conization (cone biopsy) The excision of a doughnut or cone-shaped biopsy of the uterine cervix that includes the ectocervix and endocervix; it is performed as definitive therapy for cervical intraepithelial neoplasia (CIN) 1 to III.
Patient preparation Informed consent is required. Sedatives may be required for anxious patients.
Procedure A cone biopsy is performed under local or general anesthesia with a scalpel ("cold knife") or with a CO_2 laser.
Specimen A doughnut-shaped piece of tissue corresponding to the external cervix.
Reference range Conization of the cervix is not performed in the absence of previously identified abnormalities.
Abnormal values Cervical intraepithlial neoplasia (CIN I–III), squamous cell cancer, human papilloma virus (HPV) infection, tissue margins should be free of lesions.
Cost $500–$900.
Comments Bleeding, infection, cervical stenosis, or incompetence. See *LEEP.*

Coombs test See *direct antiglobulin test, indirect antiglobulin test.*

copper Copper is an essential trace metal that is needed in several metabolic reactions in the body. Urine and plasma usually contain small amounts of free copper. Copper is increased in Wilson's disease, a rare, genetic metabolic disease common among persons of eastern European, Jewish, southern Italian, or Sicilian ancestry, or following industrial exposure to copper.
Patient preparation No preparation is required.
Procedure Copper is most commonly measured by atomic absorption spectroscopy.
Specimen Urine, less commonly plasma.
Reference range 15–60 mg/24 hours.
Abnormal values Copper is increased in Wilson's disease.
Cost $50–$100.
Comments Early detection and treatment of Wilson's disease prevents irreversible changes; treatment consists of a low copper diet and D-penicillamine.

copper sulfate test A rapid test for determining the specific gravity of blood that serves as an indirect measurement of hematocrit. It is used in the blood bank to determine blood donor acceptability. Specific gravity of 1.053, which corresponds to a hemoglobin of 12.5g/dL is a level adequate for blood donation in females; specific gravity of 1.055, which corresponds to a hemoglobin of 13.5g/dL, is adequate for male donation.

corticotropin See *adrenocorticotropic hormone.*

cortisol Cortisol is the primary glucocorticoid secreted by the adrenal cortex in response to ACTH stimulation. Cortisol is involved in metabolism of nutrients, mediation of physiologic stress, and regulation of the immune system. Heat, cold, infection, trauma, exercise, obesity, and debilitating disease influence cortisol secretion. Cortisol is secreted in a diurnal pattern with levels rising in the early morning, peaking around 8 a.m. and declining to low levels in the evening. In Cushing's syndrome, patients do not exhibit this diurnal variation.

Patient preparation No preparation is required.

Procedure Cortisol is measured by RIA, ELISA, or chemiluminescent methods.

Specimen Serum, plasma, urine. The urine specimen is a 24-hour collection that must be preserved by 20 ml 33% acetic acid or 1 g boric acid. The serum or plasma specimens must be drawn at 8 a.m. and 4 p.m. to evaluate diurnal variation.

Reference range

    Serum a.m. 5–25 µg/dL.
    Serum p.m. 2–9 µg/dL.
    Urine   30–100 µg/24 hours.

Abnormal values

    Serum increased in: pituitary overproduction, carcinoma adrenal adenoma.
    Serum decreased in: pituitary failure, adrenal gland destruction
    Urine: loss of diurnal variation suggests Cushing's syndrome.

Cost $25–$50. See *dexamethasone suppression test.*

cosyntropin test See *dexamethasone suppression test.*

C-peptide C-peptide is an inactive portion of early insulin (proinsulin) produced by the body and stored in the pancreas. It is measured in patients with hypoglycemia (low blood sugar).

Patient preparation The patient should fast for ten hours before obtaining the specimen. The patient should not have had any recent studies using radionuclides (e.g., nuclear scans).

Procedure C-peptide is measured by RIA. Glucose and insulin are measured from the same specimen.

Specimen Serum.

Reference range

    C-peptide   0.5–2.5 ng/mL.
    Insulin   20–25 µIU/mL.
    Glucose   60–115 mg/dL.

Abnormal values C-peptide and insulin are increased and glucose is decreased in islet cell tumors of the pancreas. C-peptide and glucose are decreased and insulin is increased in individuals who inject exogenous (external) insulin.
Cost $125–$200.

CPK   See *creatine phosphokinase.*

CPK-MB   See *creatine phosphokinase isoenzymes.*

C-reactive protein   A protein that is produced in the liver and named for its ability to bind the C polysaccharide of the *Streptococcus pneumoniae* cell wall. CRP is an "acute phase reactant" whose functions include complement activation, binding of T cells, inhibition of clot retraction, suppression of platelet and lymphocyte function, and enhancement of phagocytosis by neutrophils. CRP serves as a biological marker for inflammation and necrosis and is useful as a monitor of early deterioration or development of complications of therapy. CRP levels are quantified by latex agglutination and nephelometry. Because CRP rises in response to acute injury, infection, or inflammation, it is generally measured in conjunction with the erythrocyte sedimentation rate, another nonspecific marker of inflammation.
Patient preparation No preparation is required.
Procedure CRP is measured by nephelometry or turbidimetry.
Specimen Serum.
Reference range Less than 8 μg/ml.
Abnormal values
   Increased in: infection, inflammation.
Cost $15–$25.

creatine   Creatine is the end product of protein metabolism and is formed in the liver, kidneys, small intestine, and pancreas. In the muscle it combines with phosphate to form phosphocreatine—a high energy compound. During muscle contraction, some creatine enters the bloodstream.
Patient preparation No preparation is required.
Procedure Creatine is measured spectrophotometrically on an automated chemistry analyzer.
Specimen Serum.
Reference range
   Males   0.2–0.6 mg/dL.
   Females   0.6–1.0 mg/dL.
Abnormal values
   Increased in: trauma to skeletal muscle, atrophy of skeletal muscle,
      muscular dystrophy, hyperthyroidism, pregnancy, high protein intake.
Cost $75–$100.

creatine phosphokinase   (CK, CPK)   Creatine phosphokinase is the enzyme that catalyzes the creatine-creatinine metabolic pathway, which is concentrated in muscle and brain tissue. Increased levels of CPK in the serum suggest trauma to cells in these tissues.

Patient preparation No preparation is required.

Procedure CK is measured spectrophotometrically on automated chemistry analyzers.

Specimen Serum. Since the level of CPK rises to peak levels 12–24 hours after an infarction and returns to normal in 24–48 hours, the time of the specimen must be indicated.

Reference range 0–250 units/L.

Abnormal values

Increased in: myocardial infarction, muscle trauma, muscular dystrophy, cerebrovascular accident, malignancy.

Cost $15–$35. Some laboratories include CPK as part of their general chemistry profile although some regard this as unnecessary.

Comments An elevated CPK is not diagnostic of myocardial infarction. Isoenzyme determinations must be carried out for confirmation. Stress and exercise can cause elevations which are not disease related.

creatine phosphokinase isoenzymes Creatine phosphokinase has three common forms, or isoenzymes:

CK-MM	Skeletal muscle
CK-MB	Cardiac muscle
CK-BB	Brain

CK-MB is present in heart muscle and usually increased in myocardial infarction. It is also increased in muscular dystrophy, polymyositis, myoglobinuria, and occasionally in cancer (e.g., lung cancer). These other causes of elevated CK-MB must be considered when no myocardial infarction is identified. In addition to the three common forms, there are several isoforms (additional species of CK-MM and CK-MB) which can be isolated. They include macro-CPK, which consists of immunoglobulin complexes of normal isoenzymes whose clinical significance is not yet known, and mitochondrial CPK, which is found in seriously ill patients (primarily those with metastatic carcinoma) and is a recognized sign of poor prognosis.

Patient preparation No preparation is required.

Procedure The most widely used procedure and still considered the gold standard is electrophoresis. Newer immunologic assays, however, which are specific for the CK-MB isoform have proven to be more rapid and just as sensitive.

Specimen Serum.

Reference range

CK-MM	94%–100%
CK-MB	0%–6%
CK-BB	0%

Abnormal values

Increased in:

CK-MM   Muscle trauma (reflected by elevated total CPK)

CK-MB   Myocardial infarction or damage
CK-BB   Brain injury

Cost $45–$65.

Comments A single determination of CPK isoenzymes is insufficient for diagnosis because the CK-MB fraction is usually normal immediately after myocardial infarction. CK-MB begins to rise 2–4 hours after infarction, peaks between 12–24 hours, and returns to normal within 48 hours. Typically, three specimens are obtained, the first when the patient is first seen in the emergency room, another at 12 hours, and then at 24 hours. A rise and fall of levels is generally considered diagnostic of myocardial infarction. CPK isoenzyme determinations should be evaluated in conjunction with clinical findings, an electrocardiogram, and other laboratory findings such as LDH isoenzymes and AST/ALT measurements. Troponin is a new cardiac marker thought to be more specific and sensitive to myocardial infarction than CK-MB. See *troponin* in Glossary.

creatinine   Creatinine is the end product of creatine metabolism which is excreted by the kidney and thus is used to diagnose and monitor renal disease. It is sometimes measured in amniotic fluid when determining gestational age (fetal maturity index). Normal ranges vary according to the laboratory.

Patient preparation No preparation is required.

Procedure Creatinine is measured spectrophotometrically on automated chemistry analyzers.

Specimen Urine, serum, amniotic fluid.

Reference range
   Serum
      Age 1–5 years   0.3–0.5 mg/dL.
      Age 5–10 years   0.5–0.8 mg/dL.
      Males   Less than 1.2 mg/dL.
      Females   Less than 1.1 mg/dL.
   Urine
      Age 2–3 years   6–22 mg/kg/24 hours.
      Males   1–2 g/24 hours.
      Females   0.8–1.8 g/24 hours.

Abnormal values Serum creatinine increased in renal disease, urine creatinine decreased in renal disease.

Cost $10–$20. The serum test is usually part of a general chemistry profile.

Comments Both measurements are used in determining creatinine clearance.

creatinine clearance   Creatinine clearance reflects the body's ability to excrete creatinine and is used to diagnose and monitor renal function.

Patient preparation If possible, drugs should be withheld for 24 hours prior to the collection. The patient should be encouraged to drink water.

Procedure Creatinine is measured spectrophotometrically on automated chemistry analyzers.

Specimen 24-hour urine and a serum specimen obtained during the collection of the 24-hour urine specimen.
Reference range
Children   70–140 ml/min/1.73m^2
Males   85–125 ml/min/1.73m^2
Females   75–115 ml/min/1.73m^2
Abnormal values Creatinine is decreased in renal disease.
Cost $25–$50.

crithidia assay   A direct immunofluorescence test for quantifying anti-DNA antibodies in the serum of patients with systemic lupus erythematosus using *Crithidia luciliae*, a hemoflagellate with a large mitochondrion containing abundant double-stranded DNA.
Patient preparation No preparation is required other than for drawing blood.
Procedure The test if performed by indirect immunofluorescence. The patient's serum is placed on a glass slide with *Crithidia luciliae*.
Specimen Serum.
Reference range Negative; less than 1:10 dilution of serum.
Abnormal values Positive; greater than 1:10 dilution of serum.
Cost $100–$200.

CRP   See *C-reactive protein*.

cryoglobulins   Cryoglobulins are abnormal proteins present in the serum of patients with some diseases that are detected in the laboratory by chilling the serum to 32°C. Patients with cryoglobulinemia experience pain, cyanosis, and numbing of fingers and toes when they are exposed to cold. A wide range of conditions are accompanied by cryoglobulin production but may not be associated with clinical disease.
Patient preparation No preparation is required.
Procedure Cryoglobulins are detected by manually observing the effect of chilling on the serum. The formation of precipitate on chilling indicates a positive test for cryoglobulins.
Specimen Serum. Specimen must be kept warm until testing.
Reference range Negative.
Abnormal values myeloma, Waldenstrom's macroglobulinemia, chronic lymphocytic leukemia, rheumatoid arthritis, Sjögren's syndrome, systemic lupus erythematosus.
Cost $25–$45.
Comments If positive the patient must be instructed to avoid cold temperatures.

cryoglobulinemia   A condition caused by proteins that precipitate in the blood when acral parts (e.g., hands and feet) are cooled. Cryoglobulinemia is often associated with immune complex (antigen-antibody) deposits in the kidney and has been divided into three clinical forms:

Type I: Monoclonal cryoglobulinemia. Underlying disease is often malignant; IgG malignant myeloma, IgM macroglobulinemia, or lymphoma/chronic lymphocytic leukemia, rarely others (e.g., IgA nephropathy), benign monoclonal gammopathy.

Type II: Poly-monoclonal cryoglobulinemia. A complex of immunoglobulins including mixed IgM-IgG, G-G, A-G, or other combinations that may be associated with lymphoreticular disease or connective tissue disease (e.g., rheumatoid arthritis, Sjögren syndrome, mixed essential cryoglobulinemia).

Type III: Mixed polyclonal-polyclonal cryoglobulinemia. Mixtures of IgG and IgM, occasionally IgA, associated with infections; rheumatoid arthritis, SLE, Sjögren syndrome, EBV and CMV viruses, subacute bacterial infections, poststreptococcal, crescentic and membranoproliferative glomerulonephritis, diabetes mellitus, chronic active hepatitis, biliary cirrhosis.

The clinical findings include arthralgias, vascular purpuras, cold intolerance, hypertension, and congestive heart failure. The laboratory findings include decreased C4 and other complement proteins.

Patient preparation The patient should be fasting.

Procedure The specimen is refrigerated (4°C) and the amount of precipitation is measured in a special Wintrobe tube. Each millimeter of precipitation equals 1% of "cryocrit." A precipitate that forms at 4°C and dissolves at 37°C is called a cryoglobulin.

Specimen Serum.

Reference range Negative.

Abnormal values Cryoglobulins occur in: Waldenström's macroglobulinemia, myeloma, chronic active hepatitis, chronic lymphocytic leukemia, systemic lupus erythematosus, viral infections.

Cost $50–$125.

cryptococcosis A serious fungal infection caused by *Cryptococcus neoformans* that can occur in blood, lungs, spinal fluid, and other body sites.

Patient preparation No preparation is required, other than for drawing blood or obtaining cerebrospinal fluid (lumbar puncture).

Procedure The fluid (serum, cerebrospinal fluid) is analyzed by latex agglutination.

Specimen Serum, cerebrospinal fluid.

Reference range Negative.

Abnormal values Positive. The test is positive in 85%–95% of patients with cryptococcal meningitis.

Cost $50–$125.

cryptosporidia A coccidian parasite of the intestines and respiratory tract that affects many mammals. In humans, *Cryptosporidium* causes severe, chronic diarrhea in patients with AIDS and decreased immunoglobulins. It causes self-limited diarrhea in children and adults who travel to endemic areas.

Patient preparation No preparation is required.

Procedure The specimen is examined by phase contrast microscopy after

concentrating the material (including the parasites) by flotation. Fluorescent antibodies are used to increase detection rates.
Specimen Stool.
Reference range Negative.
Abnormal values Positive.
Cost $75–$125.

culdocentesis The obtention of fluid and cells from the cul-de-sac (also known as the sac of Douglas or rectouterine pouch), a space in the peritoneal cavity between the uterus and the rectum.
Patient preparation No preparation is required.
Procedure A needle is passed into the cul-de-sac to aspirate fluids and cells which are evaluated by chemical analysis and microscopic examination.
Specimen Fluid and cells.
Reference range Negative for inflammation, hemorrhage, or malignant cells.
Abnormal values red blood cells (ectopic pregnancy), pus (acute salpingitis), malignant cells (cancer).
Cost $150–$400.

culture The growth of an organism under controlled conditions in the microbiology laboratory in 2 to 15 days; it is the definitive method by which bacteria and viruses are identified. Newer molecular biology techniques being developed, particularly polymerase chain reaction (PCR), can significantly reduce this time. In addition to identification, cultures are also used to determine the most effective antibiotic for treatment by exposing the isolated organisms to various antibiotics and measuring their rate of growth. Much of this has been automated, reducing the turnaround time for this important information.
Patient preparation No preparation is required.
Procedure Specimens are obtained with swabs from an area suspected of being infected, sent to the laboratory in sterile transport media, and placed in culture media to allow growth. The most common culture is the throat swab, which is used to detect beta-streptococcus, the bacterium classically associated with "strep" throat. Blood and other body fluids can also be cultured to detect bacteria and viruses. In general, bacterial cultures take 24–48 hours to grow sufficient microorganisms for identification techniques. Viral cultures can take up to two weeks, although the recently introduced shell vial assay can identify viruses in a day's time. The longest turnaround time for culturing microorganisms is for tuberculosis, which takes six weeks.
Specimen Throat swab, urine, blood, body fluids.
Reference range No growth after an appropriate length of time (bacteria and viruses differ).
Abnormal values Any growth of an organism (above the laboratory's cutoff for contaminants) is abnormal and requires physician notification.
Cost $40–$250.

cyanocobalamin See *vitamin B₁₂*.

cyclic AMP (cyclic adenosine monophosphate, cAMP) An intracellular mediator (second messenger) of hormonal action, produced from ATP by adenylate cyclase. cAMP acts on ion channels, the guanine nucleotide regulatory system, and hormone receptors. The binding of a hormone to its receptor induces a change in G (guanosine) protein and binds GTP, forming cAMP from ATP by adenylate cyclase. This action either increases (ACTH, β-adrenergic agonists, calcitonin, corticotropin-releasing factor, dopamine, FSH, glucagon, LH, PGE1, parathyroid hormone, serotonin-5HT, TSH and vasopressin V1) or decreases (acetylcholine, a2-adrenergic agonists, angiotensin II, insulin, opiates, oxytocin, somatostatin) intracellular substances.

Because cAMP is involved in the production of parathyroid hormone, measurement of cAMP levels has been used in the differential diagnosis of hypercalcemia of hyperparathyroidism.

Patient preparation Radioisotope scans should not be performed before obtaining the specimens.

Procedure Immunoassay or high-performance liquid chromatography.

Specimen Plasma, urine. Specimens should be frozen within one hour of collection.

Reference range

Plasma	5.6–10.9 ng/ml.
Urine	112–188 mg/L.

Abnormal values

Increased in: hyperparathyroidism, hypercalcemia of malignancy.

Cost $50–75.

cystic fibrosis See *sweat test.*

cystometrography A test that measures the function of the muscles that control the emptying of the bladder; it is used to help determine the cause of bladder dysfunction. It consists of a coordinated electromyographic evaluation of the bladder sphincter, which determines bladder capacity, efficiency of the voluntary or involuntary contractions of the detrusor muscle, and the bladder's compliance (the bladder's ability to stretch when filled) and evaluates the integrity of the affector (sensory) limb of the detrusor reflex arc.

Patient preparation Informed consent is required.

Procedure Cystometrography involves the use of a catheter to determine the extent to which the bladder empties and measures the effort exerted during the process. To test thermal sensation, 30 ml of room-temperature saline solution is instilled in the bladder. Then another 30 ml of warm (40–45°C) saline solution is instilled in the bladder, and the patient is asked to report any sensations or discomfort. The 60 ml is then drained, and a saline solution or CO_2 gas is slowly introduced into the bladder by a cystometer, which allows the pressure and volume within the bladder to be recorded.

Specimen Clinical findings and data recorded by cystometry.

	Reference range	Abnormal values	Reflex
	Normal	Uninhibited neurogenic bladder	Neurogenic bladder
Urination			
Start	+	+/o	o
Stop	o	o	+
Residual			
volume	o	o	+
Sensation	+	+	o
Capacity	400–500 ml	Decreased	Decreased
Contractions	Absent	Present	Present

Modified from *Illustrated Guide to Diagnostic Tests*, Springhouse Corp., Springhouse, Pa. 1994.

Cost $250–$600.

Comments Cystometrography should not be performed in the presence of an active urinary tract infection or if the catheter cannot be passed into the urinary bladder. Although the indications for performing a cystogram are somewhat controversial, it is indicated in evaluating patients with persistent urinary incontinence or retention related to bladder pathology. See *urodynamic evaluation*. Indications include spinal cord injury and voiding defects, incontinence after prostatectomy, incontinence after surgery for incontinence (i.e., failed surgery), overflow incontinence, urgency incontinence, and sensory or motor defect of the bladder in a background of cerebrovascular accident (stroke), diabetes mellitus, multiple sclerosis, or Parkinson's disease.

cystoscopy (cystourethroscopy)   Cystoscopy is the use of a urethroscope or cystoscope equipped with a fiberoptic light source to visualize the urethra and bladder and evaluate urinary tract disease. The cystoscope also has a hollow channel to enable the urologist to take biopsies or remove small stones.

Patient preparation Informed consent is required. A sedative may be required. The patient voids before the procedure.

Procedure An endoscope (cystourethroscope) is inserted through the urethra into the bladder; the urethra and bladder are examined visually and may be photographed. Abnormalities seen may be biopsied.

Specimen Visual evaluation and biopsy, if appropriate. Urine is obtained for culture.

Reference range No abnormalities are seen.

Abnormal values Inflammation, prostatic enlargement, tumors.

Cost $300–$700.

cytology   The term cytology refers to the formal discipline in which cells are studied and the changes seen correlated with the clinical findings in patients; it also refers to the microscopic examination of body fluids for the detection of disease.

The most common specimen is a smear of cells obtained from the outer portion of the uterine cervix, commonly known as the pap smear. Cytology specimens can be obtained from various abnormal discharges, urine, cerebrospinal fluids, or sputum. The main purpose of this examination is the detection of abnormal or malignant cells. The pap smear is a normal component of a gynecological examination and is the best method to detect early, curable stages of malignancy, as well as viral, fungal, and other infections of the female genital tract. See *pap smear*.

cytomegalovirus (CMV, herpesvirus-5, HHV-5) Cytomegalovirus is a member of the herpes virus group which is global in distribution. CMV is transmitted via blood and is rarely a serious infection, although it has been linked to chronic fatigue syndrome. However, in immunocompromised patients, e.g., those with AIDS or with bone marrow transplantation, CMV infection can have serious consequences. Intrauterine infection with CMV may result in mental retardation, learning disabilities, chorioretinitis, optic atrophy, hepatospenomegaly, small size for gestational age, and thrombocytopenia. Testing in adults is generally carried out by determining the antibody levels in serum. Culture is also available for confirmation purposes but is rarely useful. Testing in neonates is done first with a screening panel known by the acronym TORCH, which corresponds to the most common neonatal infections. See *TORCH panel*.

Patient preparation No preparation is required.

Procedure CMV is measured immunologically using ELISA or chemiluminescent methods.

Specimen Serum.

Reference range

IgG	Negative, titers less than 1:16.
IgM	Negative, titers less than 1:8.

Abnormal values

IgG	Positive, titers greater than1:16 (chronic infection).
IgM	Positive, titers greater than1:8 (acute infection).

Cost $35–$55.

Comments A positive IgG test means past infection. A positive IgM test suggests a current, active infection.

cytotoxic T lymphocyte See *CD8 cell* in Glossary.

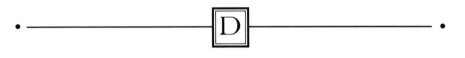

d-dimer   See *fibrin-fibrinogen degradation products.*

dehydroandrosterone   DHEA is an androgenic steroid which is secreted by both men and women. DHEA levels gradually increase during childhood and adolescence, rise rapidly after puberty, peak at age 20, and then decline.
   Patient preparation None required other than for obtaining urine or drawing blood.
   Procedure DHEA is measured by gas-liquid chromatography, radioimmunoassay, or gas chromatography-mass spectroscopy.
   Specimen 24-hour urine.
   Reference range
   Urine
      Adult male   0.1–2.0 mg/day.
      Adult female   0.1–1.5 mg/day.
      Child   Less than 0.1 mg/day.
   Serum
      Adult male   1.7–4.2 ng/mL.
      Adult female   2–5.2 ng/L.
      Pregnant female   0.5–12.5 mg/L.
   Abnormal values
      Increased in: hirsutism, polycystic ovarian syndrome, virilizing
         adrenal tumors.
      Decreased in: hyperlipidemia, psychosis, psoriasis.
   Cost $50–$100.
   Comments This test is reliable but gives equivocal results when the patient is on clomiphene, corticotropin, carbamazepine, and cephalothin.

dehydroandrosterone sulfate   DHEA-S is an androgenic steroid that is the major form of DHEA in the body and is secreted by both men and women. DHEA levels gradually increase during childhood and adolescence, rise rapidly after puberty, peak at age 20, and then decline. It has been suggested that this test should replace older tests of 17-ketosteroids in urine for estimation of adrenal C-19 steroid production.

Patient preparation No preparation is required.

Procedure DHEA-sulfate is measured by ELISA, chemiluminescence, or radioimmunoassay.

Specimen Serum.

Reference ranges

Child	0.6–2.54 µg/ml.
Adult male	2.0–3.4 µg/ml.
Adult female	
Premenopausal	0.8–3.4 µg/ml.
Postmenopausal	0.1–0.5 µg/ml.
Pregnant	0.5–12.5 µg/ml.

Abnormal values

Increased in: polycystic ovary (Stein-Leventhal) syndrome, females with hirsutism, adrenal cortex tumors, congenital adrenal hyperplasia. Decreased in: adrenal insufficiency.

Cost $75–$100.

Comments This test is reliable but gives equivocal results when the patient is on clomiphene or corticotropin.

delta-aminolevulinic acid Aminolevulinic acid is a precursor to porphyrins and normally converts to porphobilinogen through the action of the enzyme ALA-dehydrase during heme synthesis. Impaired conversion, as occurs in porphyrias and lead poisoning, causes urine ALA levels to rise before other chemical or hematologic changes occur. Measurement of ALA levels are therefore used in the diagnosis of porphyrias, hepatic, and lead poisoning.

Patient preparation See timed collection for instructions. Because certain drugs may interfere with this test, the laboratory must be notified if the patient is on any medication. A list of the interfering medications can be found in the comments section.

Procedure Delta aminolevulinic acid is measured spectrophotometrically.

Specimen A 24-hour urine specimen is collected in a light-resistant (brown) bottle containing a preservative (glacial acetic acid). Specimen must be kept refrigerated and sent to the laboratory as soon as the collection is completed.

Reference range 1.5–7.5 mg/dl/24 hours.

Cost $50–$75.

Comments Certain drugs may interfere with this test, including amiodarone, anticonvulsants, carbamazepine, phenobarbital, phenytoin, and valproic acid.

Demerol™ See *drug screening*.

dexamethasone suppression test (DST) Dexamethasone is a synthetic glucocorticoid with properties similar to those of cortisol. When given orally in low doses in normal individuals, it inhibits ACTH secretion, resulting in decreased levels of cortisol in the plasma and urine. The primary use of this test is to diagnose Cushing's syndrome, which is often due to an increase in cortisol in the circulation. Increased cortisol may in turn be due to a cortisol-secreting adrenal tumor or secondary to ectopic or paraneo-plastic ACTH secretion, which stimulates cortisol secretion. If cortisol is not reduced within the first two days after the test, an adrenal tumor is usually present. The dexamethasone suppression test has been used in the diagnosis of psychiatric diseases such as melancholia and to predict response to thera-py, although its use in this context is highly controversial.

Patient preparation Food and fluids except water and medications should be restricted for 12 hours prior to test.

Procedure In the short DST, 0.5 to 2.0 mg of dexamethasone is adminis-tered at 11 p.m., and a blood sample is collected at 8 to 9 a.m. the fol-lowing morning. In the long DST, a 24-hour urine sample is collected one day prior to the administration of dexamethasone. Dexamethasone is taken orally every six hours for two days, for each day of which a 24-hour urine specimen is collected, accompanied by blood samples taken at 8 a.m. and 4 p.m.

Specimen Both serum and urine samples are collected for this test.

Reference range
Short DST   8 a.m. plasma cortisol of 5–25 µg/dl.
Long DST   Serum cortisol 5–25 µg/dl.
Urinary free cortisol less than 20 µg/24 hours, or more than 50% reduc-tion from baseline level.

Abnormal values
Increased in: adrenal hyperplasia, adrenal tumors, ectopic ACTH, Cushing's syndrome.
Decreased in: adrenogenital syndrome, primary adrenocortical insufficiency.

Cost $30–$50 for blood measurements (each).
$30–$50 for urine measurements (each).

Comments Caffeine may cause false-positive results. Many drugs may inter-fere with test results.

differential count   See *"diff"* in Glossary.

digital rectal examination (rectal)   The insertion of a gloved index finger into the rectum by a physician or other examiner in order to palpate the prostate (to detect increased firmness) and the mucosa of the rectosigmoid colon (to identify rectal tumors).

Patient preparation No preparation is required.

Procedure The examiner places a lubricating gel on his or her gloved index finger and inserts it as far as possible into the rectum, rotating it to palpate the mucosa and underlying tissue, which in males includes the prostate.

Specimen Clinical findings.

Reference range No abnormalities identified.

Abnormal values It is used as a screening tool for identifying both lower rectosigmoid lesions and prostatic lesions (benign hypertrophy or, less commonly, adenocarcinoma).

Cost The digital rectal examination is part of a normal physical examination and is not billed as a separate procedure.

Comments Contrary to previously held beliefs, it is not necessary to have subjects return for a separate drawing of PSA specimens, as DRE does not significantly increase serum PSA levels during the immediate (i.e., 5–20 minutes) postexamination period. See *digital rectal examination*.

digital subtraction angiography (DSA) A radiographic technique that uses video equipment and computer-assisted enhancement of images obtained with conventional angiography. This technique provides a higher contrast image (at a sacrifice of decreased spatial resolution) of blood vessels than can be obtained with conventional angiography, uses less contrast, and reduces radiation exposure. It is used to study the circulation of the carotid, aortic arch, vertebral, and lower extremity. It is most useful in diagnosing cerebrovascular disease and can be used to study renal and peripheral vascular disease. Because this technique injects the dye intravenously rather than within the arteries, there is less risk and discomfort to the patient.

Patient preparation Food should be restricted for four hours; liquids are allowed.

Procedure The patient is placed in a supine position on an X-ray table. An initial series of images are taken and the injection site is cleansed. A local anesthetic is administered and a catheter is then inserted and advanced to the superior vena cava. Placement is verified by X ray, and the contrast medium (dye) together with saline are administered. After allowing time for the dye to disseminate, a second series of images are taken. The computer then digitizes the before and after images to yield an accurate picture of the dye-filled vessels. Duration of procedure is approximately 45 minutes.

Reference range Normal vasculature in areas studied.

Abnormal values Filling defects, narrowing (stenosis) of vessels, blockage (occlusion) of vessels.

Cost $1500–$2000.

Comments DSA gives a superior image of the vasculature. Movement of the patient or failure to remove radiopaque objects from X-ray field will interfere with interpretation. Risk factors include hypersensitivity to the radiocontrast medium, poor cardiac function, renal, hepatic, thyroid disease, or multiple myeloma. Because the contrast medium acts as a diuretic, the patient must increase his fluid intake for 24 hours after the procedure.

digitoxin Digitoxin is used in the same manner as digoxin but differs chemically in that digitoxin binds strongly to proteins and is therefore more slowly distributed to tissues. To achieve the same pharmacologic effect as that of digoxin, it is necessary to maintain a concentration tenfold greater than that of digoxin.

Patient preparation Same as for digoxin.
Procedure Digitoxin is measured by ELISA or RIA methods.
Specimen Serum.
Reference range 10–25 ng/ml.
Abnormal values Toxicity occurs at greater than 35 ng/ml.
Cost $45–$75.
Comments The test is reliable. Interferences are the same as for digoxin.

digoxin   Digoxin is the most widely used cardiac glycoside; it is primarily used to treat congestive heart failure and less commonly to treat atrial arrhythmias. Because cardiac arrhythmias may be induced by either too little or too much digoxin, it is common practice to measure digoxin levels and electrolytes. The specimen for digoxin levels should be drawn at least six hours after administration; otherwise, the levels will be falsely increased.

Patient preparation Because digoxin is eliminated slowly from the body, specimens are drawn six hours after the last dose of digoxin. For patients who have reached equilibrium, the specimens can be drawn anytime from six hours postadministration until prior to the next dose.
Procedure Digoxin levels are measured by a variety of methods including ELISA, EIA, RIA, and chemiluminescence.
Specimen Serum.
Reference range 0.5–2.0 ng/ml.
Abnormal values Toxicity occurs at greater than 2.0 ng/ml., panic values at greater than 3.0 ng/ml.
Cost $25–$45.
Comments Certain conditions such as renal or hepatic disease may alter test results. Incorrect timing of collection will alter interpretation of test results.

Dilantin™   See *phenytoin*.

dipstick (reagent strip)   A blotting paper impregnated with enzymes or chemicals sensitive to various parameters of clinical interest. When dipped in urine, the dipstick undergoes a color change, allowing a substance to be semiquantitatively measured, including bilirubin, glucose and reducing substances, hemoglobin, nitrates, ketones, pH, protein, hemoglobin, specific gravity, and urobilinogen. Reagent strip methodology was born in part out of the relatively low diagnostic yield of routine urinalysis. See *urinalysis*.

direct antiglobulin test (direct Coombs test)   A test used to detect autoimmune hemolytic anemias caused by antibody (immunoglobulin) and/or complement components bound to red blood cells, which occurs when immunoglobulins become sensitized to an antigen on the red blood cell's surface such as the Rh factor. Immune hemolysis may be linked to various drugs, hemolytic transfusion reaction, and hemolytic disease of the newborn (HDN). A positive Coombs test helps differentiate autoimmune and secondary immune hemolytic anemia, which can be drug-induced or associated with an underlying disease such as lymphoma.

Patient preparation Medications that may cause immune hemolytic anemia (e.g., cephalosporin, penicillin, fluoruracil, isoniazid, procainamide, quinidine, rifamipin, streptomycin, thiazides, and others) should be restricted.

Procedure Direct Coombs is a manual test in which agglutination reactions are observed.

Specimen One lavender-top tube (EDTA anticoagulated whole blood); one red-top tube (no anticoagulant).

Reference range Negative.

Abnormal values Transfusion reaction, hemolytic disease of the newborn, autoimmune hemolytic anemias.

Cost $15–$50.

Comments This test may be interfered with by hemolysis caused by rough handling. False-positive results may follow the use of many drugs (see physician for a more complete list). The test must be performed within 24 hours of obtaining sample. The direct Coombs test is performed in conjunction with the indirect Coombs test. See *indirect antiglobulin test.*

direct Coombs test   See *direct antiglobulin test.*

direct fluorescent antibody method   A technique in which a molecule of interest is detected directly, using an antibody labelled or tagged with a fluorochrome such as fluorescein-isothiocyanate; the direct test is most often used for detecting the presence of immune depositions in a histologic section (e.g., IgG or C3 complement deposits) in an epithelial basement membrane or in glomeruli. See *indirect immunofluorescence* in Glossary.

DNA hybridization   A technique for detecting the presence of a specific segment of "target" DNA.

Patient preparation None required other than obtaining blood or tissue samples.

Procedure A sample of cells is lysed (i.e., the cells' membranes are dissolved), the protein is destroyed by specific enzymes, and the DNA is extracted. The DNA, which normally exists as a double-stranded molecule, is separated (denatured) into two single strands. The single-stranded DNA is bound (immobilized) onto a blotting paper in a procedure called Southern blot hybridization, or onto tissue or cells in a procedure called in situ hybridization. In the final step a "probe" is added that is used to detect the presence of "target" DNA. The probe contains a short segment of DNA molecules that recognize and bind to the target DNA, and a "signal" molecule that allows the binding of the probe to the target. Signal molecules include radioactive phosphorus (32-phosphorus), which is recognized on an X-ray film in a procedure called autoradiography, and biotin, which is bound to enzymes that cause a color change if the probe binds to the target DNA.

Specimen Blood, tissue, cells.

Reference range No "target" DNA is detected.

Abnormal values Uses of DNA hybridization include rapid diagnosis of infection (e.g., in tissue) using in situ hybridization and detection of virus (e.g., CMV, EBV, HPV, herpes simplex virus, adenovirus, HIV-1); bacteria (e.g., enterotoxin-producing *Escherichia coli* and gonococcus); and neoplasia.

Cost $150–$500. See *HLA typing, in situ hybridization* in Glossary, *paternity testing, RFLP* in Glossary, *Southern blot* in Glossary.

do-it-yourself testing See *home testing*.

Doppler echocardiography A noninvasive imaging method for evaluating the flow of blood (hemodynamics) based on the Doppler shift principle: a change in pitch resulting from the relative motion between a source of ultrasonic waves and an observer or other collecting device. Doppler echocardiography is used to estimate transvalvular differences in pressure and calculate areas of heart valves, thereby duplicating the information provided by cardiac catheterization which it may eventually replace.

Patient preparation None required.

Procedure A transducer (a sending and receiving tube) is placed on the skin with a conductive gel, pointed toward the heart structures of interest, and an image is recorded. Doppler echocardiography is usually performed at the same time as a two-dimensional echocardiogram.

Specimen Data and images obtained.

Reference range No abnormalities in flow or reduction in valve diameters.

Abnormal values Doppler echocardiography is abnormal with alterations in the flow of blood related to valvular stenosis (narrowing) or regurgitation (backflow of blood).

Cost $200–$400.

drug screening A rapid method for identifying the presence of one or more drugs of abuse (cocaine, heroin, marijuana), usually in the urine, by one of several widely used "stat" methods including EMIT (enzyme-mediated immunologic technique) and thin-layer chromatography. The initial screening tests have become very reliable and easy to perform. When legal issues are involved, however, the processing of specimens becomes more complicated. Forensic drug screening requires that specimens be handled with very specific protocols, beginning at the time of collection. Forensic testing requires that positive results are confirmed by secondary methods which involve extensive chemical analysis. The agents screened are grouped according to their pharmacologic actions:

1. Sedative-hypnotic, e.g., benzodiazapines, methaqualone.
2. Depressant, e.g., barbituates, opiates (e.g., heroin).
3. Stimulant, e.g., amphetamines, cocaine.
4. Hallucinogens, e.g., cannabinoids (marijuana), phencyclidine (PCP).

Patient preparation Forensic drug screening requires that the specimen collection be observed by another party.

Procedure Specimen collection is extremely important in forensic testing and requires careful documentation of the chain-of-custody in the event the results are used in litigation. Each person handling the specimen documents his/her actions to ensure that the specimen remains intact and untampered.

Specimen Serum, urine, gastric fluid.

Reference range No drugs detected.

Abnormal values The detection of any drug in serum, urine, or gastric juice is abnormal. The sensitivity depends on the method used. Screening methods are less sensitive than confirmation methods.

Cost

Simple Screening	$15–$25.
Forensic	$25–$45 with additional $35–$45 if confirmation (for legal purposes) is required.

Comments

OPIATES Poppy seeds can cause false positives, but recent developments in gas chromatography-mass spectrophotometry (GC-MS) can distinguish between legal drugs and illegal opiates.

AMPHETAMINES Ephedrine and phenylpropanolamine will give positive results on screening. GC-MS will distinguish between the various drugs.

COCAINE Benzoylecgonine, the primary metabolite of cocaine, is detected by screening and GC-MS.

CANNABINOIDS (MARIJUANA) Screening procedures detect the metabolite Δ^9-tetrahydrocannabinol carboxylic acid (THC-CA) in urine. Some nonsteroidal anti-inflammatory drugs (NSAIDs) can give false-positive results with screening but GC-MS confirmation can distinguish between NSAID and THC-CA.

PHENCYCLIDINE This drug is easily detected by normal screening procedures. GC-MS is used for confirmation.

D-xylose absorption test This test is used in the differential diagnosis of malabsorption. D-xylose is a sugar not normally present in the diet which is absorbed undigested in the small intestine and passes through the liver without being metabolized. Because D-xylose is metabolically inert, blood and urine measurments of D-xylose levels reflect the absorptive capacity of the small intestine.

Patient preparation Food and liquid intake should be restricted for 12 hours (except water). Aspirin and indomethacin can interfere with test.

Procedure Fasting blood and first-voided urine are collected prior to the test. The patient is then given a 25g dose of D-xylose dissolved in 8 oz. of water, which is followed by an additional 8 oz. of water. Blood is collected two hours postingestion. All urine during the 5- or 24-hour period (depending on the test protocol) is collected. Bed rest and restriction of food and fluids (including water) are maintained throughout the test period.

Specimen Serum and urine.

Reference range

Blood	25–40 mg/dL in 2 hours.
Urine	Greater than 4 g in 5 hours.

Abnormal values

Decreased in: alcoholism, ascites, celiac disease, congestive heart failure, diabetic neuropathic diarrhea, enteritis, jejunal diverticuli (multiple), myxedema, rheumatoid arthritis, sprue, Whipple's disease.

Comments Complete collection and refrigeration of urine during collection are extremely important. Inaccurate timing of blood samples can distort results. Abdominal discomfort or diarrhea after D-xylose ingestion is common. High blood levels of D-xylose with low levels in the urine are typical of renal failure. Thus, the test should not be performed on patients with renal failure.

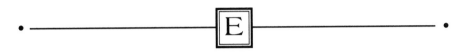

EBV See *Epstein-Barr virus*.

ECG See *electrocardiography*.

echocardiography A family of noninvasive, two-dimensional imaging techniques using Doppler ultrasonography to provide information on the size, shape, and motion of cardiac structures, pressure differences, and flow of blood through the heart and great vessels. The principle common to these methods is that blood flowing to (and through) the heart produces sound waves, some of which are reflected back (i.e., the Doppler effect) by each acoustic interface the blood encounters, which is received by a transducer. The time elapsed between the sound's transmission to the time that the echo is received is converted to a display. When a sound wave is directed at the heart at various angles, an echo reflects back from each point of contact with the heart. When a number of depth samples are taken in sequence, an imaging plane is created, allowing construction of a two-dimensional echocardiogram, which is a procedure of considerable use in evaluating pericardial and myocardial disease, ischemic and congenital heart diseases, and infectious endocarditis. Analysis of the images allows a three-dimensional image to be constructed of the heart, its valves, muscle, and even the blood as it passes through the heart. There is no radiation exposure.

Patient preparation No preparation is required.

Procedure A conductive gel is placed on the chest area of the supine patient. A transducer (an instrument that converts energy into sound and simultaneously receives sound and translates it back into energy that can be visualized) is rubbed over the heart area of the chest. The images are viewed and stored on a video recorder and an oscilliscope for evaluation.

Abnormal values Mitral valve stenosis or prolapse, aortic insufficiency, aortic stenosis, subaortic stenosis, tricuspid valve disease, pericardial effusion, congenital heart disease, enlargement of heart.

Cost $150–$300.

Comments Obese patients and patients with chronic obstructive lung disease may be difficult to examine.

echo planar imaging (MRI)   An imaging technique in which a complete planar image is obtained from one selected excitation pulse. See *MRI*.

edrophonium test   See *tensilon test.*

EEG   See *electroencephalography.*

EKG   See *electrocardiography.*

electrocardiography   The electrocardiogram (ECG, EKG) is a noninvasive test for evaluating the heart by recording the electric current passing through the heart on graph paper (electrocardiograph). The ECG is used to detect cardiac damage by evaluating alterations in flow (conduction) of electricity through the heart and can be performed while the patient is at rest or when performing specified exercises (e.g., thallium stress test). In an ECG, electrodes (leads) are placed on 12 specific sites of the body: the standard limb leads (I, II, III), the augmented limb leads (aV_R, aV_L, and aV_F), and precordial or chest leads (V_1 to V_6). The electrical activity produced by the heart's conduction system is transformed into recordings. ECG tracings consist of three major components: the P wave (atrial depolarization), the QRS complex (ventricular depolarization), and the T wave (ventricular repolarization). The ECG is used to detect the presence and location of ischemia or infarction (necrosis or death) of the myocardium (heart muscle), cardiac hypertrophy (enlargement), arrhythmias, and conduction defects. The Holter monitor is a portable ECG recording device worn by the patient for continuous monitoring of the heart's activity.
   Patient preparation No specific preparation is required.
   Procedure Electrodes are placed on the skin on various parts of the body. These electrodes cause no discomfort. The electrodes are connected to a recorder which is sensitive to the electrical conduction system of the heart. The recorder produces a graphical representation which is interpreted by a cardiologist.
   Reference range No abnormalities in waves or patterns.
   Abnormal values Myocardial infarction, arrhythmias, valve disease congenital heart disease.
   Cost $15–$100.
   Comments Although this test is performed whenever heart disease is suspected, it is advisable to have at least one ECG before the age of 40 in order to note any changes that may occur at a later date. As with all tests, the ECG is not infallable and is subject to false-negative and false-positive results. Additional testing should be carried out when clinical indications warrant.

electroencephalography   The electroencephalogram is a graphic recording of the minute electrical current produced by brain cell activity. This test is used to diagnose and manage seizure disorders. The measurements can be made while the patient is awake or asleep.

Patient preparation Because electrodes will be attached to the scalp, the patient must wash his/her hair just prior to the test in order to remove oils and chemicals. If the test is to be a sleep EEG, the patient must stay awake the night before or get very little sleep. If antiseizure medication has been prescribed, it should be taken unless the physician gives other instructions.

Procedure As many as 16–30 small electrodes are attached to the scalp with paste as the patient relaxes. The test is painless, but the patient must remain motionless. Electrical impulses from the brain are detected by the electrodes and sent to the EEG device which records the impulses (brain waves) on a continuously moving sheet of paper.

Reference range No local or general abnormalities in rhythm or waveforms are identified.

Abnormal values Seizure disorders (epilepsy), intracranial lesions, vascular lesions in brain, diminished consciousness.

Cost $50–$100.

Comments Excessive movement and drugs can interfere with accurate interpretation. Acute drug intoxication or severe hypothermia resulting in loss of consciousness causes a flat EEG.

electrolyte/fluid balance panel   A battery of laboratory tests used to detect and diagnose, in the most cost-efficient way possible, the most common imbalances of electrolytes and fluids. The panel includes measurement of sodium, potassium, chloride, pH, PCO_2, CO_2 content, osmolality in the plasma and urine, and BUN. See *organ panel* in Glossary.

electromyography (EMG)   Electromyography measures minute electrical discharges produced in skeletal muscle both at rest and during voluntary contraction and is used in the diagnosis of neuromuscular disease. The electrode for EMG is inserted through the skin, and the resulting electrical discharge or motor unit potential is recorded. Nerve conduction studies, which constitute a separate diagnostic protocol, can be performed simultaneously. Nerve conduction studies measure the speed at which nerves carry electrical signals and are often used to diagnose peripheral nerve disorders including carpal tunnel syndrome.

Patient preparation Smoking, coffee, tea, and colas are restricted for two to three hours prior to the test. Aspirin and related drugs should be discontinued five to seven days before the procedure. If a clotting problem is suspected, coagulation studies (e.g., platelet count, prothrombin time, and partial thromboplastin time) should be obtained. Needle insertion may cause discomfort.

Procedure Patient can be lying down or sitting in a chair. Needle electrodes are quickly inserted into the muscles to be tested. The muscle's electrical signal is recorded during rest and contraction. The resulting signal is

recorded on an oscilloscope. The procedure takes one to two hours.
Reference range No abnormalities at rest, with minimal muscle contraction, with full voluntary muscle contraction, or with the insertion of recording electrode needle.
Abnormal values Muscular dystrophies, glycogen storage diseases, amyotrophic lateral sclerosis, motor neuron disease, myotonia, inflammatory muscle disease, peripheral nerve disorders, endocrine myopathy, alcoholic myopathy, myasthenia gravis.

Muscle disease produces a spiked wave pattern, with the shape of the spike differing according to the disease. Weak muscles produce small waves or potentials. In myasthenia gravis, the waves disappear quickly. Nerve disease shows a decreased frequency of contractions.
Cost $400–$600.

embryoscopy An imaging technique in which an ultrasound-guided small-bore needle with an endoscope is inserted through the abdominal wall into the uterus (without violating the amniotic cavity) to view a living embryo. Embryoscopy is a new procedure that allows the early detection of major defects of the embryo (early fetus). It is performed by few obstetricians and is not performed outside major medical centers. The indications for using this technique are being developed. Unlike fetoscopy, which can only be performed in the second and third trimesters of pregnancy and carries a significant risk of fetal wastage, embryoscopy can be performed as early as six weeks after fertilization, appears to be safer, and is more informative than ultrasonography. Embryoscopy is in early stages of development, but is likely to replace fetoscopy as both a diagnostic tool (e.g., to identify gross physical defects) and therapeutic tool for performing fetal surgery and delivering gene therapy. See *fetoscopy*.

EMG See *electromyography*.

endobronchial biopsy A diagnostic procedure in which an endoscope is passed through the nose or mouth in the usual manner to visually examine the mucosa of the upper airways (oropharynx, trachea, bronchi, and upper bronchioles) and identify any physical abnormalities or lesions. If lesions are identified, an instrument, e.g., alligator forceps, cup forceps, or curette, is passed through the central channel of the endoscope and a biopsy is obtained. See *transbronchial (lung) biopsy*.
Patient preparation Informed consent is required. The patient should not consume food or liquids after midnight for a morning procedure. Routine medications can be continued. Lab work is done to exclude a clotting disorder. Testing of pulmonary function by spirometry or by measuring blood gases is performed to evaluate lung reserve and identify bronchial spasms. Premedication (narcotics or mild tranquilizers) is injected before the procedure, and atropine is given to reduce spasms, unless the patient has arrhythmias, urinary retention, or glaucoma.

Procedure A fiberoptic bronchoscope is passed through the mouth or nose, and tissue samples are removed with forceps.

Specimen Tissue from the trachea or bronchi.

Reference range No abnormalities are identified by light microscopy.

Abnormal values Benign tumors, idiopathic pulmonary fibrosis, infection, e.g., *Pneumocystics carinii* pneumonia, tuberculosis, inflammatory changes, malignant tumors, sarcoidosis.

Cost $2000–$3000.

Comments Complications include bleeding and bronchospasm.

endoscopy The visualization of the mucosal surface of the gastrointestinal tract, upper respiratory tract (oropharynx, trachea, bronchi, and upper bronchioles) and other regions of the body using an endoscope. The endoscope is a semi-rigid or flexible device that is inserted into the region of interest. It has a light source, an optical system for viewing the mucosa, a camera, and a channel that allows the insertion of sampling devices (e.g., alligator forceps, cup forceps, or curette) for obtaining biopsies or surgical instruments to perform certain types of simple (minor) surgery. The procedure is tolerated well with minimal discomfort.

Patient preparation Informed consent is required. If clotting problems are suspected, basic coagulation studies (e.g., platelet count, prothrombin time, and partial thromboplastin time) are ordered as well as a CBC to detect anemia. Fasting after midnight before the test is usually advised. For lower gastrointestinal endoscopy (colonoscopy), a cleansing enema is required to flush out stools and debris. For anxious patients, a mild sedative may be administered.

Procedure An endoscope is inserted in the appropriate body site. Photographs may be taken of any abnormalities seen. If appropriate, a biopsy is taken.

Specimen Biopsy, photographs.

Reference range No abnormalities are identified.

Abnormal values Abnormalities seen include inflammation, masses (tumors), and other anatomic changes.

Cost $700–$900.

eosinophil count The eosinophil count is generally part of the CBC (complete blood count), which is ordered separately when certain conditions, particularly allergies, are suspected. Formerly, eosinophil counts were performed manually, but now more accurate results are obtained by automated cell counters.

Patient preparation No preparation is required.

Procedure Eosinophils are counted on an automated hematology analyzer.

Specimen Whole blood (EDTA anticoagulant).

Reference range 0.3%–3.5%

Abnormal values

Increased in: allergic disorders, parasitic infections, skin disease, neoplasms.

Cost $25-$50. Usually part of a complete blood count.

epinephrine See *catecholamines.*

Epstein-Barr virus (EBV, human herpes virus-4, HHV-4) EBV virus is a DNA virus that causes infectious mononucleosis and belongs to the herpes virus family that now has eight members. EBV was first found in a Ugandan child with Burkitt's lymphoma and has since been linked to hairy leukoplakia, carcinoma of the nasopharynx, lymphomas, AIDS, and possibly also to T-cell lymphomas and Hodgkin's disease. As with hepatitis, there are several serological markers used to determine first if there is infection with EBV and also the stage of the infection.

Patient preparation No preparation is required.

Procedure Exposure to Epstein-Barr virus is measured by enzyme immunoassay.

Specimen Serum.

Reference range Patients who have not been exposed to the virus are negative for both IgG and IgM antibodies.

Abnormal values Early antigen antibody is found early in the infection and usually disappears. Viral capsid antibody-IgG is elevated during infection and remains positive; it increases dramatically during reinfection. Viral capsid antibody-IgM is elevated during infection and disappears and becomes positive with reinfection. Nuclear antibody-IgG is elevated during infection and remains positive. Nuclear antibody-IgM is elevated for four to six weeks; it becomes negative postinfection and is positive during reinfection. Epstein-Barr virus causes infectious mononucleosis and has been associated with nasopharyngeal carcinoma, Burkitt's lymphoma, and lymphomas in immunocompromised hosts, including AIDS patients.

Cost $25–$50 for a single test. $75–$100 for the complete panel.

equilibrium radionuclide angiocardiography (ERNA) A technique in which an objective signal such as the EKG is used to "gate" or physiologically control the otherwise static imaging of the cardiac blood pool. ERNA is of use in evaluating the right and left ventricles in terms of volumes as well as systolic and diastolic function and regional or global myocardial performance (e.g., myocardial infarction).

Patient preparation Any blood for tests that will be performed by radioimmunoassay must be drawn before performing the procedure.

Procedure The patient is injected with a radionuclide, e.g., technetium-99m. Multiple images of the heart are obtained, synchronized with the RR interval of the electrocardiograph. This is known as ECG-gating. The images are input into a computer that produces a moving display of the size and movements of the heart chambers and the volume of blood being passed through (the ejection fraction).

Specimen Data and images.

Reference range Normal size and motion of the heart's ventricles, with an ejection fraction of greater than 50% for the left ventricle and greater than 45% for the right ventricle.

Abnormal values Equilibrium radionuclide angiography is used to detect functional abnormalities of the heart in response to physiological stress (i.e., exercise and increased work). It is abnormal in coronary artery disease, heart failure, cardiomyopathies, and cardiotoxic drugs.

Cost $700–$1000. See *first-pass radionuclide ventriculography*.

erythrocyte count See *complete blood count, red cell count*.

erythocyte sedimentation rate (ESR, sed rate) A simple laboratory test that measures the rate at which red blood cells in well-mixed venous blood settle to the bottom of a special test tube. This serves as a nonspecific indicator of inflammation and should be performed within a few hours of obtaining the specimen. Although it is routinely ordered by many physicians, it is non-specific, and inflammation is better monitored by serial measurement of C-reactive protein. ESR is commonly used in the clinical management of patients with various rheumatic diseases, as their therapy may require frequent adjustment of medication levels.

Patient preparation No preparation is required.

Procedure This is a manual procedure in which the time required for the red blood cells to settle a specific distance is visually estimated.

Specimen Whole blood, lavender-top tube.

Reference range

Male	Older than 50 years	0–15 mm/hour.
	Younger than 50 years	0–29 mm/hour.
Female	Older than 50 years	0–25 mm/hour.
	Younger than 50 years	0–30 mm/hour.

Abnormal values

Increased in: anemia, collagen vascular disease, hyperproteinemia, neoplasia, pregnancy

Decreased in: polycythemia, microcytosis, sickle cell anemia

Cost $10–$15.

Comments Anemia and paraproteinemia invalidate the results. The test must be performed within 12 hours for valid results.

erythrocyte survival See *red cell survival (study)*.

erythropoietin Erythropoietin is a glycoprotein growth factor produced predominantly in the kidney in response to signals from an oxygen-sensitive substance, e.g., heme. It binds to receptors in erythroid precursors that mature into red blood cells. It plays an important role in regulating oxygen metabolism. It is severely decreased in end stage renal disease. Recent use of cloning technology has led to the production of synthetic hormones which are being used therapeutically in renal disease.

Patient preparation No preparation is required.

Procedure Erythropoietin is measured by RIA or ELISA methods.
Specimen Serum.
Reference range Greater than 48 IU/L.
Abnormal values

Increased in: renal transplants, ectopic production by tumors (e.g., cerebellar hemangioblastoma hepatoma, pheochromocytoma, uterine leiomyoma, renal cell carcinoma).

Decreased in: chronic inflammation, polycythemia vera, renal disease, secondary anemia, malignancy.

Cost $75–$100.

Comments Commercial kits have become available, and the costs will decrease as availability and demand increase.

esophageal acid perfusion   See *Bernstein test.*

ESR   See *erythrocyte sedimentation rate.*

estradiol   See *estrogen.*

estriol   See *estrogen.*

estrogen   Estrogens are steroid hormones produced and secreted by the ovaries and are responsible for the development of secondary female sexual characteristics and for normal menstruation. They are secreted by the follicular cells of the ovaries during the first half of the menstrual cycle, by the corpus luteum during the second or luteal phase of the cycle, and during pregnancy in response to follicle-stimulating hormone (FSH) and luteinizing hormone (LH). Slowly rising or sustained high levels of estrogens inhibit the secretion of FSH and LH. A rapid rise in estrogen occurs immediately before ovulation and appears to stimulate LH secretion. The main estrogens measured in the laboratory are estradiol, estrone, and estriol. Estradiol is used to diagnose and treat infertility. Estriol is used to analyze fetal health. See *alphafetoprotein.*

Patient preparation No preparation is required. It is important to note the phase of the menstrual cycle in which the specimen is obtained.

Procedure Estrogens are measured by RIA, ELISA, or chemiluminescence.

Specimen

Estradiol	Serum.
Estrone	Serum.
Estriol	Serum, plasma, urine.

Reference range

	ESTRADIOL TOTAL (pg/ml)	ESTRONE TOTAL (µg/L)	ESTRIOL TOTAL (urine/24 hours)
Male			
Prepuberty	2–20	*	<10 µg
Adult	10–36	*	15–40 µg

	ESTRADIOL TOTAL (pg/ml)	ESTRONE TOTAL (µg/L)	ESTRIOL TOTAL (urine/24 hours)
Female			
Prepuberty	0–100	*	<10 µg
Adult	20–300	*	15–80 µg
(not pregnant)			
Follicular phase	10–90	*	**
Midcycle	100–500	*	**
Luteal phase	50–250	*	**
Postmenopausal	10–30	*	<20 µg
Adult (pregnant)			
Less than 8 weeks	8–12	<0.5 µg/L	**
25 weeks	40–160	3.5–10 µg/L	**
Term	125–300	5–40 µg/L	**

* Estriol total is not routinely measured in males and non-pregnant women.
** Estrogens are not usually requested in these cases.

Abnormal values

Increased in: estrogen-producing tumors, precocious puberty, cirrhosis, congenital adrenal hyperplasia.

Decreased in: primary hypogonadism, Turner's syndrome, ovarian agenesis.

Cost $45–$75.

estrogen receptor   A protein in the cell nucleus that is regulated by binding to small ligands, e.g., steroid hormones, thyroid hormones, vitamin D, and retinoids. The estrogen receptor (ER) is found in high concentrations in the cytoplasm of breast, uterus, hypothalamus, and anterior hypophysis cells. Receptors are transcription factors, and extracellular estradiol diffuses across the cell membrane, binding to the estrogen receptor. The ER levels are measured by oncologists to determine a breast cancer patient's potential for response to hormonal manipulation (60% of breast cancers are "estrogen positive"). Hormonal therapy is generally less toxic than conventional chemotherapy. In breast cancer, one-half of ER-positive patients respond favorably to antiestrogen (tamoxifen citrate) therapy, in contrast to less than one-third of ER-negative patients. Tumors that are both estrogen and progesterone receptor positive respond better to hormonal therapy than those with one or no receptors. Estrogen and progesterone receptor assays help determine the prognosis and the type of therapy which will be most effective.

Patient preparation   Since these specimens are obtained at the time of surgery, preparation is that required for performing surgery.

Procedure   Estrogen receptors are currently measured histologically by specific stains and are interpreted by the pathologist.

Specimen   Specimens are tissue samples obtained either at biopsy or during surgery.

Reference range   Several assay methods are available, and each must be interpreted according to the reference range of the laboratory performing the assay. The estrogen receptor levels may be quantified by biochemical means (ER levels 10 fmol/mg of protein are positive) and semiquantified by immunocytochemical, immunohistochemical methods, gel electrophoresis, and protamine sulfate precipitation.

Cost $100–$150.

Comments It is extremely important that the surgeon request ERA and PRA analysis. The biochemical method has largely been abandoned despite the seeming advantage of quantifying the ER levels because it is difficult to transport the tissue in liquid nitrogen to the laboratory performing the test; a large amount of tissue is required, and the tissue itself must be completely malignant.

ethanol See *alcohol.*

ethyl alcohol See *alcohol.*

euglobulin clot lysis time (fibrinolysis time) A test of in vivo fibrinolysis in which diluted and acidified plasma is cooled, causing the precipitation of fibrinogen, plasminogen, plasmin, and plasminogen activator. The test is used to evaluate the time from the formation of a blood clot to its dissolution.

Patient preparation No preparation is required.

Procedure This is a manual test in which the time from the formation of a blood clot to its dissolution is visually measured.

Specimen Blood collected by venipuncture in a blue-top tube.

Reference range Normal time 140 minutes or more.

Abnormal values

   Increased in: disseminated intravascular coagulation.

   Decreased in: primary fibrinolysis.

Cost $100–$150.

excisional biopsy Any surgical procedure intended to completely remove (excise) a lesion that is being submitted for pathological evaluation. In excisional biopsies, the nature of the lesion (i.e., benign vs. malignant) is often unknown at the time of the operation, and thus the amount of normal tissue being obtained is based on clinical judgement. See *biopsy.*

exercise tolerance test (treadmill exercise test) This is the most commonly used clinical test for accurately assessing a person's risk of death from cardiovascular events. In it, the patient performs an exercise test while being monitored by electrocardiography.

exfoliative cytology The analysis of cytologic material from "accessible" organs (i.e., uterine cervix, urinary bladder, breast and nipple discharges, GI tract, respiratory tract) which is obtained noninvasively (i.e., by scraping) from hollow or tubular organs. See *aspiration cytology.*

extractable nuclear antigens (ENA) A group of antibodies that react against the Sm antigen, a nonhistone nucleoprotein devoid of nucleic acid (after Smith, a patient with the antigen), and ribonucleoprotein (RNP), an antibody now known as anti-U1 small nuclear RNP; anti-Sm antibodies are relatively specific for lupus erythematosus. RNP are common in mixed connective tissue disease, demonstrating a "speckled" pattern of immunofluorescence.

Patient preparation No preparation is required.

Procedure ENA are measured by ELISA methodologies.

Reference range Negative.

Abnormal values ENAs are present in mixed connective tissue disease, scleroderma, Sjögren's syndrome, and systemic lupus erythematosus.

Cost $35–$50.

extrinsic factor See *vitamin B₁₂*.

F

factor I   See *coagulation studies.*

factor II   See *coagulation studies.*

factor V   See *coagulation studies.*

factor VII   See *coagulation studies.*

factor VIII   See *coagulation studies.*

factor VIII-related antigen   See *von Willebrand factor.*

factor IX   See *coagulation studies.*

factor X   See *coagulation studies.*

factor XI   See *coagulation studies.*

factor XII   See *coagulation studies.*

factor XIII   See *coagulation studies.*

fasting blood sugar   See *glucose.*

FDP   See *fibrin-fibrinogen degradation products.*

febrile agglutinins   Febrile agglutinins are used to detect antibodies to specific bacterial antigens such as *Salmonella* H, *Salmonella* O, *Salmonella* A, B, C, D, and E; *Proteus* antigens, OX-19, OS-K, and OX-2; *Brucella* antigen, and *Francisella tularensis* antigen. The test identifies agglutinins in the sera of patients with persistent fever who are suspected of having a bacterial infection.

   Patient preparation No preparation is required.

Procedure Febrile agglutinins are measured by latex agglutination assays.
Specimen Serum. Titers on a single specimen have no clinical utility; specimens should be taken during the acute phase and convalescent phase of an infection.
Reference range Less than a fourfold increase in titer in paired sera.
Abnormal values Greater than a fourfold increase in titer in the paired sera suggests infection and must be followed by specific diagnostic testing to determine the cause of the abnormal values.
Cost $25–$50.
Comments There are many cross reactions that make interpretation difficult. The test is considered obsolete, as more specific serological tests are now available.

ferritin Ferritin is the major iron storage protein found in reticuloendothelial cells which is normally present in small amounts in serum. In healthy adults, serum ferritin levels are directly related to the amount of available iron stored in the body. When all available sites on the ferritin molecule are filled, ferritin is 23% iron by weight and is the only test needed to diagnose iron-deficiency anemia. It is a recent analyte which can be measured quite accurately. Although it is usually used in conjunction with iron and iron binding studies, it is a more accurate test and can be utilized to screen for iron deficiency.
Patient preparation No preparation is required.
Procedure Ferritin is measured by ELISA, EIA, chemiluminescence, and RIA.
Specimen Serum.
Reference range

Males	33–236 ng/ml.
Females	
Under age 40	11–122 ng/ml.
Over age 40	12–263 ng/ml.

Abnormal values
Decreased in: hypochromic, microcytic anemias, iron-deficiency anemia.
Increased in: iron overload, hemochromatosis, inflammation, malignancy.
Cost $25–$45.
Comments Elevated ferritin levels may be associated with increased risk of myocardial infarction. In infants receiving iron therapy, ferritin measurements are unreliable. A bone marrow aspiration and biopsy may be required in the face of low-normal ferritin and low serum iron in the anemia of chronic disease, or low-normal ferritin in the presence of liver disease.

fetal hemoglobin An "immature" hemoglobin (Hb), composed of two α and two γ chains, that usually disappears in the neonatal period. Normally, the finding of red blood cells with fetal hemoglobin in the maternal circulation implies fetal-maternal hemorrhage, which is measured by the Kleihauer-

Betke test (a test that determines the number of RBCs with fetal Hb, a value of importance if the infant is Rh-postive and the mother is Rh-negative and requires Rh immune globulin to prevent sensitization against the fetal red blood cell antigens).

Patient preparation No preparation is required.

Procedure Fetal hemoglobin is measured by electrophoretic methods.

Reference range Less than 2% in normal adults.

Abnormal values Fetal hemoglobin is increased in thalassemia and hereditary persistence of fetal hemoglobin.

Cost $45–$65.

fetal monitoring   A test of the fetus' physiologic status which usually takes place in a hospital. There are two types of fetal monitoring, indirect and direct. In indirect fetal monitoring, electrodes are placed on the abdominal skin over the uterus to detect the fetal heartbeat and uterine contractions. Direct fetal monitoring involves the placing of an electrode directly on the fetus while it is in the uterus; this is done after the membranes around the fetus have ruptured. Formerly limited to high-risk pregnancies, fetal monitoring has become a common procedure that has been linked to a decrease in labor-related death and disability. A consequence of fetal monitoring is that there is an increased possibility the obstetrician will perform a cesarean section.

Patient preparation For external monitoring, there is no preparation. The patient may be asked to eat a meal prior to the test to increase the activity of the fetus. The patient must be still during the procedure. For direct monitoring, the patient is prepared for a vaginal examination. The patient may experience mild discomfort when the uterine catheter and scalp electrode are inserted.

Procedure External: An electronic transducer and a cardiotachometer are placed on the abdomen above the fetus to monitor fetal vital signs and uterine contractions. Direct: A catheter with an electrode attached is introduced into the cervix, pressed firmly against the fetal scalp, and rotated to insert the electrode into the scalp. Measurements are then recorded on various instruments, and the results are analyzed by the physician.

Reference range Fetal heart rhythm (FHR) ranges from 120–160 beats/minute with a variability of 5–25 beats/minute from the baseline.

Abnormal values The purpose of this test is to monitor fetal heart rate, measure frequency and pressure of uterine contractions, and to evaluate fetal health. Abnormalities in the FHR can be the result of many conditions and must be evaluated by a physician.

Cost $400–$600.

fetoscopy   An imaging technique in which an ultrasound-guided, 3 mm in diameter needle with an endoscope is inserted through the abdominal wall into the uterus to view a living fetus. Fetoscopy can be performed in the second and third trimesters of pregnancy and carries a significant risk of fetal wastage that can be caused by the rupture of fetal membranes. See *embryoscopy*.

fiberoptic bronchoscopy See *bronchoscopy, bronchial brushings, bronchial washings*.

fibrin-fibrinogen degradation products (FDPs, fibrin splits) Fibrinogen degradation products are polypeptide fragments that are generated by enzymes when the body tries to dissolve blood clots in the form of thrombosis. Unchecked primary fibrinolysis occurs in intravascular lesions associated with pathological fibrinolysis or various extravascular conditions. An excessive amount of FDPs is usually due to disseminated intravascular coagulation (DIC).
   Patient preparation No preparation is required.
   Procedure FDP are measured using automated coagulation instruments.
   Specimen Plasma in a special tube containing thrombin and an antifibrinolytic agent. Tube must be filled properly for accurate results.
   Reference range Less than or equal to 10 µg/ml.
   Abnormal values
      Increased in: intravascular lesions, deep vein thrombosis,
         disseminated intravascular coagulation, pulmonary
         thromboembolism, extravascular conditions, allograft rejection,
         glomerular disease, hematomas, liver disease, neoplasia,
         obstetric complications (e.g., abruptio placentae, eclampsia,
         retained dead fetus), sepsis, severe liver disease.
   Cost $25–$50.

fibrin split products See *fibrin-fibrinogen degradation products*.

fibrinogen (coagulation factor I) An insoluble glycoprotein present in the plasma that is necessary for normal platelet function and wound healing; it is converted into fibrin in the common pathway of coagulation. Fibrin in turn provides the physical scaffolding for the permanent hemostatic plug. Each of the three constituent chains of the fibrinogen molecule is encoded by three closely linked genes located on long arm of chromosome 4. The fibrinogen dimer is assembled in the endoplasmic reticulum of liver cells, where much is retained and degraded. Fibrinogen is one of the so-called acute phase reactants which may be markedly increased in various types of nonspecific stimuli, e.g., inflammation.
   Patient preparation No preparation is required.
   Procedure Fibrinogen is measured on an automated coagulation instrument.
   Reference range 165–410 mg/dL.
   Abnormal values
      Increased in: Hyperfibrinogenemia.
      Decreased in: Afibrinogenemia.
   Cost $45–$65.

fibrinolysis time   See *euglobulin clot lysis time.*

fine needle aspiration (FNA)   A method of diagnostic cytology and pathology using a thin or skinny (from 18- to 23-gauge) needle to obtain cells and minute tissue fragments for examination by light microscopy. The sites selected for FNAs are often guided by radiologists with fluoroscopy, computed tomography, or MRI.

fine needle aspiration biopsy (FNAB)   A minute sample of tissue which is obtained by FNA; lesions identified in children include thyroglossal duct cyst, sialadenitis, lymphangioma, granulomatous lymphadenitis, lymphomas, neuroblastoma, Wilms' tumor, sarcomas, eosinophilic granuloma, and others. In adults, virtually any lump or bump (especially of internal organs that cannot be readily biopsied by an open procedure, e.g., liver, periaortic lesions) can be "FNABed" to obtain diagnostic material. The FNAB may be performed in concert with radiologists who can help the pathologist guide the needle to the exact location of the lesion using various imaging modalities, including fluoroscopy, CT, and MRI.

fine needle biopsy   See *biopsy.*

first-pass radionuclide angiocardiography   A technique used in cardiology to obtain images of the heart during the transit of a radiopharmaceutical (e.g., ^{99m}Tc pertechnate) through the central circulation. The high-velocity components of the radiopharmaceutical's passage through the heart are recorded in a brief timespan and analyzed quantitatively. The method requires a digital gamma camera able to rapidly and accurately capture images. Because the information is recorded in eight to ten heartbeats (cardiac cycles), the presence of arrhythmias or premature beats invalidates the study. FPRA may be performed prior to equilibrium studies and is regarded by some physicians as being the method of choice in evaluating right ventricular function and ventricular ejection fraction. FPRA is more complicated and performed less frequently than equilibrium radionuclide angiography (ERNA); it is more accurate than EKG-gated ejection fraction studies. See *equilibrium radionuclide angiocardiography.*

first-pass radionuclide ventriculography   A technique in which there is a brief sampling of radionuclide data as the labeled bolus passes through the heart; it is assumed that the mixing of the radioactive label (usually ^{99m}Tc) with the blood is virtually complete, and the changes in the count rates are directly proportional to volumetric changes. Because all of the data is acquired in eight to ten cardiac cycles, the presence of rhythmic abnormalities would invalidate the data. This technique is used to evaluate the right and left ventricles in terms of volumes, systolic and diastolic function, and regional or global myocardial performance (e.g., myocardial infarction).

flexible bronchoscopy See *bronchoscopy, bronchial brushings, bronchial washings.*

flexible fiberoptic sigmoidoscopy See *sigmoidoscopy.*

fluorescein angiography A technique used to diagnose chorioretinal disease based on the enhancement of anatomic and vascular details in the retina after intravenous injection of fluorescein. Fluorescein angiography is an integral tool in evaluating retinal disease because it can precisely delineate abnormal areas; it clearly demonstrates certain defects (e.g., choroidal neovascularization, proliferative diabetic retinopathy, and light toxicity) and thus is useful in planning laser therapy for vascular lesions of the retina.
Patient preparation The patient's pupils are dilated with a mydriatic agent.
Procedure Once the fluorescein, a dye, passes into the choroidal and retinal circulation, the pattern of its distribution can be viewed and photographed with a fundus camera as a function of its intrinsic fluorescence.
Specimen Photographs of retina.
Reference range Normal flow of blood through retinal blood vessels.
Abnormal values Defects seen include changes of diabetes (proliferative diabetic retinopathy), new blood vessel formation, and photo damage.
Cost $400–$600.

fluorescent in situ hybridization See *FISH* in Glossary.

fluorescent treponemal antibody absorption test (FTA-ABS) A highly sensitive 96%–97% serological test for the diagnosis of congenital, secondary, and tertiary neurosyphilis. FTA is used to confirm the presence of *Treponema pallidum,* the causative agent in syphilis, when the RPR screening test is positive.
Patient preparation No preparation is required.
Procedure After reacting the patient's serum with sensitized cells, a fluorescent dye which reacts with the complex formed is viewed through a fluorescent microscope.
Specimen Serum, cerebrospinal fluid (CSF).
Reference range Negative.
Abnormal values Syphilis, neurosyphilis (CSF positive).
Cost $10–$25.
Comments In most states, a positive FTA-ABS test must be reported to the local department of health. There are, however, many conditions which may cause false positives. Approximately 2% of the general population have a false-positive reaction.

foam stability index (foam stability test, shake test) A semiquantitative bedside test for determining fetal lung maturity. The index is based on the stability of bubbles when amniotic fluid is shaken in test tubes with increasing concentrations (42%–58%) of ethanol which reduces the foaming or bubbling action of phosphatidyl choline. Each tube is shaken vigorously; the higher the concentration of alcohol in which the bubbles are maintained, the more mature the lungs.

Patient preparation See *amniocentesis* for preparation.

Procedure A sample of amniotic fluid is shaken vigorously, and the formation of bubbles is observed.

Reference range Formation of a complete ring of bubbles is a positive result and indicates pulmonary maturity.

Abnormal values Negative results indicate a high risk of respiratory distress syndrome.

Cost Test is done as part of the amniocentesis and carries no additional charge.

folic acid   Folic acid is a general term for a water-soluble vitamin that cannot be synthesized by mammals. Folic acid is part of a normal diet and is present in raw fruits and vegetables, kidney and liver, and can be destroyed by extensive cooking. Folic acid deficiency, like that of vitamin B_{12}, causes megaloblastic anemia, which is characterized by low numbers of enlarged RBCs.

Patient preparation No preparation is required.

Procedure Folic acid is measured using ELISA, RIA or chemiluminescence.

Specimen Whole blood (EDTA), serum. Serum folate is not stable; therefore, the serum must be separated and frozen as soon as possible after drawing the specimen.

Reference range

Red blood cell folate	125–600 ng/ml.
Serum folate	Greater than 2 ng/ml.

Abnormal values

    Decreased in: alcoholism, malabsorption, certain anticonvulsant medications.

Cost $10–$15.

Comments Folic acid analysis is normally part of an anemia panel including vitamin B_{12} and ferritin and is used primarily to determine the type and cause of anemia.

follicle-stimulating hormone (FSH)   A hormone secreted by the pituitary gland that stimulates development of the follicle during the menstrual cycle. Its measurement is usually used to determine the cause of infertility, gonadal failure, and menstrual disturbances. Levels vary with age and time of the menstrual cycle.

Patient preparation No preparation is required.

Procedure FSH is measured by ELISA, chemiluminescence, or RIA.

Specimen Serum.

Reference range

Prepuberty children	Less than 22 mIU/L.
Males	Less than 22 mIU/L.
Females	
Nonmidcycle	Less than 20 mIU/L.

| Midcycle | Less than 40 mIU/L. |
| Postmenopausal | 40–160 mIU/L. |

Abnormal values
  Increased in: hypogonadism, anorchidism, gonadal failure,
    menopause, Klinefelter's syndrome, alcoholism, castration.
  Decreased in: pituitary (hypophysis) failure, hypothalamic failure.
Cost $25–$50.
Comments Since FSH levels are quite variable, single determinations have little value, and serial determinations yield more reliable information. FSH is usually measured in conjunction with LH (luteinizing hormone) and prolactin.

free catecholamine test (urinary free catecholamine test)   This laboratory test measures the concentrations of the free (i.e., unbound, nonmetabolized) catecholamines, epinephrine and norepinephrine, that are excreted in the urine in a 24-hour period. In normal individuals, the free catecholamines represent 2%–4% of the total catecholamine production.
  Patient preparation No preparation is required, other than for obtaining a 24-hour urine specimen.
  Procedure Free catecholamines are measured by fluorometry.
  Specimen 24-hour urine.
  Reference range Less than 100 µg/24 hours, of which 80 µg is norepinephrine and 20 µg is epinephrine.
  Abnormal values Increased epinephrine and/or norepinephrine may be seen in neuroendocrine tumors, including pheochromocytoma and neuroblastoma.
  Cost $20–$30. See *total catecholamine test.*

free T4 (free thyroxine index, FT₄I, T7 assay, T12 assay)   Free T4 is the amount of thyroxine not bound to thyroid-binding globulin. It has been measured as an index but there is now a direct measurement available which gives more accurate results than the calculation.
  Patient preparation No preparation is required.
  Procedure Free T4 is measured by ELISA, chemiluminescence, or RIA.
  Specimen Serum.
  Reference range 0.9–2.3 ng/dL.
  Abnormal values
    Increased in: hyperthyroidism, factitious hyperthyroidism,
      false increases occur with heparin therapy.
    Decreased in: hypothyroidism, false decreases occur with phenytoin
      and valproic acid therapy.
  Cost $45–$65.

frozen section   A rapid diagnostic procedure performed on tissue obtained intraoperatively where the tissue is frozen in a synthetic material, sectioned with a cryostat, stained with hematoxylin and eosin, and viewed with a light microscope, allowing a rapid diagnosis of a pathologic tissue. The technique provides the surgeon with information necessary to guide therapy and to determine the extent of further surgery at the time of surgical procedure; the information obtained from a "frozen" includes (1) differentiating between benign and malignant, (2) determining the type of malignancy, e.g., lymphoma versus carcinoma, (3) evaluating tissue margins for involvement by malignancy, e.g., basal cell carcinomas, (4) determining the adequacy of tissue for further studies after the patient is closed, and (5) determining the type of tissue, e.g., differentiating lymphoid tissue from parathyroid gland. "Quick sections" shorten the turnaround time for a diagnosis from one to three days to 15 minutes, but the disadvantage is that the tissue is suboptimal because it contains freezing artefact and is thus more difficult to interpret than paraffin-embedded tissue. In nonpalpable mammographically identified lesions of the breast, FS diagnosis has a sensitivity of 92% and specificity of greater than 99%.

FTA-ABS See *fluorescent treponemal antibody absorption*.

fundoscopy (fundoscopic examination)   The fundus is the back part of the eyeball. It is examined with an ophthalmoscope. This is an instrument equipped with a lens and a light which allows the physician to readily see the major parts of the eye when the pupil is dilated. This examination is a standard part of an eye exam. Physicians may also examine the fundus when there are indications of diabetes, hypertension, or atherosclerosis. The fundoscopic examination, when carried out by an experienced physician, can detect early signs of hypertension, diabetes, and other diseases.

galactose Galactose is a sugar (aldohexose) present in milk, sugar beets, and seaweed; it is a constituent of lactose, gangliosides, and mucoproteins. Galactosemia is an inherited condition caused by a deficiency of various enzymes. Clinical findings include cataracts, mental retardation, hepatosplenomegaly, cirrhosis, and Fanconi syndrome. Laboratory findings include hypergalactosemia, albuminuria, aminoaciduria, galactosuria, proteinuria, and tyrosyluria.

gallium scan A radioscintillation imaging method in which ^{67}Gallium citrate ($T_{1/2}$, 25 days) is injected intravenously, and images of its pattern of distribution are obtained. Once injected the gallium binds primarily to transferrin and to any tissue that also concentrates lactoferrin. The gallium scan was formerly used to localize abscesses, osteomyelitis, and other infections; it is currently used for staging of lymphomas, lung carcinoma, hepatoma, melanoma, metastases (to bone, brain, lung), head and neck, and gastrointestinal and genitourinary neoplasia.

Patient preparation Patient is given a high-fiber diet. Just prior to the test, the patient is given a laxative or cleansing enema.

Procedure The gallium-67 is given intravenously. The patient is then asked to return at various times. A laxative may be given to help remove unnecessary radioactivity from the bowel. A special camera is used to record images over the abdomen, chest, or other areas where infection is suspected.

Reference range Gallium activity is normally demonstrated in the liver, spleen, bones, and large bowel.

Abnormal values Inflammatory lesions and malignancy.

Cost $500–$700.

gamma glutamyl transferase (GGT) An enzyme that is very sensitive to biliary obstruction and catalyzes the transfer of a γ-glutamyl group from glutathione or γ-glutamyl peptide to another peptide or amino acid. GGT is located on the cell membrane and microsomal fractions and is involved in amino acid transport across cell membranes. It is most abundant in the liver but is also present in the kidney and pancreas. It is used in the diagnosis of liver disease and is especially sensitive to alcohol intake.

Patient preparation No special preparation is required.

Procedure Gamma glutamyl is measured by a spectrophotometer.

Specimen Serum.

Reference range

Males	15–85 units/L.
Females	5–55 units/L.

Abnormal values

Increased in: hepatoma, pancreatic carcinoma, carcinoma metastatic to liver, chronic alcoholism, cirrhosis, hepatitis.

Cost $15–$25; it may be part of a general chemistry panel.

Comments Although elevated in alcoholism, some heavy drinkers do not have increased levels. It is more sensitive than other liver enzymes but gives better information when used in conjunction with the other liver enzymes AST, ALT, ALP, and bilirubin.

gastric analysis Gastric analysis involves the insertion of a tube into the stomach to obtain gastric fluid which is then analyzed to determine its acidity. Gastric fluid contains water, electrolytes, hydrochloric acid, mucin, pepsin, gastrin, and intrinsic factor (necessary to absorb vitamin B_{12}). Because of new technology using gastroscopes, gastric analysis is no longer frequently performed.

gastrin Gastrin is a hormone secreted in the stomach and pancreas. It aids digestion by stimulating gastric acid production, and secretion of pepsin and intrinsic factor.

Patient preparation No preparation is required.

Procedure Gastrin is measured by radioimmunoassay.

Specimen Serum.

Reference range

Fasting	Up to 100 pg/ml.
Postprandial	95–140 pg/ml.

Abnormal values

Increased in: achlorhydria, duodenal ulcer, extensive stomach cancer, gastrinoma, Zollinger-Ellison syndrome.

Cost $45–$75. See *secretin injection test*.

Comments If gastrin is not markedly elevated and gastrinoma is suspected, secretin stimulation can be used to verify suspicions. Many gastric conditions cause mild elevations of gastrin and must be ruled out.

gene amplification The increase in copy numbers of a gene, an event associated with cellular oncogenes in malignancy, where the copy number is a crude indicator of tumor aggressiveness.

general health screen A battery of tests performed on serum that is considered to be the most cost-effective means of determining a person's basic state of health; the screen includes albumin, alkaline phosphatase, AST (GOT), BUN/creatinine, calcium, total bilirubin, cholesterol, glucose, K⁺, LDH, total protein, Na⁺, triglycerides, and uric acid. See *executive profile* in Glossary, *organ panel* in Glossary.

germ tube test   The germ tube is a short projection on a germinating spore of *Candida albicans* that appears after three hours of incubation at 37°C on an appropriate culture medium. It is a rapid bench test that allows a presumptive diagnosis of *C. albicans*.

GGT See *gamma glutamyl transferase.*

Giardia lamblia   The most common protozoan parasite affecting the human small intestine.
   Patient preparation Specimens are obtained with either a warm saline or Fleet phosphosoda enema.
   Procedure The stool specimen is examined microscopically.
   Specimen Stool.
   Reference range Negative.
   Abnormal Values Histologic changes induced by *G. lamblia* infection in the small intestine range from near-normal to villus atrophy and/or crypt elongation with a variable inflammatory response. See *parasite identification.*
   Cost $50–$75.

glomerular filtration rate   See *creatinine clearance.*

glucagon   A polypeptide hormone produced by the pancreatic islet α cells that opposes the action of insulin; activates hepatic phosphorylase; decreases gastric motility, secretion, and muscle mass; and increases ketogenesis and hepatic incorporation of amino acids and urinary excretion of sodium and potassium. It is found in very high levels in glucagonoma, a tumor of the pancreas.
   Patient preparation No special preparation is necessary.
   Procedure Glucagon is measured by RIA methods.
   Specimen Plasma. The specimen is drawn into a chilled lavender-top tube and delivered to the laboratory immediately. If this is not possible the plasma should be separated and frozen immediately.
   Reference range Less than or equal to 60 pg/ml.
   Abnormal values
      Increased in: acute pancreatitis, diabetic ketoacidosis, giant cell bronchiogenic carcinoma, glucagonoma, hepatic cirrhosis, hypoglycemia, stress, uremia.
      Decreased in: chronic pancreatitis, cystic fibrosis.
   Cost $50–$75.
   Comments The glucagon suppression test is essentially the same as a glu-

cose tolerance test except the analyte measured is glucagon. In a normal test, glucagon secretion is suppressed. In a patient with glucagonoma, there is no suppression of glucagon secretion.

glucose   Glucose is the principal sugar in the body, the metabolism of which provides most of the body's energy. Glucose is largely present in the form of two sugars (formally known as disaccharides) linked to each other by specific chemical bonds. Sucrose is formed from glucose and fructose, lactose from glucose and galactose, maltose from two glucoses and is the complex polysaccharide starch. Disaccharides are broken down into monosaccharide by the enzymes lactase, maltase, and sucrase that are specific for each disaccharide. Starch is broken down by amylase secreted by the pancreas and salivary glands. Several hormones are involved in the regulation of glucose metabolism; the most well-studied is insulin, which is secreted by the pancreas. Although glucose is an essential source of energy needed to maintain proper body functions, it must be carefully regulated. Excess glucose (hyperglycemia), a pivotal finding in diabetes mellitus, can cause irreparable harm. On the other hand, decreased glucose (hypoglycemia) will cause metabolic shutdown because of a lack of energy. Glucose is one of the most commonly measured analytes and is generally part of any chemistry screening panel. A fasting glucose (i.e., no solid food for 12 hours prior to the taking of the specimen) is used as the initial screening test. An abnormal fasting level is then followed by some type of glucose tolerance test.

Patient preparation The patient must fast for 12 hours prior to the drawing of the specimen.

Procedure Glucose is measured spectrophotometrically on automated chemistry instruments.

Specimen Plasma drawn in a gray-top tube (oxalate/fluoride anticoagulant) is the preferred specimen. This anticoagulant stops glucose metabolism and therefore stabilizes glucose levels. Serum can be used but metabolism can occur causing falsely decreased levels if not analyzed within a short time.

Reference range

Premature infants	40–65 mg/dL.
0–2 years	60–110 mg/dL.
2 years to adult	62–115 mg/dL.

(Normal range increases over age 50)

Abnormal values

Increased in: coma, diabetes mellitus, hyperthyroidism, obesity.

Decreased in: galactosemia, hypopituitarism, insulinoma.

Cost $5–$10 when performed as a single test.

Comments An elevated result should be repeated or followed by a postprandial glucose (a specimen taken within a specified time of a normal meal). If these tests are abnormal a glucose tolerance test is recommended.

glucose-6-phosphate dehydrogenase   Glucose-6-phosphate dehydrogenase

(G-6-PD) is an NADP$^+$ enzyme that catalyzes a reaction of the pentose phosphate pathway of RBC metabolism, which helps RBCs resist oxidant stress. Deficiency of this enzyme causes hemolysis (bursting of the RBCs and release of hemoglobin into the plasma). The common form of this enzyme is called the B variant and is present in 99% of Caucasians in the United States. The A variant differs from the B variant by a single amino acid. Approximately 20% of black females and 16% of black males have the B variant. G-6-PD deficiency is caused by a defect on the X chromosome.

Patient preparation No special preparation is required.

Procedure Both the qualitative and quantitative methods are measured spectrophotometrically. This is a manual method.

Specimen Whole blood drawn in lavender-, green-, or yellow-top tubes.

Reference range 8.2–8.4 IU/g hemoglobin.

Abnormal values Hereditary G-6-PD deficiency. Mutations responsible for the deficient state can be identified by use of molecular biologic techniques.

Cost $25–$50.

glucose tolerance test (GTT)   The glucose tolerance test is a standardized test that measures the body's response to an oral (challenge) dose of glucose. It is primarily used to support or exclude the diagnosis of diabetes mellitus. The GTT may be performed in individuals with symptoms (e.g., increased fasting glucose level, hypertriglycerdemia, neuropathy, impotence, glycosuria) that are suggestive of diabetes mellitus. In pregnancy, GTT is used to diagnose gestational diabetes. In the most commonly used GTT, 100 g of glucose is ingested by a fasting individual, which stimulates insulin secretion; the peak glucose levels in normal subjects are reached within one hour; in diabetics, the peak is reached after two to three hours and the peak glucose level is much higher.

Patient preparation It is important for the patient to eat an adequate, well-balanced diet for three days prior to the test. The patient must abstain from smoking, eating and drinking (except water) for 12 hours prior to the test.

Procedure Glucose is the analyte being measured. It is measured spectrophotometrically on automated chemistry instruments.

Specimen Plasma (gray-top, sodium fluoride tube). Baseline (fasting) blood and urine specimens are obtained, after which a glucose-rich drink is administered. The volume of the "cola" administered is dependent on the patient's age: children receive 1.75 g/kg body weight up to 75g, and the usual adult dose is 75 g. For presumed gestational diabetes the dose is 100 g, which follows a gestational diabetes screening test of 50 g glucose. After ingesting the "cola," blood and urine specimens are drawn at 30, 60, 90, and 120 minutes. In the gestational diabetes screening test, a single blood specimen is drawn at 60 minutes postingestion. It is imperative that the times of specimen drawing be clearly marked on the tubes so the laboratory can properly process the specimens, and a reliable interpretation of the glucose tolerance curve can be made.

Reference range

Fasting	60–115 mg/dL.
One hour	Less than 184 mg/dL.
Two hours	Less than 138 mg/dL.
Gestational screen	Less than 140 mg/dL.

Cost $30–$50.

Comments If the test is being done in a laboratory's patient service center, the glucose in the urine is measured by a dipstick before administering the concentrated glucose drink. If the dipstick is positive, the patient's physician is contacted for instructions. Patients with known diabetes mellitus or fasting glucose of greater than 140 mg/dL on two consecutive occasions should not undergo the GTT. Because of the cola's high glucose concentration, emesis (vomiting) is occasionally a problem. The test should be delayed for 24 hours before attempting the readminister the test.

glycosylated hemoglobin (glycated hemoglobin, hemoglobin A1c, HbA_{1c}) A general term for any of four distinct fractions of hemoglobin A (HbA_{1a1}, HbA_{1a2}, HbA_{1b}, HbA_{1c}) to which D-glucose binds irreversibly in the red blood cell. Because this complex extends over the life of the RBC, its concentration in the blood reflects the amount of glucose in the circulation. Therefore, the concentration of HbA_{1c} (the most commonly measured of the fractions) is used to determine long-term glucose control in diabetes, especially in insulin-dependent diabetics whose glucose levels are labile.

Patient preparation No special preparation is necessary.

Procedure The most common method is liquid chromatography. Differential spectrophotometric methods have been introduced and are now widely used because they can be performed on automated chemistry instruments.

Specimen Whole blood (lavender- or gray-top tube).

Reference range

Non-diabetics	4%–7%
Well-controlled diabetes	Less than 9%

Cost $25–$35.

Comments As a rule, HbA_{1c} is not measured more often than at four- to six-week intervals. Elevated hemoglobin F can interfere with some methods for measuring HbA_{1c}. This should be evaluated if an unexpectedly elevated result is obtained.

gonorrhea Gonorrhea is a sexually transmitted disease caused by the bacterium *Neisseria gonorrhoeae* which commonly affects the genitourinary tract in the form of pelvic inflammatory disease, salpingitis, and urethral involvement. Hematogenous spread may result in arthritis and inflammation of the liver or heart. Because of the dangers associated with untreated *N. gonorrhoeae* infections, it is imperative that the laboratory use the proper methods for detection. The standard for detecting *N. gonorrhoeae* is culturing the organism in the laboratory, using a swab of the infected site (e.g., vaginal, cervical, throat, anal, or urethral) as the specimen. The main problem with cultures is the organism's viability. If the specimen is not cultured within a short time or is exposed to adverse conditions, the culture may be false negative. Enzyme-linked immunoassays have been used but are not reliable when specimens are obtained from sources other than the vagina, cervix, or urethra. DNA probes are the method of choice today but still must be performed from a swab. In the near future, PCR amplification techniques will be available. These testing modalities will allow the use of urine as the specimen, making screening of males and females much easier.

Patient Preparation No special preparation is required.

Procedure A special swab provided by the laboratory is used to obtain the specimen from the affected site. The swab is then placed in a transport tube containing a solution which promotes the stability and growth of the organism. Testing is carried out by culture, ELISA procedures, or DNA probe procedures. PCR amplification methods are not widely available at this time.

Specimen Swab.

Reference range Negative.

Abnormal values Infection by *N. gonorrhoeae*.

Cost

Culture	$25–$35.
ELISA	$25–$35.
DNA Probe	$35–$50.

Comments Although culture is considered the most specific of the methods, improper transportation of the specimen will cause the bacteria to die, thereby yielding false-negative results. ELISA and DNA probe procedures are not dependent on the presence of live organisms.

growth hormone (hGH, GH, Somatotropin) Human growth hormone is produced in the pituitary gland (anterior hypophysis) and is secreted in episodic bursts, most prominently during early sleep. Growth hormone's most conspicuous effects occur during growth phases of infancy and early childhood. Measurement of hGH is usually carried out to detect deficiencies in growing children. Growth hormone deficiencies can lead to dwarfism in children, while an excess of growth hormone can lead to gigantism in children and acromegaly in adults.

Patient preparation Patient should observe an overnight fast and have complete rest for 30 minutes prior to the test.

Specimen Serum. The specimen should be separated, and the serum frozen prior to transportation to the laboratory.

Reference range

Children	Less than 20 ng/ml.
Adult, male	Less than 5 ng/ml.
Adult, female	Less than 10 ng/ml.

Abnormal values

Increased in: gigantism in children, acromegaly in adults, hypoglycemia, vigorous exercise.

Decreased in: dwarfism in children.

Cost $50–$75.

Comments Synthetic GH is now available for treating GH deficiency. It has also been used illicitly by athletes to promote growth of muscle tissue.

guaiac test   See *occult blood testing.*

Guthrie screening test   A test formerly used to detect increased levels of phenylalanine, which inhibits the growth of *Bacillus subtilis* at serum levels above 4.0 mg/dL, which are levels seen in phenylketonuria, a disease that causes mental retardation in children. Phenylalanine in now measured by a fluorometric ninhydrin method. See *phenylalanine.*

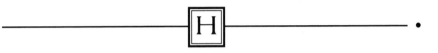

Hageman factor   See *fibrinogen*.

hair analysis   The use of scalp hair as primary analytical specimen. Hair can be analyzed to detect chronic poisoning by heavy metals (e.g., arsenic, lead, and mercury) or to determine the adequacy of zinc in the diet, using flame photometry. Samples of hair may be used to detect chronic drug abuse, which has certain advantages as it is nonintrusive, clean, difficult to cheat on, and provides a long-term "record" of drug ingestion.

Patient preparation None required. The hair must be clean for analysis.

Procedure Once removed, the hair can be analyzed by GC/MS (gas chromatography-mass spectroscopy), EIA (enzyme immunoassay), or RIA (radioimmunoassay).

Specimen Hair.

Reference range Negative for heavy metals. Negative for drugs of abuse.

Abnormal values Amphetamines, cocaine, and heroin can be detected; the limits of detection are 10 pg/mg to 10 ng of hair.

Cost $50–$200.

Comments Differences in drug levels determined by the testing are based on race (Asians absorb the most, Caucasians the least), hair color (dark hair absorbs more), and environmental contamination (e.g., passive absorption of cocaine may occur in children of drug-abusing parents). Hair analysis is believed by some providers of alternative health care to be of use in evaluating a person's health and nutritional status by measuring protein and vitamin levels. Given the variability of the interlaboratory and intralaboratory results, this form of hair analysis is believed by mainstream medical practitioners to be in the domain of quackery.

Ham test (acidified serum test)   A test used to determine the susceptibility of red blood cells to hemolysis (rupture), which is markedly increased in paroxysmal nocturnal hemoglobinuria (PNH). In acidified serum, complement is activated by the alternate pathway, binds to red blood cells, and lyses the PNH cells which are very sensitive to complement activation. A positive

Ham test also occurs in the rare condition congenital dyserythropoietic anemia type II, also known as HEMPAS.

Patient Preparation No special preparation is required.

Specimen Whole blood (EDTA anticoagulant).

Reference range No hemolysis.

Abnormal values Hemolytic anemia, paroxysmal nocturnal hemoglobinuria (PNH), congenital dyserythropoietic anemia type II.

Cost $25–$50.

Comments False positives can occur in other hematologic diseases. A recent transfusion will obscure the results.

haptoglobin   A protein in the circulation that migrates in the α_2 portion of serum subjected to electrophoresis. Haptoglobin is an acute phase reactant that increases in the serum in response to acute inflammation or infection, stress, or necrosis (death of tissue). Its major role is to bind hemoglobin released from red blood cells that undergo natural cell death, preventing the accumulation of hemoglobin in the plasma. After the iron has been removed, the haptoglobin-bound hemoglobin is eliminated by the reticuloendothelial (monocyte-phagocytic) system.

Patient Preparation No special preparation is required.

Specimen Serum.

Reference range 40–180 mg/dL.

Abnormal values

    Decreased in: megaloblastic anemia, infectious mononucleosis, hematoma, congenital (primarily blacks and Asians).

    Increased in: acute infection, inflammation, malignancy.

Cost $25–$50.

hCG   See *human chorionic gonadotropin.*

HCT   See *hematocrit.*

HDL   See *high-density lipoprotein(s).*

HDL-cholesterol   The cholesterol that is bound to high-density lipoprotein. Increased HDL-C and HDL-C:total cholesterol ratios are associated with increased longevity and decreased morbidity and mortality from myocardial infarction.

Patient preparation Patient should fast for 12 hours prior to drawing the specimen.

Procedure In the most common methodology, HDL-C is separated from the other forms of cholesterol by differential precipitation or solubility. The cholesterol remaining in solution is then measured spectrophotometrically on automated chemistry analyzers. The classical method of differential ultracentrifugation is very time consuming, costly, and rarely used method impractical in the clinical laboratory.

Abnormal values
   Male 15–65 years   Less than 35 mg/dL is a coronary risk factor.
   Female 15–65 years Less than 40 mg/dL is a coronary risk factor.
Cost $15–$30.

HDL/LDL ratio   The ratio of cholesterol carried by high-density lipoprotein to that carried by low-density lipoprotein, which allows a rapid risk stratification for atherosclerosis-related cardiac disease; the HDL/LDL ratio is decreased by saturated fatty acid.

hearing (function) test (pure tone audiometry)   Sound is heard in two ways: by its intensity (loudness) and by its tone. Both are measured in hearing tests, as are ability to hear sound through air (air conduction) and bone (bone conduction). Hearing is evaluated with an audiometer, an instrument that emits precise sounds of various tones and intensities; the patient's range of hearing (measured in cycles per second) at upper and lower limits of tones and intensities is recorded. The human ear can detect sounds in the range of 16–16,000 cps; many animals can hear tones above 50,000 cps, well beyond the range of human hearing. Intensity is measured in decibels. A whisper is in the range of 20 db. Usual home or office background noise is in the range of 60 db. Loud rock and roll music is usually above 120 db. Constant exposure to sounds louder than 85 db can cause hearing loss. Air and bone conduction studies are used to determine problems with the eardrum, middle ear, and ear-nerve disease. In these studies, the patient listens through earphones connected to the audiometer. For air conduction studies, various sounds are used. In bone conduction studies, an attachment from the earphones is applied to the bone behind the ear.

Helicobacter pylori   A gently curved bacillus, *H. pylori*, is held responsible for most cases of gastritis and is present in 10%–50% of healthy young persons and up to 60% of those 60 years or older. 90% of patients with stomach cancer have been infected by *H. pylori*. *H. pylori* may be spread by intrafamilial contacts and is increasingly implicated in duodenal ulcers which may respond to antibiotics. *H. pylori* has also been linked to the development of gastric and duodenal ulcers, hypertrophic gastropathy, gastric adenocarcinoma, and more recently to gastric non-Hodgkin's lymphoma.
   Patient preparation No special preparation is necessary.
   Procedure Antibodies to *H. pylori* are measured by ELISA procedures. To confirm the presence of *H. Pylori*, some physicians carry out an endoscopic biopsy for pathological examination. However this practice is decreasing as the serological tests become more specific and sensitive.
   Reference range Negative.
   Abnormal values No *H. Pylori* are seen in stomach biopsies of normal individuals.
   Cost $800–$1000.

helper:suppressor ratio   The ratio of CD4 helper T cells (T lymphocytes) to CD8 suppressor T cells, normally 1.5–2.0. In AIDS this ratio is the single best monitor of the patient's clinical status, where less than 0.5 is commonly seen, and values of 0.1 or less presage fulminant clinical deterioration. The helper to suppressor ratio is most commonly determined by flow cytometry. See *T and B cells.*

hematocrit   Hematocrit is defined as the percentage of whole blood that corresponds to red blood cells (erythrocytes). There are two basic methods for this determination. The automated method is more commonly performed and is a calculated hematocrit rather than a direct measurement. It is determined by the formula MCV **x** red blood cell number, where MCV is the average volume of red blood cells. The second method for determining the hematocrit is the manual (or direct) method. In the manual method the blood is centrifuged to separate the cells and plasma, and the percentage of red blood cells is determined visually. The manual method is used when the amount of blood is insufficient for automated determination (e.g., pediatric or elderly patients).

Patient preparation No special preparation is required, other than for drawing blood.

Procedure The hematocrit is determined by spinning (centrifuging) the blood and measuring the percentage of red blood cells.

Specimen The specimen for the automated methods is whole blood drawn in lavender-top containers (EDTA anticoagulant). The specimen for the manual method is usually obtained from a fingerstick and collected in a heparin-treated glass capillary tube.

Reference range

Children age 2	35%–44%
Children age 6	31%–43%
Female adult	35%–47%
Male adult	42%–52%

Abnormal values

Increased in: polycythemia.

Decreased in: anemia, hemolytic anemia, blood loss.

Cost $25–$50. Usually part of a CBC.

Comments The manual method generally yields results 2%–3% higher than the automated methods.

hemizona assay   This test evaluates the ability of sperm to bind to or penetrate human egg zona, which is compared to a known fertile donor; the hemizona assay provides an alternative to the sperm penetration assay (SPA). The assay may be performed in addition to the SPA and like the SPA, may correlate with the results of in vitro fertilization and indicate a male factor in infertility. See *sperm penetration assay.*

hemoglobin   Hemoglobin is a protein that is the major constituent of red blood cells. The primary role of hemoglobin is to transport oxygen as well as buffer the carbon dioxide produced by respiration. There are several forms of hemoglobin. Hemoglobin F is formed in the fetus and is the major hemoglobin until birth. At birth up to 30% of the hemoglobin is hemoglobin A. In adults, hemoglobin is primarily hemoglobin A with small amounts of hemoglobins F and A_2. Hemoglobin defects are inherited and termed hemoglobinopathies. Altered hemoglobins often do not have the same oxygen-carrying capacity as hemoglobin A. In individuals with partial defects (traits) of hemoglobin, hemoglobin exists in both the normal and the altered state, and those with the trait often do not exhibit overt symptoms. Hemoglobin variants are detected by hemoglobin electrophoresis. The most common hemoglobinopathies and their hemoglobins are:

Sickle cell	Hgb S
Sickle/C disease	Hgb S, Hgb C
Hemoglobin C disease	Hgb C
Thalassemia major	Hgb F
Thalassemia minor	Hgb A2

Patient preparation No special preparation is necessary.

Procedure Hemoglobin is measured spectrophotometrically on automated hematology analyzers.

Specimen Blood collected in a lavender-top container (EDTA anticoagulant).

Reference range

Birth	15.3–18.9 g/dL.
Infant	11.3–12.5 g/dL.
Female adult	12.7–14.7 g/dL.
Male adult	14.4–16.6 g/dL.

Abnormal values

Increased in: polycythemia.

Decreased in: anemia, hemolytic anemia, blood loss.

Cost $25–$50. Usually part of a CBC.

Comments Hyperlipidemia can cause falsely elevated results.

hemoglobin electrophoresis A method used in most laboratories to screen for hemoglobinopathies. Red blood cells are lysed, releasing the hemoglobin from the cells; a small portion of the lysate is applied to a separation medium, either cellulose acetate sheets or agarose gels. The hemoglobins are separated by applying an electric current to the gel. The major hemoglobins are isolated and identified by using buffers of varying pH. Newer techniques include isoelectric focusing, capillary electrophoresis, and high-pressure liquid chromatography. The latter techniques are used mainly when unusual (e.g., unstable) hemoglobins are suspected.

Patient preparation No special preparation is necessary, other than for drawing blood.

Procedure Hemoglobin is obtained from broken-down red blood cells, placed in an acid or alkaline solution, and subjected to an electric current; this causes the hemoglobins to move to specific locations on an agar gel, which is used to detect broad types of hemoglobin.

Specimen Whole blood collected in a lavender-top tube (EDTA anticoagulant).

Reference range See *hemoglobin.*

Cost $45–$75, depending on the presence of an unusual hemoglobin.

hemoglobin S test See *sickle cell test.*

hepatitis See Glossary.

hepatitis A virus (HAV)   An acute, rarely fatal disease of global distribution caused by a picornavirus; hepatitis A is a common cause of morbidity in many countries. Approximately 30% of the U.S. population has evidence of previous infection. Hepatitis A virus is most often transmitted by the oral-fecal route and is often caused by the consumption of contaminated food. This can include shellfish or food prepared by infected virus carriers who do not follow appropriate sanitary practices such as hand washing. The clinical findings include fever, nonspecific gastrointestinal malaise, hepatosplenomegaly, jaundice, and itching. The disease duration is four to six weeks and is followed by full recovery. Antibody formation provides protection against repeated infection. The laboratory findings include increased transaminases and darkened urine due to increased bilirubin. Two virus-specific antibodies can be detected: the IgM antibody against HAV and the IgG antibody against HAV. The IgM antibody can be detected within a few days of onset and usually disappears within six weeks. It is commonly known as the acute-phase antibody. The IgG antibody is usually detected five to six weeks post onset and is positive for life. Given the usual (oral-fecal) route of transmission, certain groups are at high risk, including travelers, military personnel, institutionalized persons, children in day care centers, other children and adolescents, Native Americans, raw shellfish eaters, and those engaging in high-risk sexual practices.

Patient preparation No special preparation is required.

Procedure Hepatitis markers are measured by ELISA.

Specimen Serum is the preferred specimen; heparinized plasma may be used.

Reference range Negative for both IgG and IgM antibodies.

Abnormal values Presence of either IgG or IgM anti-hepatitis A antibodies.

Cost $45–$65.

Comments In general, the laboratory measures total antibody against HAV. If this test is positive, IgM hepatitis A antibodies are measured in order to determine if the positive test is due to active or past infection.

hepatitis B virus (HBV)   Hepatitis B virus is a small, highly contagious DNA virus that is transferred from person to person by the exchange of body fluids (e.g., blood, semen). HBV was a major health hazard of blood transfusions prior to the availability of specific serologic tests, which are highly sensitive and now performed on all donated blood. HBV remains a public health hazard because it is also a sexually transmitted disease. The symptoms of HBV infection are quite varied and range from minor aches and pains to death. There are several stages of the disease: acute, convalescent, and chronic. The stages are determined by the presence of various viral antigens and antibodies to viral antigens in the blood.

Patient preparation No special preparation is required.

Procedure Hepatitis markers are measured by ELISA.

Specimen Serum is the preferred specimen. False positives may occur with heparinized plasma.

Reference range Negative for all markers; in vaccinated individuals, antiHBsAb is positive.

Abnormal values Positive results denote acute or past exposure to the virus.

Cost The cost varies with the tests requested; in general, tests are not performed as individual tests, but as panels tailored to the needs of the patient.

Comments Newer tests (e.g., polymerase chain reaction) may be used in special cases and can detect minute amounts of viral DNA. These tests are not FDA approved but can be very helpful in cases where HCV infection is suspected but the test results yield questionable results.

hepatitis C virus (HCV)   Hepatitis C virus is another virus that primarily infects the liver and is believed to play a role in causing liver cancer. As with hepatitis B, HCV is transmitted through body fluids such as blood and semen and can be transmitted vertically (from mother to infant). HCV was formerly linked to non-A, non-B hepatitis because no specific test was available and its presence was deduced by negative results for hepatitis A and B. Testing for HCV has been available for less than 10 years. Current screening tests detect antibodies formed against the virus, but should be verified or confirmed with the so-called RIBA test because false-positive results are relatively common. Polymerase chain reaction (PCR) tests have been developed for this virus and are used primarily to follow the course of interferon therapy. There are some instances where hepatitis C infection is suspected and the screening test is positive. In these cases, the PCR methodology can yield important information.

Patient preparation No special preparation is required.

Procedure Hepatitis markers are measured by ELISA.

Specimen Serum.

Reference range Negative for all tests.

Abnormal values A positive result denotes current or past infection.

Cost The screening test is usually performed as part of a hepatitis diagnostic panel and costs vary depending on the contents of the panel. RIBA costs $50–$75; PCR is currently performed only in specialized laboratories and costs $125–$150.

hepatitis D virus (hepatitis delta, delta agent, HDV)   The HDV virus is an incomplete RNA virus that was once thought to require helper activity from HBV. HDV is no longer considered a defective virus, because it can reproduce in absence of HBV coinfection, although production of hepatic disease may require HBV synergy. Patients with HDV are usually positive for HBsAg, HBcAb and HBe. HDV is often associated with fulminant hepatitis and cirrhosis (cirrhosis develops in 60%–70% of HDV-infected patients) and is endemic in many parts of the world.

Patient preparation No special preparation is required.
Procedure Hepatitis markers are measured by ELISA.
Specimen Serum.
Reference range Negative.
Abnormal values A positive result denotes active infection.
Cost $35–$50.
Comments Most laboratories will not perform the testing for HDV if the patient tests negative for hepatitis B antigen.

herpes virus A family of DNA viruses with prolonged dormancy lasting up to years; seven (and possibly eight) human herpesviruses (HHV) have been identified.

Patient preparation No special preparation is required.
Procedure Herpesvirus is detected by culture. Antibodies to herpesvirus are detected by immunoassay.
Specimen Serum is the specimen of choice for immunoassays. Cultures are usually performed from swabs taken from infected sites and require the appropriate transport medium to maintain viral viability.
Reference range Negative.
Cost
    ELISA $25–$100 depending on the number of tests required.
    Culture $50–$100.

heroin See *drug screening*.

hexosaminidase A family of four enzymes involved in the metabolism of gangliosides (water-soluble glycolipids most prevalent in the brain). Hexosaminidase A deficiency is linked to Tay-Sachs disease, an autosomal recessive condition that affects Ashkenazi Jews. Tay-Sachs disease is characterized by an accumulation of gangliosides in the lysosomes of the brain, which results in hypotonia, increased sensitivity to sound (hyperacusis), mental retardation, and death by age two to three. Because of the high prevalence (more than 1 in 30) among Ashkenazis of the gene that encodes defective hexosaminidase A, testing for the enzyme prior to marriage is virtually mandatory and has resulted in the disappearance of Tay-Sachs disease. A deficiency of hexosaminidase A and B results in Sandhoff's disease, a condition that is clinically identical to Tay-Sachs disease, but is panethnic, i.e., affects all ethnic groups equally.

Patient preparation No special preparation is required.

Procedure Hexosaminidase is measured spectrophotometrically.
Specimen Serum from red-top tube.
Reference range See the laboratory report.
Abnormal values Absence of hexosaminidase A suggests Tay-Sachs disease. Absence of hexosaminidase A and B suggests Sandhoff's disease.
Cost $75–$125.

Hgb See *hemoglobin.*

HGSIL See *high-grade squamous intraepithelial lesion* in Glossary.

5-HIAA See *5-hydroxyindole acetic acid.*

high-density lipoprotein(s) (HDL) A heterogeneous class of molecules found in the blood which includes proteins (33% by weight), cholesterol (30%), phospholipids (29%), triglycerides (8%), cholesterol esters, and apolipoproteins. HDL is involved in the transportation of cholesterol from the intestine. The larger the HDL molecule, the more efficient the lipid transportation and, by extension, breakdown of lipids. HDL levels are the single most important predictor of coronary heart disease (CHD) given that several risk factors for CHD (e.g., smoking, obesity, and lack of exercise) may lower HDL; HDL has an inverse relation with VLDL and LDL (lipoproteins known to be atherogenic); and HDL may interfere with atherogenesis by promoting reverse cholesterol transport or preventing aggregation of LDL particles in the arterial wall. Small HDL molecules (HDL$_3$) are metabolically "early" forms, are more prominent in alcoholics, and have a reverse relationship with the risk of CHD and atherosclerosis. High levels of HDL are "protective" and reduce the risk of atherosclerosis while low levels are associated with an increased risk of arterial disease. Most physicians order a group of tests commonly known as lipid profile to determine risk status; the tests measure cholesterol, triglycerides, HDL, and LDL. Some physicians may also measure serum levels of apolipoproteins A and B, although the usefulness of these latter tests is unknown.
Patient preparation No special preparation is necessary, other than for drawing blood.
Specimen Serum.
Reference range

Low risk	40 mg/dL.
Intermediate risk	35–40 mg/dL.
High risk	Less than 35 mg/dL.

Cost $35–$45 when ordered alone. See *apolipoproteins.*

high-performance liquid chromatography See *HPLC* in Glossary.

high-resolution computed tomography A computed tomographic (CT) study at slice (collimation scan interval) widths of 4 mm or less, which is narrower than the usual 1 to 3 cm interval slices obtained in conventional CT imaging. HRCT is the optimal technique for evaluating interstitial lung disease and emphysema and is preferred to conventional CT in detecting subpleural nodules, small linear densities, "honeycombing," and bronchiectasis and is of use in any body region where great detail is desired. See *spiral computed tomography.*

His bundle electrocardiography A relatively recent and sophisticated means of recording the electrical activity of the heart. In this clinical test, the bipolar cardiac catheter electrode system is used to record His bundle activity, study the cardiac physiology of patients with recurrent arrhythmias, optimize pacemaker implantation, and to differentiate true atrioventricular (AV) blocks from pseudo-AV blocks.

Patient preparation The patient is placed in a supine position on a special X-ray table and prepared for the insertion of a catheter.

Procedure EKG electrodes are placed on the limbs. A local anesthetic is injected and a J-tip electrode is introduced into the femoral vein. Recordings are made as the electrode passes through the heart valves.

Reference range The physician must interpret the recordings along with other diagnostic test results.

Cost $250–$500.

histocompatibility antigens See *HLA typing.*

histoplasmosis Infection with the fungus *Histoplasma capsulatum* which is regionally endemic in the Ohio and Mississippi River valleys, the Caribbean, and Central and South America. Histoplasmosis results from inhalation of dust, particularly from chicken houses, bat-infested caves, and pigeon droppings that contain the spores of *Histoplasma capsulatum.* The clinical findings in histoplasmosis range from asymptomatic to an acute respiratory illness that may evolve to chronic cavitary lung infection (the lesions of which may undergo calcification), disseminated disease with fever, hepatosplenomegaly, lymphadenopathy, and multiorgan involvement. The diagnosis of histoplasmosis is based on serological testing with complement fixation, immunodiffusion, or latex particle agglutination for antibodies. It is important to review the patient's travel history.

Patient preparation No special preparation is required.

Procedure Antibodies are detected by ELISA and IFA.

Specimen Serum.

Reference range Negative.

Abnormal values A positive result suggests exposure to histoplasmosis.

Cost $45–$75.

Comments Recent histoplasma skin testing causes transiently elevated antibody titers; it is essential that patients be questioned about past exposure to skin test antigens.

HIV-1 (human immunodeficiency virus, HTLV-III, human T-cell lympho-trophic virus, type III, AIDS-related virus, ARV) The retrovirus that is intimately linked to AIDS (acquired immunodeficiency syndrome) and widely believed to be the most likely cause of AIDS. See *acquired immunodeficiency syndrome.*

HLA typing Human leukocyte antigens (HLA) are present on the surface of lymphocytes. These antigens are essential to immunity and determine the degree of compatibility between transplant donors and recipients. Incompatible HLA-A, HLA-B, HLA-C, or HLA-D may cause unsuccessful tissue transplantation. There are many antigenic determinants, and one set of each antigen is inherited from each parent, which makes HLA typing useful in determining parentage. There is a high incidence of specific HLA types linked to specific diseases, but these findings have little diagnostic significance. HLA testing is best used as an adjunct to diagnosis of such diseases.

Patient preparation No special preparation is required.

Procedure HLA antibodies are measured by immunoassay.

Specimen Whole blood collected in an ACD tube.

Reference range HLA typing is not a test that gives standard results.

Abnormal values Diseases associated with certain types of HLAs:

HLA-DR5	Hashimoto's thyroiditis
HLA-B27	Ankylosing spondylitis
HLA-B8 & Dw3	Graves' disease
HLA-B8	chronic autoimmune hepatitis, celiac disease, myasthenia gravis
HLA-Dw3	Addison's disease, Sjögren syndrome, dermatitis herpetiformis, systemic lupus erythematosus.
HLA-B27, Bw2	multiple sclerosis

Cost $125–$300.

Comments A recent blood transfusion will interfere with accurate results.

homovanillic acid (HVA) Homovanillic acid is a metabolite of dopamine, which is used to synthesize epinephrine and norepinephrine. Dopamine is broken down in the liver to form homovanillic acid, which is excreted in the urine. HVA is generally measured along with the major catecholamines and other catecholamine metabolites.

Patient preparation Restrictions on medication intake may be indicated. The ordering physician must determine the restrictions.

Procedure HVA is measured by HPLC methods.

Specimen 24-hour urine specimen. Specimen must be preserved with 6N HCl.

Reference range

Age in years	mg/mg creatinine
15–17	0.5–2
10–15	0.25–12
5–10	0.5–9
2–5	0.5–13.5

1–2	4–23
0–1	1.2–35

Abnormal values Increased in neuroblastoma and ganglioneuroma.

Cost $50–$75.

Comments Many drugs can affect HVA levels. Drug restrictions must be followed for accurate results to be obtained.

hot scan See *hot nodule* in Glossary.

hPL See *human placental lactogen.*

HPV (human papillomavirus) A potentially premalignant virus which is most prevalent in those with the greatest number of sexual partners. 65 genotypes of HPV (a genotype is considered distinct if it has less than 50% DNA sequence similarity or "homology" with its closest relative) have been described. HPV can be identified within cells (by the technique of in situ hybridization) in skin tumors that are benign (e.g., condyloma acuminatum), malignant (e.g., squamous cell carcinoma of the anus, penis, and uterine cervix), or of uncertain clinical behavior (e.g., inverted papillomas of the nasopharynx). HPV types 6 and 11 are not considered premalignant, while HPV types 16, 18, 31, 33, and 35 are associated with cervical dysplasia, CIN, and anogenital cancer. A majority of women with HPV, especially 16 and 18, develop CIN-II to CIN-III. The mechanism for malignant degeneration occurrences is unclear. See *cervical intraepithelial neoplasia.*

HSIL See *high-grade squamous intraepithelial lesion* in Glossary.

human chorionic gonadotropin (hCG) Chorionic gonadotropin is a hormone synthesized and secreted by the placenta. It has an alpha chain of amino acids that is structurally similar to TSH, FSH, and LH. There are several immunoassays for hCG that detect either the intact molecule or the beta subunit. Both forms can detect early pregnancy, and assays for either are used in all pregnancy testing kits. The beta subunit of the hCG molecule is elevated in both pregnancy and various types of cancer. The intact hCG molecule is thought to be more specific of pregnancy. Levels of hCG increase during the first trimester of pregnancy, peak around the tenth week, then fall to less than 10% of the first trimester peak levels. Persistent elevation of hCG usually means trophoblastic disease (i.e., neoplastic disease of placental origin). In most normal pregnancies, it is not necessary to serially quantitate hCG levels.

Patient preparation No special preparation is required.

Procedure HCG is measured by RIA, EIA, and chemiluminescence.

Specimen Urine or serum; urine is primarily used as an early screen for pregnancy, and serum is used to confirm and follow high-risk (nonroutine) pregnancies.

Reference range
Urine   More than 25 mIU/ml suggests pregnancy.
Serum nonpregnant   Less than 5 mIU/ml.

Abnormal values
Increased in: multiple gestation; polyhydramnios; eclampsia; erythroblastosis fetalis; trophoblastic disease (e.g., hydatidiform moles, choriocarcinoma, and placental site trophoblastic tumor); tumors producing either the β subunit or both α and β subunits, measured by ELISA or RIA; ectopic elevation of hCG may occur with cancer of the stomach, liver, pancreas, breast, kidney, lungs, and adrenal cortex; seminoma; leukemia; lymphoma; melanoma.
Decreased in: ectopic pregnancy.

Cost
Urine $10–$30.
Serum $35–$55.

human placental lactogen (chorionic somatomammotropin, human placental lactogen, hPL)   Human placental lactogen is a hormone produced at the time of the implantation of the fertilized egg and secreted by the placenta. hPL regulates and coordinates fetal growth and metabolism and maternal metabolism, which exerts its effects on the mother, causing relative insulin resistance and increased levels of circulating free fatty acids. hPL is thought to optimize metabolism of nutrients by the fetus in the first half of pregnancy. In the second half of pregnancy there is little correlation between hPL levels and fetal well-being. Human placental lactogen stimulates the production of milk and enlargement of breasts and is somatotopic and luteotropic. Urine and plasma HPL levels reflect placental size and tend to be high in diabetic mothers.

Specimen Serum.

Reference range Varies with duration of gestation, rising with gestation to plateau at about 37 weeks (10 µg/ml).

Males   Less than 0.5 mg/ml.
Nonpregnant females   Less than 0.5 mg/ml.
Weeks of gestation
  5–27   Less than 4.6 mcg/ml.
  28–31   2.4–6.1 mcg/ml.
  32–35   3.7–7.7 mcg/ml.
  36–term   5–8.6 mcg/ml.

Abnormal values
Increased in: diabetes mellitus, Rh isoimmunization, hydatiform mole, choriocarcinoma.
Decreased in: postmaturity syndrome, retarded growth, toxemia of pregnancy, threatened abortion.

Critical value Less than 4 µg/ml after 30 weeks gestation.

Cost $60–$120.

Comments Chorionic gonadotropim levels and estrogen levels are more useful than hPL in evaluating pregnancy, although hPL may supplement other laboratory tests.

HVA   See *homovanillic acid.*

17-hydroxycorticosteroid (17-OHC)   A general term for any steroid hormone formed in the adrenal gland by action of 17-hydroxylase, which includes cortisol, cortisone, 11-deoxycortisol, and tetrahydro derivatives. Urinary excretion of 17-hydroxycorticosteroids is a rough guide of both the functional status of the adrenal gland and the rate of catabolism.
   Patient preparation All drugs should be withheld for several days prior to the collection, if possible without doing harm to the patient. Stress should be avoided.
   Procedure 17-OHC is measured by RIA methods.
   Specimen 24-hour urine collection with HCl or acetic acid as preservative.
   Reference range
      Less than age 8   Less than 1.5 mg/24 hours.
      8–12 years old   Less than 4.5 mg/24 hours.
      Adult females   4.5–12.0 mg/24 hours.
      Adult males   2.5–10.0 mg/24 hours.
   Abnormal values
      Increased in: Cushing's syndrome, ectopic ACTH syndrome, obesity, pancreatitis, pregnancy, stress.
      Decreased in: Addison's disease, adrenogenital syndrome, pituitary insufficiency.
   Cost $50–$75.
   Comments The availability of more reliable methods for serum or urine cortisol makes this test less useful.

5-hydroxyindole acetic acid (5-HIAA)   A compound that is a metabolite of the tryptophan-serotonin metabolic pathway which is excreted in the urine. 5-HIAA may be markedly (25–50 fold normal) elevated in carcinoid tumors, in particular of the midgut (less commonly of the lung and ovary). Carcinoid tumors may be first suspected in patients with features of the so-called carcinoid syndrome, e.g., bronchoconstriction, diarrhea, flushing, right-sided heart lesions, and facial telangiectasia.
   Patient preparation The patient being tested for 5-HIAA must avoid exposure to certain foods (e.g., avocados, bananas, chocolate, eggplant, plantains, pineapples, plums, tomatoes, walnuts) and drugs (e.g., acetaminophen, salicylates, phenacetin, cough syrup containing glyceryl guaiacolate, imipramine, isoniazid, naproxen, mephenesin, methocarbamol, monamine oxidase inhibitors, methenamine, methyldopa, phenothiazines) for 48 hours or more before collecting the urine.
   Procedure 5-HIAA is measured colorimetrically on an automated chemistry analyzer.
   Specimen 24-hour urine. The specimen must be preserved with glacial

acetic acid, HCl, or boric acid. Laboratory instructions must be followed for accurate determinations.

Reference range 1–9 mg/24 hours.

Abnormal values:

Increased in: carcinoid syndrome, Hartnup's disease, nontropical sprue, certain psychiatric conditions.

Decreased in: massive resections of the gastrointestinal tract, renal insufficiency, phenylketonuria.

Cost $50–$75.

Comments It is imperative that specimen collection instructions be closely followed in order to avoid false-positive results.

17-hydroxyprogesterone This analyte is a precursor to cortisol, a critical metabolic building block, which is in turn the precursor for the major steroids produced by the adrenal cortex. 17-hydroxyprogesterone may be markedly increased in patients with the autosomal recessive 21-hydroxylase deficiency, which is the most common cause of congenital adrenal hyperplasia, a condition characterized by virilization of females and wasting of salt by the kidneys.

Patient preparation No special preparation is required.

Procedure 17-hydroxyprogesterone is measured by RIA procedures.

Specimen Serum, plasma, amniotic fluid. Specimen must be separated from the blood within four hours.

Reference range

Male	50–200ng/dL.
Female	Follicular phase 20–80 ng/dL.
Luteal phase	100–300 ng/dL.
Postmenopausal	Less than 50 ng/dL.

Abnormal values

Increased in: congenital adrenal hyperplasia, hirsutism, infertility, adrenal tumors, ovarian tumors.

Cost $50–$75.

Comments Because 17-hydroxyprogesterone deficiency can be life threatening, early diagnosis and therapy are essential.

hydroxyproline Hydroxyproline is an amino acid that is a major constituent of collagen. Because collagen is the only protein that contains appreciable amounts of hydroxyproline, an increase of hyroxyproline in the urine indicates increased turnover of bone matrix, which is most often caused by osteoporosis.

Patient preparation No special preparation is required.

Procedure Hydroxyproline is measured by HPLC.

Specimen 24-hour urine collection with 10 ml of toluene as the preservative.

Reference range

Male	15–45 mg/24 hours.
Female	7–25 mg/24 hours.

Abnormal values
Increased in: acute osteomyelitis, bone tumors, burns (severe), congenital hyperphosphatasia, fibrous dysplasia, healing fractures, hyperparathyroidism, hyperthyroidism, osteomalacia, Paget's disease of bone, rickets.
Cost $50–$75.

hysterosalpingography (uterography, hysterography)   A diagnostic procedure in which radiocontrast is instilled in the uterine cavity and fallopian tubes, followed by fluoroscopic examination or obtention of a plain film. Hysterosalpingography is used in evaluating infertility (e.g., to determine the patency of the fallopian tubes) and has been used to identify lesions of the uterine cavity, including submucosal leiomyomas, endocervical and endometrial polyps, congenital malformations of the uterus, including septal defects (e.g., uterus didelphys) or uterine hypoplasia, pelvic tuberculosis, and as an adjuvant in the diagnosis of endometrial cancer.

hysteroscopy   The visual examination of the uterine cavity using a flexible fiberoptic instrument known as a hysteroscope. Hysteroscopy is used to evaluate abnormal uterine bleeding, to identify and resect various lesions of the uterine cavity, including uterine synechiae and septae, submucosal leiomyomas, endocervical and endometrial polyps, IUDs (intrauterine devices), and for endometrial ablation. It may be used in conjunction with other procedures including curettage and laparoscopy. Because the uterine cavity is small and lined with a thin layer of endometrium, it must first be distended with saline or dextran or insufflated with carbon dioxide. If the hysteroscopy is largely diagnostic in nature, it can be performed with local anesthesia (e.g., intravenous sedation and paracervical block). Extensive manipulation and or resection requires regional or general anesthesia. Failure of hysteroscopy may occur in cervical stenosis, inadequate distension of the uterine cavity, bleeding, and excess mucus secretion. Complications include perforation, bleeding, and infection.
Patient preparation The patient lies on an examining table, and the vagina and cervix are cleansed.
Procedure The hysteroscope tubing is inserted and the uterine cavity is visualized through the flexible fiberoptics. The physician may photograph an unusual finding for later review.
Abnormal values Intrauterine adhesions, uterine tumors, foreign bodies, congenital malformations, traumatic injuries, occlusions, fistulas.
Cost $300–$500.

imaging The term imaging is used in two different areas of diagnostic medicine, pathology and radiology. A key component in pathology imaging is the ability to record, transmit, and store images of pathological lesions. In radiology, imaging refers to the production of noninvasive images of body regions through the use of ionizing radiation (e.g., CT or mammography) or electromagnetic radiation (e.g., MRI or ultrasonography) with or without radiocontrast medium. The information obtained may then be analyzed by a computer to produce a two-dimensional display; the information provided may be anatomic (CT, MRI, mammography, ultrasonography), metabolic (PET-positron emission tomography, SPECT-single photon emission computed tomography,) or data on electrical activity (SQUID).

immunoelectrophoresis (IEP)   A technique used to detect abnormal proteins (immunoglobulins) in body fluids (e.g., serum or urine). IEP is used to evaluate monoclonal gammopathies. A new technique called immunofixation electrophoresis (IEF) is replacing IEP. IEF takes less time to perform and is much easier to interpret.

Patient preparation No special preparation is required.

Procedure The fluid of interest is electrophoresed on a gel and then allowed to react, via diffusion, with antibodies to various immunoglobulins (including IgA, IgG, IgM, and the immunoglobulin light chains kappa and lambda). If abnormal immunoglobulins are present in the specimen, they appear as extra arcs on the gel.

Specimen Serum or urine.

Reference range No abnormal arcs detected.

Abnormal values multiple myeloma, Waldenström's disease (or macroglobulinemia), amyloidosis, collagen diseases, malignant lymphoma, dysgammaglobulinemic states.

Cost $50–$75.

Comments IEP is not a quantitative test. It is being replaced by immunofixation electrophoresis which is more sensitive, easier to interpret, and provides a more rapid turnaround.

147

immunofixation electrophoresis (IFE) A technique used to characterize monoclonal gammopathies. IFE combines high-resolution protein electrophoresis with immunoprecipitation. IFE is most often requested to evaluate a monoclonal immunoglobulin detected in protein electrophoresis. Specific light and heavy chains of monoclonal proteins can also be characterized by this method.

Patient preparation No special preparation is necessary, other than for drawing blood.

Procedure The serum is subjected to electrophoresis. The proteins and immunoglobulins separate according to their electrical charge. Specific antibodies are poured on the gel which bind to the immunoglobulins; a stain is applied to highlight and identify them.

Specimen Serum or urine.

Reference range No abnormal bands are detected.

Abnormal values Monoclonal gammopathies, multiple myeloma, malignant lymphoma, amyloidosis, dysgammaglobulinemic states.

Cost $35–$50.

Comments Because of ease of interpretation and more rapid turnaround time, IFE is replacing IEP as the method of choice in evaluating monoclonal gammopathies.

immunoglobulins Immunoglobulins are highly specific molecules produced by the immune system's B lymphocytes in response to a foreign substance (antigen). They are composed of two identical light and two identical heavy chains which have constant and variable regions, the latter of which are critical for the recognition of the antigen to which they are capable of binding. Immunoglobulins can be defined as

1. Idiotypes, which are immunoglobulins that have been evoked by a particular antigenic site or epitope.
2. Isotypes, which are immunoglobulin subtypes (IgG, IgA, IgM, IgD, IgE) that all normal individuals have.
3. Allotypes, which are subtypes shared by population groups, e.g., with racial differences.

Immunoglobulin (antibody) levels are an indirect marker of the status of the immune system. Immunoglobulins form against specific antigens (e.g., hepatitis, CMV, EBV) and other infectious agents. Recent infection is usually characterized by an increase in specific IgM antibodies against the pathogen of interest. With prior infection, there is an elevation of IgG antibodies to the pathogen.

impedence plethysmography A noninvasive method that measures the changes in electrical resistance between two electrical probes. IP indicates the changes in the volume of different regions of the body as may be seen in obstruction to venous outflow. IP was the most widely used method for the diagnosis of deep vein thrombosis but has been superseded by B-mode ultrasonography, which is more accurate. See *plethysmography, ultrasonography.*

indirect antiglobulin test (indirect Coombs test)   This test detects sensitization of red blood cells in vitro (i.e., outside of living cells) and screens for the presence of unexpected antibodies in the first trimester of pregnancy or before transfusing blood.
  Patient preparation No special preparation is required.
  Procedure This is a manual test in which clumping of red blood cells is visualized to determine whether or not a reaction has taken place.
  Specimen Serum in a red-top tube, i.e., without anticoagulant.
  Reference range Negative.
  Abnormal values Presence of unknown antibodies.
  Cost $25–$50.
  Comments Usually part of a pretransfusion panel or blood type workup. A positive test requires further analysis to identify the antibodies. The direct Coombs test is performed in conjunction with the indirect Coombs test. See *direct antiglobulin test.*

indirect Coombs test See *indirect antiglobulin test.*

insecticide poisoning Insecticides are working tools of agriculture, and acute overdose either through accident or intent (i.e., suicide) is not uncommon. In rural communities, insecticide poisoning constitutes a significant minority of the visits to the emergency room. Insecticides are of two broad categories: the newer cholinesterase inhibitors and the older organochlorine compounds (e.g., DDT and chlordane) that have either been taken off the market or fallen into disuse. The cholinesterase inhibitors are divided into organophosphates which are esters of phosphoric acid or thiophosphoric acid, and carbamates, which are synthetic derivatives of carbamic acid. Despite their significant chemical differences, they both block the transmission of neural impulses.
  Patient preparation No special preparation is required.
  Procedure Organophosphates are measured in urine by gas-liquid chromatography.
  Specimen Urine, frozen until analysis.
  Reference range Less than 0.1 mg/L.
  Abnormal values Greater than 0.1 mg/L.
  Cost $75–$150.
  Comments Signs and symptoms of organophosphate poisoning include drooling, defecation, lacrimation, urinary incontinence, pupillary constriction, bradycardia, bronchoconstriction, muscle twitching, respiratory and/or cardiovascular depression, and possibly respiratory death. Carbamates are less efficient at penetrating the CNS and thus are not as dangerous as the organophosphate insecticides. Diagnosis requires history

of exposure, signs and symptoms, and measurement of acetylcholinesterase in the red blood cells and serum, which falls to 50% or less of normal levels. The clinical signs and symptoms of organophosphate poisoning generally do not occur until acetylcholinesterase has fallen to less than 20% of normal.

in situ carcinoma See *carcinoma in situ* in Glossary.

insulin Insulin is a protein hormone composed of two polypetide chains joined by disulfide bonds. It is produced by the β islet cells of the pancreas. Insulin's actions can be divided into those that occur within seconds, minutes, or hours. Insulin facilitates the uptake and storage of glucose by muscle, fat, and neutrophils and promotes the storage and utilization of glucose. In healthy individuals, the insulin levels parallel the rise and fall of glucose in the blood. Diabetes mellitus is the result of either a deficiency of insulin or resistance to its effects.

Patient preparation No special preparation is required.

Procedure Insulin is measured by EIA or RIA methods.

Specimen Serum, which must be kept cold until analysis.

Reference range 0–25 μU/ml; insulin is normal in noninsulin-dependent diabetes mellitus.

Abnormal values Insulin is decreased in insulin-dependent diabetes mellitus.

Cost $50–$75.

Comments C-peptide is a product of insulin metabolism. It is used to determine the functioning of the islet cells and is measured in patients with suspected surreptitious injection of insulin.

insulin tolerance test A provocation type test in which administration of insulin is followed by serial measurement of human growth hormone (hGH) and adrenocorticotropic hormone (ACTH). Insulin evokes a decrease in glucose (hypoglycemic), which stimulates hGH and ACTH in persons with pituitary or adrenal hypofunction. See *glucose tolerance test.*

Patient preparation Patient must fast for 10 to 12 hours before the test.

Procedure Early in the morning (between 6 a.m. and 8 a.m.) specimens are obtained for basal levels of glucose, hGH, and ACTH. Insulin is then administered intravenously at the appropriate dose over a period of two minutes or less. Blood samples are drawn at 30, 45, 60, and 90 minutes after administering the insulin.

Specimen

Glucose	Plasma (gray-top tube, sodium fluoride anticoagulant).
hGH	Plasma (green-top tube, sodium heparin anticoagulant).
ACTH	Plasma (green-top tube, sodium heparin anticoagulant).

Reference range A 10–20 ng/dL increase of hGH and ACTH over baseline levels. Peak levels occur at 60–90 minutes.

Abnormal values hGH and/or ACTH deficiency.

Cost $75–$100.

Comments This test is performed in a clinical setting; intravenous glucose should be available in case of severe hypoglycemia.

intraocular pressure See *tonometry.*

intravenous digital subtraction angiography See *digital subtraction angiography.*

intrinsic factor Intrinsic factor is a vitamin B_{12}-binding glycoprotein produced in the parietal cells of the stomach that is essential for the absorption of vitamin B_{12}. Intrinsic factor secretion closely parallels the secretion of hydrochloric acid and is stimulated by histamine, gastrin, and methionine. It usually greatly exceeds that required for vitamin B_{12} absorption. Megaloblastic (also known as pernicious) anemia may be due to any condition that results in decreased intrinsic factor, e.g., low gastric acid production or agents that reduce gastric acid secretion by blocking parietal cell receptors, such as H_2-blockers or anti-intrinsic factor antibodies.

iron iron-binding capacity, total iron-binding capacity, TIBC Iron is an essential mineral that is bound to hemoglobin and responsible for the transportation of oxygen. The term "total iron" (the adjective "total" is rarely used in practice) is the amount of iron actually present in the serum. In contrast, the term "total iron-binding capacity" indicates the amount of iron that could be present in the circulation (i.e., be bound by the existing carrier proteins in the serum) and is a chemical approximation of the amount of transferrin (the protein responsible for the transportation of iron in the blood). There are now direct measurements of transferrin available but they are not widely used. Iron and TIBC are often part of a general chemistry panel which can be performed on highly automated instruments currently available. See *transferrin.*

Patient preparation Patient must fast for at least 12 hours prior to the test. Because iron is generally lower in the evening, morning specimens are preferred. Recent iron therapy or blood transfusion yields false-positive results.
Procedure Iron and iron-binding capacity are measured spectrophotometrically on automated chemistry analyzers.
Specimen Serum.
Reference range

Adult males	50–160 µg/dL.
Adult females	45–150 µg/dL.
Iron-binding capacity	250–350 µg/dL.
Percent saturation	20%–50%.

Abnormal values
   Increased in: hemochromatosis.
   Decreased in: periods of increased need (e.g., growth, pregnancy), hemorrhage, menstrual disorders, i.e., when excessive, deficient iron in

diet (e.g., vegetarians, milk-fed infants), postgastrectomy.
Cost $35–$50.

Ivy bleeding time A quantitative coagulation assay measuring the platelet and vascular response to a standardized skin wound.
Patient preparation No special preparation is required.
Procedure A sphygmomanometer (blood pressure cuff) is placed around the upper arm and inflated to 40 mm Hg pressure. A 5 mm incision is made on the flexor surface of the forearm, and the time required to stop bleeding is then measured.
Reference range 1–6 minutes.
Abnormal values
   Increased in: Bernard-Soulier disease, Glanzmann's thrombasthenia, platelet defects, e.g., thrombocytopenia, storage pool disease, vascular defects (Ehlers-Danlos disease, von Willebrand's disease).
Cost $50–$75.

K

ketogenic steroids   These are metabolites of cortisol, pregnanetriol, and other adrenocortical steroids which are usually part of a general screen that measures other analytes. Specific tests are required to provide more definitive information in the presence of an abnormality identified by the screening process.

Patient preparation   Patient must not be under stress or taking ACTH.

Procedure Ketogenic steroids are measured by spectrophotometric methods.

Specimen A 24-hour urine collection. The receptacle must have a preservative, most commonly 6N HCl, to maintain the pH between 4 and 6.

Reference range

Infants to 11 years	0.1–4 mg/24 hours.
11–14 years	2–9 mg/24 hours.
Men	4–14 mg/24 hours.
Women	2–12 mg/24 hours.

Abnormal values

Increased in: Cushing's syndrome, congenital adrenal hyperplasia, adrenal carcinoma or adenoma.

Decreased in: panhypopituitarism, congenital hypothyroidism (cretinism), general wasting.

ketone body (ketone)   One of three organic molecules (acetone, acetoacetate, β-hydroxybutyrate) with a carbonyl group (C=O). Formation of ketone bodies is a physiological defense in starvation, diabetes mellitus, and defective carbohydrate metabolism. In diabetes, fatty acid levels are very high because the lack of insulin prevents glucose from being used to produce energy, and the body's metabolic needs are met by fatty acids. Ketone bodies are products of incomplete fat metabolism, are present in acidosis, and are present in the serum and urine in uncontrolled diabetes mellitus.

Patient preparation No special preparation is required.

Procedure Ketone bodies are measured by gas-liquid chromatography.

Specimen Urine (random), serum.

Reference range Negative.

Abnormal values Positive in ketoacidosis.
Cost $75–$100.

ketones See *urinalysis.*

17-ketosteroids A general term for the "male" hormones which are primarily produced by the testes and adrenal cortex; they include androsterone, dehydroepiandrosterone-DHEA, epiandrosterone, etiocholanolone, 11-keto- and 11-β-hydroxyandrosterone, and 11-keto- and 11-β-hydroxyetiocholanolone. This test is used primarily to evaluate testicular or adrenal function.

Patient preparation No special preparation is necessary.
Procedure 17-ketosteroids are measured by spectrophotometric and gas chromatographic methods.
Specimen A 24-hour urine collection which has been preserved with 6N HCl. The pH must be between 4 and 7.
Reference range

Male, urine	8–20 mg/day.
Female, urine	6–15 mg/day.

Abnormal values
Increased in: adrenal or testicular tumors or hyperplasia, pregnancy, physical or mental stress, polycystic ovarian disease.
Decreased in: adrenal hypofunction (primary or secondary), Klinefelter's syndrome, castration, hypothyroidism, anorexia nervosa.
Cost $75–$90.

17-ketosteroids, fractionated A battery of assays used to evaluate adrenal function.

Patient preparation No special preparation is required.
Procedure The individual analytes are quantified by gas chromatography.
Specimen A 24-hour urine collection which has been preserved with 6N HCl. The pH must be between 4 and 7.
Reference ranges

STEROID	ADULT MALE	ADULT FEMALE	MALE (age 10–15)	FEMALE (age 10–15)	BOTH SEXES (age 0–9)
Androsterone	2.2–5	0.5–2.4	0.2–2	0.2–2.5	<1.0
Dehydroepiandrosterone	0–2.3	0–1.2	<0.4	<0.4	<0.2
Etiocholanolone	1.9–4.7	1.1–3	0.1–1.6	0.7–3	<1.0
11-Hydroxyandrosterone	0.5–1.3	0.2–0.6	0.1–1.1	0.2–1	<1.0
11-Hydroxyetiocholanolone	0.3–0.7	0.2–0.6	<0.3	0.1–0.5	<0.5
11-Ketoandrosterone	0–0.1	0–0.2	<0.1	<0.1	<0.1
11-Ketoetiocholanolone	0.2–0.7	0.2–0.6	0.2–0.6	0.1–0.6	<0.7
Pregnanediol	0.6–1.6	0.2–2.4	0.1–0.7	0.1–1.2	<0.5
Pregnanetriol	0.6–1.3	0.1–1	0.2–0.6	0.1–0.6	<0.3
5-Pregnanetriol	0–0.3	0–0.3	<0.3	<0.3	<0.211
Ketopregnanetriol	0–0.2	0–0.4	<0.3	<0.2	<0.2

Units are in mg/dL

Abnormal values This test is used to evaluate adrenal and gonadal function and may be used to monitor cortisol therapy.
Cost $150–$200.
Comments This test should only be performed if the total 17-ketosteroid levels are abnormal.

17-ketosteroids, total Measurement of all the 17-ketosteroids as a group is used as a screen. If the total is increased, each individual steroid is analyzed separately (fractionated 17-ketosteroids) in the much more expensive fractionation procedure.
Patient preparation No special preparation is required.
Procedure Total 17-ketosteroids are measured by spectrophotometric methods.
Specimen A 24-hour urine collection with 6N HCl as preservative.
Reference range

0–11 years	0.1–3 mg/24 hours.
11–14 years	2–7 mg/24 hours.
Men	6–21 mg/24 hours.
Women	4–17 mg/24 hours.

Abnormal values
  Increased in: adrenal hyperplasia, carcinoma, adenoma, adrenogenital syndrome.
  Decreased in: Addison's disease, panhypopituitarism, eunuchoidism.
Cost $40–$60.

kidney biopsy See *renal biopsy.*

kidney stone analysis (renal calculus) Kidney stones develop when crystallizable substances that are normally present in the urine become too concentrated, reach a state of supersaturation, and precipitate in the form of crystals. Kidney stones are clinically characterized by colicky pain, hematuria, and ureteral or renal pelvic obstruction, which may facilitate infection or lead to hydronephrosis. In the laboratory the composition of stones is determined in order to allow the physician to develop a preventive diet for the patient. Approximately 5% of women and 10% of men will have at least one stone by age 70. The types of stones suffered tend to run in families. Some are associated with other conditions such as bowel disease, ileal bypass, or renal tubule defects. There are several common types of stones:
  1. CALCIUM STONES These account for 75%–85% of all stones, are most commonly found in men, and are composed of calcium oxalate, carbonate, or phosphate. They can be controlled by altering the diet.
  2. URIC ACID STONES A type of stone that is most commonly found in men. Approximately 50% of those with uric acid stones also have gout.
  3. CYSTINE STONES A type of stone that is most commonly formed in those with the hereditary disease cystinuria.
  4. MAGNESIUM AMMONIUM PHOSPHATE STONES (Struvite stones) A

type of stone most commonly formed in women which results from urinary tract infection with bacteria (e.g., *Proteus* species) that produce specificenzymes. Stuvite stones can become very large, fill the renal pelvis, develop a staghorn appearance, obstruct the urinary tract, and cause kidney damage.

Patient preparation No special preparation is necessary.

Procedure Stones are analyzed by infrared spectroscopy and biochemical analysis.

Specimen The stones are obtained either by surgery or by a patient who collects a stone after passing it during urination.

Cost $100–$400. The cost depends on the complexity of the stone. Simple calcium oxalate stones are relatively easy to analyze by light microscopy or optical crystallography. More "exotic" stones may require the use of X-ray diffraction.

Kleihauer-Betke test   A staining method that identifies the presence of fetal hemoglobin (HbF) in red blood cells, based on the relative resistance of fetal hemoglobin to alkaline buffer elution. The Kleihauer-Betke test is most commonly used to differentiate between fetal and maternal red blood cells in the mother's circulation or in amniotic fluid. Fetal red blood cells are red and refractile after alkaline buffer treatment and eosin staining, while maternal cells appear as red cell ghosts lacking hemoglobin. The Kleihauer-Betke test is used to estimate the volume of transplacental hemorrhage in mothers with Rh immune disease and the amount of Rh immune globulin that should be administered to the mother to reduce sensitization to Rh factor and to the child to reduce the incidence of Rh factor-induced hemolytic disease of the newborn.

Patient preparation No special preparation is required.

Procedure Blood is placed in an acidic solution and a blood smear is made on a microscope slide. Fetal cells will show preservation of hemoglobin staining, whereas adult cells will appear as ghosts. The relative percentage of stained to unstained cells is determined.

Specimen Whole blood drawn in a lavender-top tube.

Reference range See laboratory report.

Abnormal values Elevated results are found in transplacental hemorrhage.

Cost $45–$75.

Comments The results of this test are used to calculate the dosage of Rhlg (RhoGam).

L

lactate dehydrogenase (LDH)   Lactate dehydrogenase is an enzyme present in the cytoplasm of all cells; it catalyzes the interconversion of lactate and pyruvate. Measurement of total LDH activity is used to screen for liver, muscle, and myocardial disease. This enzyme is normally part of a routine chemistry profile which includes several enzymes used to distinguish between various disease states. It is not used as a stand-alone diagnostic tool but in combination with other tests.

Patient preparation No special preparation is necessary.

Procedure LDH is measured by spectrophotometric methods on automated chemistry analyzers.

Specimen Serum.

Reference range 94–250 U/L (values vary widely between laboratories and are method dependent). When comparing results from different laboratories it is important to note the specific reference range listed.

Abnormal values
  Increased in: liver disease, neoplasia, pulmonary infarction,
    myocardial infarction, hemolysis.

Cost $15–$30. The test is usually part of a routine chemistry profile.

Comments In myocardial infarction, levels of LDH rise, peak at 48 hours, then slowly return to normal. The cardiac-specific isoenzyme is used to follow this trend rather than the total activity.

lactate dehydrogenase isoenzymes   An enzyme tetramer composed of two different 34 kD subunits, H (heart) and M (muscle), which are separable by electrophoresis. The HHHH tetramer (LD_1) is the most rapidly migrating or anodic fraction and has an electrophoretic mobility in the α_1 region of an electrophoresis gel; the slowest migrating or cathodic fraction is composed of the MMMM tetramer (LD_5) and migrates to the gamma (γ) region in a serum protein electrophoretic gel. There are thus five major forms (isoenzymes) of lactic dehydrogenase which are numbered sequentially; each is related to a tissue in which it predominates.

  LD_1 Heart and red blood cells

LD$_2$	Heart and red blood cells
LD$_3$	Platelets, lungs, and skeletal muscle
LD$_4$	Liver and skeletal muscle
LD$_5$	Liver and skeletal muscle

In general, total LD levels rise with various forms of tissue injury and is measured as a screen for nonspecific enzyme abnormalities. If it is elevated, as it usually is in myocardial infarction, the serum is separated into isoenzyme fractions, which localizes the abnormality to a particular tissue. Normally LD$_1$ is greater than LD$_2$; with cardiac damage LD$_2$ becomes more prominent. Electrophoresis was the first methodology used to evaluate LDH isoenzymes but had the drawback of a relatively long turnaround time. A new method, immunoinhibition, has been developed to measure changes in the LD$_1$/LD$_2$ ratio. It is automated and results are available in less than one hour. As with CPK isoenzymes, the enzymes levels rise and fall, and for true diagnostic specificity, squential specimens are preferred. LD is elevated for a longer period than CPK isoenzymes and can be positive after CPK isoenzymes (e.g., CPK-MB) have returned to normal. It is not necessary for the total LDH levels to be elevated in order to use isoenzyme fractionation for diagnostic purposes.

Patient preparation No special preparation is necessary.

Procedure The isoenzymes are separated and analyzed electrophoretically.

Specimen Serum.

Reference range

LD$_1$	22%–36%
LD$_2$	35%–46%
LD$_3$	13%–26%
LD$_4$	3%–10%
LD$_5$	2%–12%

Abnormal values

Markedly increased: myocardial infarction, megaloblastic anemia, severe hypoxia.

Moderately increased: chronic myelocytic leukemia, hemolytic anemia.

Mildly increased: liver disease, hepatitis, hepatobiliary obstruction, cirrhosis, delirium tremens.

Cost $50–$75.

lactic acid (lactate)   Lactic acid is present in the blood as lactate. It is an intermediary product of carbohydrate metabolism derived from muscle cells and red blood cells. The enzyme lactic dehydrogenase (LDH) catalyzes the interconversion of lactate and pyruvate. During excercise, lactate increases, and LDH maintains the proper balance between lactate and pyruvate. Oxygen deprivation results in the blockage of metabolism of pyruvate and causes increased lactate levels (lactic acidosis). Untreated lactic acidosis leads to coma and death.

Patient preparation No special preparation is necessary. Hand clenching or any undue physical stress should be avoided.

Procedure Lactic acid is measured spectrophotometrically.

Specimen Whole blood (arterial or venous) or plasma. A gray-top tube with sodium fluoride as anticoagulant is used.

Reference range

Venous   4.5–19.8 mg/dL.
Arterial   4.5–14.4 mg/dL.

Abnormal values

Increased in: congestive heart failure, dehydration, hypoxia, poisoning, renal disease, shock, any disease that causes oxygen depletion in tissues.

Cost $45–$60.

lactogenic hormone   See *prolactin*.

lactose tolerance test   A clinical test for lactase deficiency in which 100 g of lactose (a disaccharide composed of glucose and galactose) is administered orally, and serum glucose is monitored. Lactose intolerance is presumed to exist if the glucose levels rise less than 20 mg/dL. Extreme lactose deficiency results in osmotic diarrhea.

Patient preparation The patient should fast for eight hours before testing. No gum chewing or smoking is allowed during the test.

Procedure A fasting glucose specimen is drawn. The 100 g of lactose is mixed with water or orange juice and consumed by the patient. Blood specimens are drawn 30, 60, 120, 180, and 240 minutes after the drink is consumed. These specimens are analyzed for glucose.

Specimen The samples are drawn in gray-top tubes containing oxalate and fluoride.

Reference range An increase in plasma glucose of greater than 20–30 mg/dL.

Abnormal values An increase in plasma glucose of less than 20 mg/dL over the fasting level, with symptoms, is considered abnormal and is evidence for lactase deficiency.

Cost $80–$100.

Comments A trial of withdrawal from lactose-containing food is advocated before the lactose tolerance test. This test may produce diarrhea and cramps.

LAP   See *leukocyte alkaline phosphatase*.

laparoscopy   The laparoscope is a small, flexible instrument equipped with an optical lens. It is used diagnostically to view various internal organs and obtain biopsies from the liver, ovaries, and elsewhere by inserting it through a small incision in the anterior abdominal wall. It can also be used therapeutically to perform procedures such as lysis of adhesions, tubal sterilization, remove foreign bodies, and to fulgurate implants of endometriosis. The test is used to aid in diagnosing the cause of pelvic pain, visualizing the liver, evaluating pelvic masses, and obtaining biopsy material. For most diagnostic and therapeutic uses, laparoscopy has replaced laparotomy. Laparotomy is reserved for instances when more extensive surgery is being considered.

Patient preparation This is an operative procedure and is generally carried out in a hospital setting.

Procedure This procedure is done under local or general anesthetic. It involves insufflating the peritoneal cavity with carbon dioxide or nitrous oxide to distend the abdominal wall and provide an organ-free space for insertion.

Cost $4000–$5000.

laryngeal electromyography   A technique analogous to conventional electromyography. It is used to differentiate nerve from muscle disorders, determine the site of a neurogenic lesion (i.e., upper vs. lower neurons), and to differentiate organic from functional defects. Laryngeal electromyography is used to evaluate patients with vocal cord dysfunction, including those with tremor, myoclonus, pyramidal and extrapyramidal disorders, and primary muscular disorders, allowing the delineation of specific (superior vs. recurrent laryngeal) nerve involvement and the provision of prognostic information.

laryngoscopy   The laryngoscope is a small, flexible fiberoptic tube similar in its basic design to other endoscopes. It is threaded down the throat and used to view laryngeal structures. The purpose of this procedure is to detect lesions, strictures, or foreign bodies in the larynx.

Patient preparation The patient is placed in a supine position or is sitting in a chair. The patient's throat and mouth are sprayed with local anesthetic; general anesthesia is rarely required.

Procedure The patient's head is positioned and held as the physician introduces the laryngoscope through the patient's mouth. The larynx is examined for abnormalities; tissues or secretions may be removed for further study. Minor surgery (e.g., removal of polyps or nodules) may be performed.

Cost $200–$400.

Comments Discomfort is common during the procedure.

laryngostroboscopy   A technique for examining the vocal fold's vibratory function and assessing the effectiveness of medical, surgical, and speech therapy. It is used to evaluate voice complaints in singers (e.g., vocal fold paralysis), dysphonia in the absence of obvious lesions, laryngeal lesions that result in a pathologic voice and to assess mucosal hygiene and provide feedback on the results of phonosurgery.

LATS   See *long-acting thyroid stimulator* in Glossary.

latex fixation test   See *latex agglutination test* in Glossary.

laxative screen (laxative survey)   A battery of tests performed in specialized reference laboratories using an array of diagnostic modalities (e.g., spectrophotometry and TLC of urine or stool supernatant) to identify anthraquinones, bisacodyl, phenophthalein, castor oil, mineral oil, magnesium, phosphate, and components of laxatives, which are commonly abused and thus need to be ruled out/in as a cause of chronic diarrhea.

LDL   See *low-density lipoprotein.*

LDL-cholesterol   Cholesterol that is carried in the circulation by LDL (low-density lipoprotein) which, when elevated, is a major risk factor for atherosclerosis. Until recently the only way of determining LDL-cholesterol in the clinical laboratory was with the Friedenwald calculation. The situation has changed with commercial availability of the LDL-DIRECT™.

LE cell preparation   A test used to evaluate autoimmune diseases, specifically systemic lupus erythematosus, which is useful in the diagnosis of "lupoid" hepatitis. Because antinuclear antibodies are of greater diagnostic utility, the less sensitive LE prep has been phased out, although it continues to be used by some physicians in diagnosing lupus erythematosus.
   Patient preparation No special preparation is required.
   Procedure Heparinized blood is gently agitated with glass beads, releasing neutrophil nuclei which are then incubated with antinuclear protein in the serum; the "glassy" appearance of LE bodies results from homogenization of the chromatin; these bodies are then phagocytosed by the remaining neutrophils.
   Specimen Whole blood. Heparin anticoagulated blood is the specimen of choice. EDTA anticoagulated blood may cause false-negative results.
   Reference range Not detected.
   Cost $25–$50.

lecithin:sphingomyelin ratio   See *L/S ratio.*

LEEP (loop electrosurgical excision procedure)   A recently introduced therapy for treating cervical and vulvar lesions that uses a high-frequency, low-voltage, alternating current that minimizes thermal damage while preserving good hemostatic properties; LEEPs are most commonly used to treat condylomas and cervical intraepithelial neoplasia (CIN) and are popular because they can be performed in an office setting with a lower equipment cost, minimal damage to surrounding tissue, and low comorbidity. See *cervical intraepithelial neoplasia, conization, HPV.*

leucine aminopeptidase   A liver enzyme that is increased in hepatobiliary disease but not in bone disease. Gamma-glutamyl transpeptidase (GGT) and 5-neucleotidase are more frequently used than leucine aminopeptidase. Leucine aminopeptidase has not proven to be a reliable marker or organ-specific disease and is not commonly requested.

Patient preparation No special preparation is required.

Procedure This enzyme is measured by spectrophotometric methods.

Specimen Serum, ascitic fluid.

Reference range 12–33 IU/L (method dependent, see laboratory reference range when comparing results).

Abnormal values

Increased in: biliary cirrhosis, obstructive jaundice, tumors metastatic to the liver, choledocholithiasis, pancreatic carcinoma, pancreatitis, third trimester of pregnancy.

Cost $50–$70.

Comments This test is not readily available; GGT and 5-NT are more commonly used in the evaluation of hepatobiliary disease.

leukocyte alkaline phosphatase See *neutrophil alkaline phosphatase.*

leukocyte count See *complete blood count.*

leukocyte migration inhibition assay See *macrophage migration inhibition test.*

LFT See *liver function test(s)* in Glossary.

LH See *luteinizing hormone.*

lipase (triacylglycerol acylhydrolase) A pancreatic enzyme that hydrolyses glycerol esters of long chain fatty acids. Pancreatic lipase cleaves the outer ester linkages of long chain fatty acids and is elevated only in pancreatitis (markedly so in acute pancreatitis) and pancreatic duct obstruction. Serum lipase is usually normal in patients with elevated serum amylase without pancreatitis and in those who have peptic ulcers, salivary adenitis, inflammatory bowel disease, intestinal obstruction, and macroamylasemia. Lipase and amylase are elevated in acute pancreatitis, but the elevation of lipase is more prolonged.

Patient preparation No special preparation is required.

Procedure Lipase is measured spectrophotometrically.

Specimen Serum; specimens from dialysis patients must be obtained prior to treatment.

Reference range Less than 200 units/L

Abnormal values

Increased in: pancreatitis, primary biliary cirrhosis, chronic renal failure.

Cost $30–$40.

Comments Lipase should be measured in conjunction with amylase for better diagnostic value.

lipids Dietary lipids are emulsified by bile and absorbed in the small intestine. Excessive excretion of lipids (steatorrhea) may occur with various digestive and absorptive disorders.

Patient preparation Patient must refrain from alcohol and maintain a high-fat diet for three days prior to collection.

Specimen 72-hour stool. Waxed collection containers should not be used; specimens must be kept refrigerated and tightly covered.

Reference range Less than 7g/24 hours

Abnormal values

> Increased in: pancreatic insufficiency, cystic fibrosis, chronic pancreatitis, pancreatic obstruction, hepatic disease, biliary obstruction, celiac disease, intestinal fistula, small intestine diverticula.

Cost

Qualitative	$40–$60.
Quantitative	$90–$110.

Comments Although the qualitative method can give an indication of steatorrhea, the quantitative method is more definitive.

lipoprotein electrophoresis Electrophoresis is a method by which large molecules are separated by electrical charge on a support medium. Lipoprotein electrophoresis is used to determine types of lipid patterns. Direct quantification of LDL, HDL, cholesterol, and triglycerides anticipate that lipoprotein electrophoresis will be "retired" as a diagnostic tool. The electrophoretic patterns obtained by lipoprotein electrophoresis are classified as phenotype I through V. The following is a list of the symptoms associated with each phenotype.

PHENOTYPE I Early vascular disease absent, abdominal pain, deficient lipoprotein lipase, eruptive xanthomas, lipemia retinalis.

PHENOTYPE II Early severe vascular disease, familial trait is autosomal-dominant, homozygotes are severely affected.

PHENOTYPE III Accelerated vascular disease, adult onset, diet, lipid-lowering drugs very effective, abnormal glucose tolerance.

PHENOTYPE IV Accelerated vascular disease, adult onset, weight loss lowers VLDL, high-fat diet may convert to type V.

PHENOTYPE V Abdominal pain, weight loss does not lower VLDL, pancreatitis, abnormal glucose tolerance, vascular disease not associated

Patient preparation Patient should fast for 12 hours prior to collection.

Procedure Electrophoresis.

Specimen Serum.

Reference range See laboratory report.

Cost $40–$50.

lithium Lithium carbonate is used to treat biploar (manic-depressive) disease by blocking neurotransmission in the brain. Levels must be carefully monitored as the difference between therapeutic and toxic range is very narrow.

Patient preparation No special preparation is required.

Procedure Lithium is measured using ion-selective electrodes that are specific for lithium.
Specimen Serum.
Reference range 0.6–1.2 mEq/L.
Abnormal values Greater than 1.5 mEq/L is toxic; above 4 mEq/L may be fatal.
Cost $40–$50.

loop-o-gram A radiocontrast study in which a catheter is introduced into an ileal conduit to evaluate the presence of residual or recurrent cancer of the transitional epithelium of the bladder. Ileal conduits are usually created surgically as a urinary diversion in patients who have had significant resections of the urinary bladder, e.g., for bladder cancer.

low-density lipoprotein (LDL) Ultracentrifugation and electrophoresis were, until recently, the only methods which could be used to directly measure LDL. The most common method for measuring LDL was a calculation based on the levels of cholesterol, HDL, and triglycerides. This calculation gives erroneous results if the triglyceride results are greater than 400 mg/dL. Recently a newer method which involves the differential extraction of the LDL-cholesterol from the other lipoprotein-cholesterol fractions.
Patient preparation No special preparation is required. However, if this is done as part of a lipid profile including triglycerides, a 12-hour fast is necessary.
Procedure Most laboratories utilize the differential separation of LDL-cholesterol spectrophotometrically on an automated chemistry analyzer.
Specimen Serum.
Reference range Results are generally reported as relative risk of coronary artery disease.

Less than 100 mg/dL	Normal risk.
100–130 mg/dL	Elevated risk.
Greater than 130 mg/dL	High risk.

Abnormal values Elevated levels of LDL-cholesterol (bad cholesterol) indicate risk of coronary and artery disease.
Cost $50–$70.

L/S ratio The ratio of lecithin (phosphatidyl choline) to sphingomyelin, a parameter used to determine infant lung maturity and predict the infant's ability to survive without developing respiratory distress. Surface-active lecithin appears in the amniotic fluid at 24–26 gestational weeks; sphingomyelin is similarly produced but remains relatively constant. Before the 32nd week, the L/S ratio is less than 1.5, but after the 34th week, the L/S ratio is more than than 2.0, which corresponds to an adequate level of surfactant for extra-uterine pulmonary function. L/S ratio may be determined by thin-layer chromatography and by two-dimensional chromatography, the latter of which has fewer false negatives. See *biophysical profile, lung profile.*

Patient preparation Preparation is the same as that for amniocentesis.
Procedure L/S ratio is determined by thin-layer chromatography.
Specimen Amniotic fluid.
Reference range Greater than 2.0 at 34 weeks.
Abnormal values Low levels at 34 weeks indicate high risk for respiratory distress syndrome.
Cost $75–$125.

lumbar puncture (spinal tap)   A diagnostic procedure in which a very long needle is inserted into the subarachnoid space between the third and fourth lumbar vertebrae in order to obtain cerebrospinal fluid (CSF). A lumbar puncture can be used to evaluate intracranial pressure.
Patient preparation Informed consent is required. If a clotting disorder is suspected, basic coagulation studies (e.g., platelet count, partial thromboplastin time, and plothrombin time) should be obtained.
Procedure The procedure is performed in the hospital at bedside. A long needle is inserted at the L4–L5 vertebral interspace and subarachnoid (cerebrospinal) fluid is obtained. The fluid is sent to the laboratory for analysis of chemistries (i.e., glucose, proteins), to microbiology for culture, and to pathology to evaluate the cells.
Specimen Cerebrospinal fluid.
Reference range No abnormalities.
Abnormal values Increased white blood cells indicate infection or malignancy. If meningitis is present, the white blood cells will be neutrophils (polymorpholnuclear leukocytes). If leukemia is present, white blood cells will be lymphocytes or abnormal granulocytes.
Cost $50–$150.

lumbar thermography   See *thermography* in Glossary.

lumpectomy (segmental mastectomy)   A cosmetically acceptable surgical procedure for excising breast cancer, which in early (less than 4.0 cm) breast carcinoma combined with radiotherapy offers a 90% five-year survival; some data suggest that a lumpectomy with axillary lymph node dissection may be as effective as a mastectomy in treating breast cancer. Because survival hinges on complete removal of the cancer, the pathologist's role is critical. If he or she finds cancer at the lumpectomy's margins, further and usually more aggressive therapy is required, usually in the form of higher doses of radiation or performance of a radical mastectomy.
Patient preparation Informed consent is required. It is common practice to include in the consent form permission for the surgeon to perform a more extensive procedure (e.g., a mastectomy) if the tumor is found to be extensive. Baseline coagulation studies (platelet count, partial thromboplastin time, and prothrombin time), complete blood count, and routine chemistries including electrolytes (potassium, sodium, calcium, bicarbonate) and glucose are obtained.

Procedure Most lumpectomies are performed under general anesthesia. The tissue is removed and sent to pathology for examination, which may include a frozen section examination. The tissue is also evaluated for the presence of estrogen and progesterone receptors.
Specimen Tissue.
Reference range A lumpectomy is only performed when the diagnosis of malignancy has been previously established.
Abnormal values Cancer. There are various types, including in situ, ductal, and lobular carcinoma.
Cost $1500–$3000. Surgeon, anesthesiologist, and hospital fees can substantially increase the costs.

lung profile A two-dimensional chromatograph from an acetone-precipitated lipid extract of bloody amniotic fluid. A lung profile allows determination of relative amounts of lecithin, sphingomyelin, phosphatidyl glycerol, phosphatidyl inositol and phosphatidyl serine (measured by densitometry after charring) and in experienced hands allows determination of fetal lung maturity; in the presence of phosphatidyl glycerol, neonatal respiratory distress syndrome does not occur. See *L/S ratio, pulmonary function test, organ panel* in Glossary.

lung volumes A group of air "compartments" into which the lung may be functionally divided into:
EXPIRATORY RESERVE CAPACITY The maximum volume of air that can be voluntarily exhaled.
FUNCTIONAL RESIDUAL CAPACITY Volume left in the lungs at the end of a normal breath which is not normally part of the subdivisions.
INSPIRATORY CAPACITY The maximum volume that can be inhaled.
INSPIRATORY RESERVE CAPACITY The maximum volume that can be inhaled above the tidal volume.
TIDAL VOLUME The normal to-and-fro respiratory exchange of 500 cc.; vital capacity is the maximum amount of exhalable air; after a full inspiration, which added to the residual volume, is the total lung capacity.
TOTAL LUNG CAPACITY The entire volume of the lung, circa 5 liters.
VITAL CAPACITY The maximum volume that can be inhaled and exhaled. See *pulmonary function test, spirometry.*

lupus anticoagulant (lupus inhibitor) A generic term for IgG or IgM class antibodies that arise spontaneously in patients with lupus erythematosus (LE) and are directed against various components of coagulation factors. While these antibodies produce in vitro interference with phospholipid-dependent coagulation, e.g., activated partial thromboplastin time (aPTT) and kaolin clotting time assays in specimens from patients with LE, they do not produce in vivo coagulopathy in the absence of other platelet defects or coagulation defects or in the presence of drug-induced antibodies. Lupus anticoagulants have also been identified in patients with HIV, deep vein thrombosis, and others. Lupus anticoagulants may be present if patient:control clotting time is 1.5 times normal at a dilution of 1:1000 and the altered aPTT is corrected by 1:1 mix with normal plasma. Lupus anticoagulants include anticardiolipin and other antiphospholipid antibodies. See *anticardiolipin antibodies*.

lupus erythematosus test   See *LE cell preparation*.

luteinizing hormone   (LH)   Luteinizing hormone is a glycoprotein hormone secreted by the anterior pituitary gland. In females, LH is secreted cyclically along with follicle-stimulating hormone (FSH). The cyclic release is responsible for ovulation and transforms the ovarian follicle into the corpus luteum, which produces progesterone and estrogens. In males, continuous release of LH stimulates the cells of the testes to release testosterone. LH levels are almost invariably requested with FSH to diagnose infertility in females. In males, LH controls the secretion of testosterone and is measured in a workup for testicular dysfunction. LH and FSH act in concert to stimulate and maintain spermatogenesis.

Patient preparation No special preparation is required.

Procedure LH is measured by RIA, EIA, or chemiluminescence.

Specimen Serum.

Reference range

Children	4–20 mIU/ml.
Adult male	7–24 mIU/ml.
Adult female	
Follicular phase	5–15 mIU/ml.
Midcycle	30–60 mIU/ml.
Luteal phase	5–15 mIU/ml.

Abnormal values

Increased in: castration, ovarian failure, postmenopausal.

Decreased in: hypogonadic states.

Cost $80–$90.

Comments LH is usually measured along with FSH and prolactin. All levels of these hormones must be evaluated in relation to the menstrual cycle to be of any value.

Lyme disease   Lyme disease is caused by *Borrelia burgdorferi*, a spirochete that is transmitted to humans via the deer tick *Ixodes dammini*. The disease responds to proper antibiotic therapy but can become chronic. There are three laboratory tests currently available for the diagnosis of Lyme disease: serology, Western blot, and PCR (polymerase chain reaction). The serologic test is the initial screening test used when Lyme disease is suspected or if a tick bite has been noted. The serologic tests measure antibodies (IgM and IgG) and are very sensitive but often false positive. The methods used include ELISA, immunofluorescence assay, solid-phase fluorescence immunoassay. Agreement among laboratories as to whether a subject has Lyme antibodies when tested by indirect fluorescent antibody (IFA) or

ELISA is low and lacks standardization. The Western blot test is a more specific test but is less sensitive and is used to confirm positive serologic tests. PCR is a new technology and is used primarily in difficult cases and in detecting the DNA of the spirochete in joint fluid or CSF. Nonspecific laboratory findings in Lyme disease include increased ESR, IgM, and cryoglobulins, decreased C3 and C4, and increased IgG and IgM antibody titers to *B. burgdorferi*. Histologic stains of involved tissue (Warthin-Starry and Dieterle) have a low diagnostic yield; definitive diagnosis requires identification of IgG antibodies to *B. recurrentis* by the Western immunoblot. The clinical findings in Lyme disease are divided into the following stages:

STAGE I. Rash stage, which presents as a solitary reddish papule and plaque with centrifugal expansion (up to 20 cm), peripheral induration, and central clearing, persisting for months to years.

STAGE II. Cardiovascular (myocarditis, pericarditis, transient atrioventricular block, ventricular dysfunction); neurological (Bell's palsy, meningoencephalitis, optic atrophy, polyneuritis) symptoms.

STAGE III. Migratory polyarthritis; Lyme disease may be accompanied by headache, stiff neck, fever, and malaise that subsequently manifest as migratory polyarthritis, intermittent oligoarthritis, chronic arthritis of the knees, chronic meningoencephalitis, cranial or peripheral neuropathy, migratory musculoskeletal pains, and cardiac abnormalities.

Patient preparation No special preparation is required.

Procedure Lyme testing is carried out by ELISA and confirmation is done by Western blot.

Specimen Serum.

Reference range Negative.

Abnormal values In a person with Lyme disease, the indirect fluorescence antibody screening test is positive. This must be confirmed by the Western blot method, which detects specific protein "bands." According to some experts, the diagnosis of Lyme disease requires that at least five of the ten bands be present in the patient's serum.

Cost

Lyme serology	$80–$100.
Western blot	$140–$170.
PCR	$240–$280.

Comments The serologic test and Western blot both differentiate the acute phase antibodies (IgM) from the chronic phase antibodies (IgG). The PCR test detects the DNA of the spirochete directly. It is the last test used because it is difficult and expensive.

lymphangiography Lymphangiography consists of a radiologic examination of the lymphatic system in which an oil-based radiocontrast medium is injected into the foot or hand. The feet are used to examine the lymphatic circulation of the legs, inguinal and iliac regions, and retroperitoneum to the thoracic duct. Injection into the hands allows the visualization of the axillary and supraclavicular lymphatic circulation and lymph nodes. Lymphangiography is used primarily to diagnose and monitor treatment of lymphomas.

Patient preparation The injection site is sterilized with alcohol and other antiseptics.

Procedure The oil-based radiocontrast medium is injected into the prepared foot or hand veins. Fluoroscopy is used to monitor the filling of the lymphatic vessels.

Abnormal values Insufficient or incomplete filling of lymph nodes suggest the presence of obstruction, often in the form of lymphomas or other lymphatic or metastatic tumors.

Comments The patient may experience tenderness at the injection site. The patient should be assessed for signs of hypersensitivity reactions during the procedure. If it is done as an outpatient procedure, the patient should be accompanied by a friend or relative.

lymphocyte proliferation test See *mitogenic assay.*

lymphocyte typing (T and B cells) Lymphocytes can be separated into two basic classes of cells: T cells (helper or suppressor lymphocytes) and B cells. These cells are intimately involved in the immune response to foreign antigens such as bacteria, viruses, and nonhomogenic proteins. The laboratory can quantify various antigenic markers on the cells using monoclonal antibodies and flow cytometry. The data resulting from these studies can be used to measure and monitor immune dysfunction. T and B cell studies provide a means of monitoring the effectiveness of therapy used in AIDS patients which is often empirical. Many types of leukemia can be specifically diagnosed by determining lymphocyte markers, resulting in more effective use of chemotherapy. These tests are relatively expensive and are used mainly after a presumptive diagnosis has been made.

Patient preparation No special preparation is required.

Procedure Flow cytometry is used to measure T and B cells.

Specimen Whole blood (using heparin as the anticoagulant). The specimens must remain at room temperature. Tests can also be carried out on tissue specimens such as bone marrow.

Cost $90–$600 depending on the extensiveness of the test battery.

Comments There is no universal menu of testing. Each laboratory performs markers in groups of panels designed to give the most information using the minimum number of markers.

lymphocytotoxicity assay A complement-mediated assay commonly used in HLA (human leukocyte antigen) typing laboratories. This assay tests for the presence of cytotoxic antibodies in the serum of the potential recipient that are capable of reacting with the lymphocytes of the potential donor. See *mixed lymphocyte culture.*

lysozyme (muramidase) A low-molecular weight enzyme that is present in a wide variety of body fluids, particularly in tears and salivary glands.

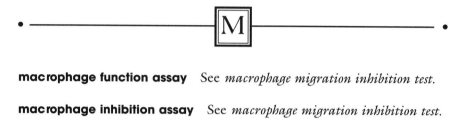

macrophage function assay   See *macrophage migration inhibition test.*

macrophage inhibition assay   See *macrophage migration inhibition test.*

macrophage migration inhibition test (macrophage inhibition assay, migration inhibition assay, leukocyte migration inhibition test)   A test that is based on the observation that normal lymphocytes produce immune-enhancing factors known as lymphokines (MIF) monocyte/macrophage inhibitory factor and (LIF) leukocyte inhibitory factor after lymphocytes have been stimulated with common antigens to which they have been exposed or "sensitized." Although this correlates well with immune competence and is one of the best tests for delayed type hypersensitivity, it is subjective, poorly standardized, and used primarily in research. With availability of ELISA tests, DNA analysis, and cell surface markers, this test has been largely abandoned.

Patient preparation No preparation is required, other than for drawing blood or obtaining tissue from the spleen or lymph nodes.

Procedure Lymphocytes are washed and separated from the plasma by centrifugation and exposed to the mitogens/antigens (e.g., streptokinase-streptodornase, *Candida* antigen, PPD, concanavalin A, phytohemagglutinin, pokeweed mitogen). Migration inhibitory factor (MIF) is then assayed using guinea pig macrophages or human monocytes. The fluid above the lymphocytes is used to determine the inhibition of migration on a sample of macrophages that have not been previously stimulated.

Specimen Whole blood drawn in yellow-top or green-top tubes. The test must usually be scheduled in advance.

Reference range Less than 15% inhibition of migration.

Abnormal values Greater than 20% inhibition of macrophage migration is abnormal in various immunodeficiency states, e.g., AIDS, DiGeorge syndrome, Wiskott-Aldrich syndrome, and others.

Cost $150–$250.

magnesium (Mg⁺⁺)   An intracellular ion required for many metabolic processes that involve carbohydrates, proteins, and nucleic acids. When magnesium is bound to the high-energy compound known as ATP, it acts as a cofactor in enzymatic reactions and is important in neuromuscular activity. Magnesium levels may be requested in patients with malabsorption, patients on low-protein, low-calorie diets, or patients with dehydration and renal failure.

Patient preparation No preparation is required, other than for drawing blood or obtaining urine.

Procedure Magnesium is measured by atomic absorption spectrophotometry.

Specimen Serum, urine.

Reference range

Serum	1.5–2.3 mg/dl.
Urine	7.3–12.2 mg/dl.

Abnormal values

Decreased in: alcohol abuse, burns (severe), dehydration, diabetic ketoacidosis, diarrhea, hyperaldosteronism (primary aldosteronism) hypercalcemia, hypokalemia hypoparathyroidism, post-bowel resection, malabsorption, malnutrition, pancreatitis (acute) renal insufficiency, drugs (e.g., amphotericin B, calcium gluconate, diuretics, insulin, neomycin).

Increased in: adrenocortical insufficiency (Addison's disease), diabetes mellitus (uncontrolled), leukemia, hypothyroidism, renal failure, therapy with magnesium-based antacids and laxatives.

Cost $30–$40.

magnetic resonance imaging See *MRI.*

major crossmatch A test used in the blood bank, which consists of placing a sample of a blood donor's red blood cells in a test tube with a sample of the patient's serum to detect the presence of antibodies. If the patient has antibodies that react against the donor cells, they are incompatible in terms of their blood groups. This could result in a major hemolytic transfusion reaction, in which the donor's red blood cells are destroyed in the patient, who might die from the reaction. A minor crossmatch consists of testing the patient's red blood cells against a potential donor's serum to detect the presence of incompatibility of the ABO blood group and other major antigenic groups.

Patient preparation No preparation is required, other than for drawing blood.

Procedure The procedure consists of mixing red blood cells from the donor with serum from the recipient in a test tube.

Specimen Blood collected in a red-top tube.

Reference range No incompatibility.

Abnormal values Agglutination or clumping of cells in the test tube indicates a mismatch between the serum of the recipient (or donor) and the red blood cells of the donor (or recipient).

Cost $45–$65.

malaria Malaria is one of the most common infectious diseases in the world. In developed nations, malaria is rarely seen except in immigrants or people who have traveled to malaria-endemic countries. Its parasite is transmitted to humans through the bite of the *Anopheles* mosquito. There are four species of malarial parasites: *Plasmodium falciparum*, also known as malignant malaria, is the most dangerous; *P. vivax, P. ovale,* and *P. malariae* are less lethal. The parasites migrate into the blood in two- to three-day cycles. When the parasites and other related debris burst from the red blood cells, the patient develops a fever. The diagnosis of malaria is most easily made from microscopic examination of bloodsmears obtained at the onset of symptoms. Proper therapy depends upon identification of the specific type of malaria parasite.

Patient preparation No preparation is required, other than for drawing blood.

Procedure The procedure consists of examining a "thick" smear of peripheral blood by light microscopy for the presence of plasmodial parasites.

Specimen Fresh EDTA-anticoagulated blood. Blood smears must be prepared quickly for optimal resolution.

Reference range No abnormalities are seen.

Abnormal findings The parasites may have banana-like and ring-like shapes when examined by microscopy.

Cost $40–$60.

malathion See *insecticide poisoning.*

malonate test A color test that evelutes the ability of bacteria to use malonate as a source of carbon. The test can differentiate among the coliform bacteria, which belong to the *Enterobacteriaceae* family and may cause gastroenteritis and upper respiratory tract infections.

Patient preparation No preparation is required, other than for obtaining urine, stool cultures, a throat swab, or sputum.

Procedure The specimen is placed in a test tube filled with malonate broth, and the presence of color changes are evaluated.

Specimen Urine, stool, throat swab, sputum.

Reference range The fluid in the tube remains green.

Abnormal values The fluid turns blue in the presence of *Klebsiella pneumoniae.*

Cost $25–$45.

mammography The radiologic examinaton of the breast using a device designed specifically for obtaining images of the breast. Mammography is the single best noninvasive procedure for detecting breast cancer. The false-negative rate is 10%–15%. The radiation dose during the usual mammographic study is 0.025–0.035 rem, which is very low, and thought by experts to be of little long-term significance. The American Cancer Society and the National Cancer Institute have recommended regular self-examination of the female breast after age 20, a baseline mammogram between ages 35 and 40, and annual or biennial mammograms thereafter. The frequency with which mammograms should be obtained is a function of the individual's relative risk factors for breast cancer (e.g., first-degree relative with breast cancer, African-American, and late age of first pregnancy). After age 50, annual screening mammography has been recommended; 24% of biopsies of nonpalpable breast masses with calcification have breast cancer. See *breast biopsy, cancer screen, lumpectomy*.

Patient preparation The patient should not use perfume, powder, or deodorant in the region before the procedure. Mammography is more difficult in obese patients.

Procedure The procedure consists of obtaining a radiologic image of each breast by compressing it between a film/screen cassette plate, and a mobile plastic compression paddle.

Reference range The normal breast has a dark gray radiologic appearance which corresponds to fat; it is punctuated by whitish areas and bands which correspond to fibrous and glandular tissues.

Abnormal values The most characteristic mammographic finding in cancer is the presence of finely-stippled microcalcifications, which appear as white dots between the size of a pinhead and a pencil point. Suspicious geographic-shaped densities are also characteristic of cancer in a mammogram. Other findings are thought to be less reliable.

Cost $75–$100.

Comments A consensus development panel, convened in 1997 by the National Institutes of Health, reached the controversial conclusion that not every woman in her 40s should undergo routine mammographic screening.

manganese A mineral present in trace amounts in several enzymes (e.g., arginase and cholinesterase), which is ingested in the diet with unrefined grains, leafy green vegetables, and nuts. Toxic levels are the result of industrial exposure to manganese-laden fumes and dusts in the manufacture of steel and dry cell batteries.

Patient preparation No preparation is required, other than for drawing blood.

Procedure Manganese is measured by atomic absorption spectrophotometry.

Specimen Serum, urine collected in a metal-free container, hair.

Reference range
 Serum 0.04–1.4 µg/dl.
 Urine Less than 2.0 µg/L.

Abnormal values
 Serum Greater than 0.10 µg/dL.
 Urine Greater than 10 µg/L.

Cost Blood $140–$160; urine $70–$90.

Mantoux test A test used to diagnose tuberculosis, based on hypersensitivity to tuberculin, a concentrated preparation of the tuberculosis antigen known as PPD (purified protein derivative).

Patient preparation No preparation is required, other than a small injection.

Procedure A short needle is used to inject PPD in the superficial skin. The immune response to the injected tuberculin is interpreted between 48 and 72 hours by a physician or other health professional.

Reference range An increased firmness of less than 10 millimeters at the site of injection is interpreted as negative.

Abnormal values An increased firmness of greater than 20 millimeters in diameter at the site of injection is positive.

Cost $15–$25.

Comments True negatives mean that the individual does not have tuberculosis. False-negative results may occur in patients with AIDS, sarcoidosis, viral infection, steroid therapy, and defects in the immune system. See *prick test.*

marijuana ("pot," "weed")   The leaves from the hemp plant *Cannabis sativa,* which are smoked, producing a hallucinogenic effect due to neurochemical Δ^9-tetrahydrocannabinol (THC). Marijuana is inhaled differently than tobacco, in order to maximize THC absorption and elicit the desired "high." The subject prolongs inhalation, markedly increasing carbon monoxide and tar levels. Most testing for marijuana is done for legal reasons, such as the testing of employees or impaired drivers suspected of using marijuana or other substances of abuse.

Patient preparation No preparation is required, other than for obtaining urine.

Procedure Various laboratory methods can be used to identify THC, including enzyme immunoassay and thin-layer chromatography.

Specimen Urine.

Reference range Negative.

Abnormal values THC and its breakdown products are detectable in the urine as early as one hour after smoking and for up to 72 hours or more.

Cost $40–$60.

match test   A simple screening test of the lung's exhaling capacity and expiratory airway obstruction, in which a lighted match is held at 10 to 15 cm from the open mouth. Failure to blow out the match after six attempts indicates a maximum breathing capacity below 40 liters/minute and a maximum midexpiratory flow rate of less than 0.6 liters/second. Patients with advanced emphysema often fail the match test. See *pulmonary function test.*

maturation index (squamous cell index)   A crude technique used to evaluate a woman's hormonal status, which is based on the ratio of the three major covering (epithelial) cells, the parabasal, intermediate, and superficial squames seen on a Pap smear. Among the patterns seen in the maturation index are the progesterone, midcycle, ovulation, and primary amenorrhea patterns. It is absolutely reliable in only two situations: marked estrogen effect, as seen in normal menstruating women, and complete absence of estrogen, as seen in postmenopausal women. The maturation index cannot be evaluated in cervical inflammation, drugs that alter squamous maturation, (e.g., tetracycline, digitalis, thyroid hormone), and local surgery, including conization. Because the woman's hormonal status can now be far more easily and accurately determined by directly measuring the serum levels of progesterone, estrogen, luteinizing hormone, and follicle-stimulating hormone, the maturation index has waned in popularity. See *acetowhite lesion, colposcopy.*

maximum acid output (MAO) A measurement of the maximal amount of hydrogen ions that can be secreted by the stomach. The MAO is defined as the sum of four 15-minute acid outputs, after either pentagastrin or histamine stimulation. The MAO reflects the number of acid-secreting cells that are present in a person's stomach and is a function of the person's sex, body weight, lean body mass, and age. MAO is markedly increased in the Zollinger-Ellison syndrome and conditions of increased gastrin production. MAO is measured from the gastric juice and ranges from 5–40 mEq/hour (5–40 mmol of titratable acid/hour). See *pentagastrin test, secretin injection test.*

maximum breathing capacity See *maximum voluntary ventilation.*

maximum voluntary ventilation (maximum breathing capacity) A clinical test that is a nonspecific indicator of the function of a person's airways, lung tissue, thoracic cage, and respiratory muscles. It is used to evaluate preoperative pulmonary function, pulmonary disability, and prediction of ventilatory reserve, it is commonly decreased in smokers. The MVV test induces a sharp decrease in carbon dioxide (hypocapnia) and alkalosis, which often causes dizziness and lightheadedness.
  Patient preparation The patient should not eat three hours before the test.
  Procedure The patient breathes the maximum possible number of times in a determined period of time; a spirometer measures the volume of ventilation in liters per minute.
  Specimen The respiratory rates should be consistently between 90 and 120 breaths per minute, and measured for 10 to 15 seconds.
  Reference range The MVV should be greater than 80% of that predicted for the person's age.
  Abnormal values The severity of breathing impairment is mild if the MVV is 65%–80% of that predicted for age, moderate if 50%–64%, severe if 35%–49%, and intense if less than 34%.
  Cost $200–300. See *pulmonary function test.*

MBC See *minimum bactericidal concentration* in Glossary.

MCH See *mean cell (corpuscular) hemoglobin.*

MCHC See *mean cell hemoglobin concentration.*

mean cell (corpuscular) hemoglobin (MCH) A measurement of the amount of hemoglobin in an individual red blood cell.

Patient preparation No preparation is required, other than for drawing blood.

Procedure The MCH is measured by an automated hematology analyzer, e.g., a Coulter counter.

Specimen Blood.

Reference range 26–34 pg per red blood cell.

Abnormal values The MCH is decreased in microcytic anemia, which is often caused by iron deficiency. The MCH is increased in macrocytic anemia, e.g., megaloblastic anemia, which is due to vitamin B_{12} or folic acid deficiency.

Cost The MCH is performed as part of a routine CBC and is not billed separately. The cost of a CBC ranges from $15 to $35. See *complete blood count, red cell indices.*

mean cell hemoglobin concentration (MCHC)   A value that is derived on automated red blood cell counters.

Patient preparation No preparation is required, other than for drawing blood.

Procedure The MCHC is measured by an automated hematology analyzer, e.g., a Coulter counter.

Specimen Blood.

Reference range 31–36 g/dL.

Abnormal values The MCHC is decreased in microcytic anemia, which is often caused by iron deficiency. The MCHC is normal or decreased in macrocytic anemia, e.g., megaloblastic anemia, which is usually due to vitamin B_{12} or folic acid deficiency.

Cost The MCHC is performed as part of a routine CBC and is not billed separately. The cost of a CBC ranges from $15 to $35. See *complete blood count, red cell indices.*

mean cell volume (MCV)   A calculated value for the average volume of peripheral red blood cells.

Patient preparation None other than that for drawing blood.

Procedure The information needed to calculate the MCV is produced by an automated hematology analyzer, e.g., a Coulter counter.

Specimen Blood.

Reference range 80–100 femtoliter/cell.

Abnormal values The MCV is decreased in microcytic anemia, which is often caused by iron deficiency; it is increased in macrocytic anemia, e.g., megaloblastic anemia, which is usually due to vitamin B_{12} or folic acid deficiency.

Cost The MCV is performed as part of a routine CBC and is not billed separately. The cost of a CBC ranges from $15 to $35. See *complete blood count, red cell indices.*

measles (rubeola)   An extremely contagious viral infection, which is characterized by high fever, lethargy, cough, conjunctivitis, coryza, and a maculopapular rash. Measles is primarily a disease of children; it is prevented by proper vaccination. Because the virus is airborne, it spreads rapidly among schoolchildren. The diagnosis of measles is usually established by its typical clinical history and epidemiologic evidence (i.e., if other children have the same complaints), or less commonly by direct microscopic examination of the cells obtained from a scraping of the oral cavity.

Patient preparation No preparation is required; measles is a clinical diagnosis but may be confirmed by scrapings or cells from the oral cavity.

Specimen Cells from mouth.

Reference range The cells from the mouth are unremarkable by microscopy.

Abnormal values Microscopy reveals typical "giant" cells. The cells can also be examined for these changes by fluorescence microscopy. White blood cells, especially the lymphocytes, are often decreased. There is also an increased immunoglobulin M (IgM) antibody against measles in the acute phase of disease. As it resolves, the IgM falls and the immunoglobulin G rises, indicating the presence of a protective immune response.

Cost $50–$75.

mediastinoscopy   An invasive surgical procedure in which a flexible endoscope is inserted into the superior mediastinum through a hole in the chest wall, and the regional structures (lungs, lymph nodes, pericardium) are examined visually to detect the presence of masses, neoplasms, or other lesions. If structural abnormalites are identified, they are biopsied and sent to a laboratory to determine whether the tissue is benign or malignant and if the patient requires further therapy. Mediastinoscopy is also performed as part of a "staging procedure" when the patient is known to have a malignancy. In such cases, it is used to determine how far the tumor has spread, which will determine the type of therapy recommended by the oncologist.

Patient preparation Food cannot be ingested eight hours before the procedure. Mediastinoscopy is a moderately invasive procedure, which can be performed under local anesthesia. Informed consent and hospital admission are required. Before the procedure, oral intake should be limited to clear liquids, and baseline coagulation studies, platelet count, potassium level, X ray(s), and an electrocardiogram should be in the chart. Vital signs should be documented. Full emergency equipment (e.g., defibrillator, intubation devices, epinephrine, atropine, antiarrhythmic agents, and oxygen) should be available, and a thoracic surgery team should be notified.

Procedure The procedure consists of the insertion of a flexible endoscope, which has a central channel that allows the obtention of masses or lesions to be biopsied.

Specimen Small tissue fragments.

Reference range The normal mediastinum has no visible lesions.

Abnormal values Fresh blood and inflammatory or malignant masses may be seen.

Cost $500–3000. See *endoscopy*.

melena See *occult blood testing*.

mercaptoethanol agglutination inhibition test A laboratory test used to separate IgG from IgM as the cause of an agglutination reaction. When a person is exposed to a bacteria or virus, the immune system responds by producing immunoglobulins, which are at first relatively nonspecific and often immunoglobulin M; if the infection is chronic, the IgG is more elevated than the IgM. Treating IgM antibodies with mercaptoethanol abolishes its agglutination reaction and ability to bind complement.

Patient preparation No preparation is required, other than for drawing blood.

Procedure The test is based on 2-mercaptoethanol's ability to disrupt IgM molecules. The patient's serum is incubated with 2-mercaptoethanol, and the intensity of the agglutination reaction is measured.

Specimen Serum.

Cost No cost associated with this test, because it is a necessary component when performing immunoelectrophoresis.

mercury A highly toxic heavy metal that is used in a wide range of household products (e.g., as a fungicide in latex paints) and can be absorbed through the skin, or by the lungs when vaporized. Inorganic mercury may cause nausea, diarrhea, and renal toxicity. Organic mercury causes neuromuscular changes in the form of loss of coordination, muscle pain, and behavior that suggests mental disorders (the name "mad hatter disease" was coined because those who made felt hats suffered long-term exposure to mercury and were often "mad").

Patient preparation No preparation is required, other than for drawing blood.

Procedure Mercury can be identified by a simple "spot" test and quantified by using the technique of atomic absorption spectrophotometry.

Specimen Whole blood collected in a heavy, metal-free EDTA container. 24–hour urine collected in an acid-washed plastic container.

Reference range

Blood	0.02–0.08 µg/ml.
Urine	10–50 µg/24 hrs.

Abnormal values

Blood	Greater than 0.1 µg/ml.
Urine	Greater than 100 µg/24 hrs.

Cost $95–110.

Comments Mercury preparations used in health care have minimal toxicity, and mercury-based agents used in diuretics, topical antiseptics, and dental amalgams are thought to be relatively safe. The practice of removing dental amalgams as suggested by some practitioners of alternative medicine is believed by toxicologists to cause a marked short-term increase in a person's mercury levels and is not recommended by mainstream physicians or dentists.

metabisulfite test A laboratory screening test for sickle cell anemia, which primarily affects blacks, but is also rarely seen in those whose ancestors originated in the Mediterranean.

Patient preparation No preparation is required, other than for drawing blood.

Procedure Sodium metabisulfite, a reducing agent, is added to a sample of blood.

Specimen Blood.

Reference range The red blood cells do not change shape.

Abnormal values When exposed to the reduced oxygen environment induced by metabisulfite, red blood cells with a high content of hemoglobin S (which is responsible for sickle cell anemia), hemoglobin C Harlem, and hemoglobin I will change from the usual rounded discoid shape to crescent-shaped or sickled red blood cells.

Cost $25–$50.

metanephrines (urine) Any of a number of breakdown products of exogenous or endogenous catecholamines, which are small molecules known as neurotransmitters. Metanephrines are increased in certain relatively uncommon tumors.

Patient preparation The specimen should be collected with the patient at rest and, if possible, not currently receiving any medications.

Procedure The specimen is determined by the Pisano method which detects color changes after processing the specimen.

Specimen Urine collected for 24 hours in a bottle that has a small amount of acid in it.

Reference range Adults 0.25–0.8 mg/day or 0.05–1.20 µg/mg of creatinine.

Abnormal values

  Increased in: neuroblastoma, which is most common in children, pheochomocytoma, stress, sepsis. Falsely increased metanephrines may be due to high dietary intake of bananas, coffee, tea, chocolate, drugs (e.g., chlopromazine, corticosteroids, L-dopa, dopamine, hydralazine, imipramine, nalidixic acids, phenobarbital, phenyle phrine, tetracycline). Falsely decreased metanephrines may be due to drugs (e.g., clonidine, guanethidine, propranolol, reserpine, theophylline).

Cost $110–$130.

Comments Measurement of total metanephrines provides the highest number of true positive results for pheochromocytoma and is a "first choice" screening test. Positive results should be confirmed with urinary catecholamine fractionation. See *catecholamines.*

methanol (methyl alcohol, wood alcohol) A highly toxic alcohol used as an industrial solvent and in canned fuel and antifreeze. It may be used like ethanol (the usual drinking alcohol) as an inebrient by indigent alcoholics. It is metabolized to produce formaldehyde and formate, which cause the blood to become more acid. This may damage the optic nerve and cause blindness.

Patient preparation No preparation is required, other than for drawing the appropriate specimen.

Procedure Methanol can be detected by color changes and measured by gas-liquid chromatography.

Specimen Serum, plasma, urine, gastric juice. The containers must be kept tightly sealed.

Reference range Negative.

Abnormal values Serum concentrations of greater than 200 mg/L are toxic.

Cost $70–$75.

Comments The ingestion of as little as 15 milliliters has been fatal.

methotrexate (MTX)   A widely used but toxic anti-tumor drug, which may be used alone to cure certain malignancies or in combination with other agents to treat leukemias; lymphomas; head, neck, ovarian, and small-cell carcinomas; osteosarcoma; and medulloblastoma. It may also be used to treat nonmalignant conditions, e.g., recalcitrant ("stubborn") psoriasis, rheumatoid arthritis, and graft-versus-host disease, which occurs in patients who have received organ transplants. Methotrexate may interfere with aspirin, sulfonamides, phenytoin, ethanol, and anticoagulants. It requires careful calculation of dosage given its toxic side effects, which include nausea, vomiting, anorexia, inflammation of the mouth, stomatitis, central nervous system changes, hypersensitivity, hepatocellular damage, ocular irritation, and nephrotoxicity. Dose-limiting myelotoxicity may appear shortly after beginning therapy.

Patient preparation No preparation is required, other than for drawing blood.

Procedure Methotrexate is measured by enzyme-linked immunoassay, radioimmunoassay, and high-performance liquid chromatography.

Specimen Serum, plasma.

Reference range The therapeutic concentrations are variable.

Abnormal values Greater than 9.1 ng/ml, or 454 ng/ml 48 hours after high-dose therapy.

Cost $70–$90.

metyrapone test   A diagnostic tool used by endocrinologists to evaluate the hypothalamus-pituitary-adrenal "axis," particularly defects in pituitary gland activity. Metyrapone decreases the negative feedback of ACTH synthesis by the pituitary gland. The patient's adrenals must be able to respond to ACTH.

Patient preparation Steroids, if being administered, should be discontinued before the test.

Procedure Metyrapone is administered the night before the specimen is collected. 11-deoxycortisol and cortisol are measured in a specimen collected in the morning.

Reference range 11-deoxycortisol is increased to more than 7 mg/dl. Cortisol is decreased to less than 10mg/dl.

Abnormal values The metyrapone test is used to identify Cushing's syndrome, adrenal cortical tumors, and ectopic ACTH syndrome, especially when an excess of corticosteroids may be due to internal production by tumors.
Cost $130–$150.
Comments This test should not be performed in patients with adrenal insufficiency, as it further decreases the levels of steroids.

MHPG   See *catecholamines, metanephrines (urine).*

MIC   See *minimum inhibitory concentration* in Glossary.

microhematuria   See *microscopic hematuria* in Glossary.

MIF test   See *macrophage migration inhibition test.*

milk intolerance   See *lactose tolerance test.*

mini-mental test   A brief and simplified clinical test of a person's mental status. Each correct answer in the following series of questions is given one point for a total score of 30.
ORIENTATION IN TIME Year, season, month, date, day—total 5 points.
ORIENTATION IN SPACE Country, state, county, town, place, hospital ward—5 points.
COGNITION Serial sevens (x 5) or spell "world" backwards—5 points.
SHORT RECALL Name three objects—total 3 points.
MEMORY Rename three above objects—3 points.
FOLLOW A THREE-PART COMMAND Take a paper, fold it, put it on the floor—3 points.
COMMON OBJECT RECOGNITION Name two familiar objects—2 points.
RECOGNITION OF COMMON PHRASE "No ifs, ands, or buts"—1 point.
READ AND OBEY Close your eyes—1 point.
WRITE SIMPLE SENTENCE—1 point.
COPY DRAWING Intersecting pentagons—1 point.
A person with a change in mental status and a score of greater than 27 points most often has affective depression. Patients who are depressed and have cognitive impairment have scores of about 20 and those with true dementia often have scores of less than 10.
Cost $50–$75.

Minnesota Multiphasic Personality Inventory (MMPI)   A true-false test for evaluating an individual's psychological and personality "profile," which is widely used both in the United States and internationally. The MMPI consists of more than 500 questions administered to those over age 15, which are used to stratify 14 personalities from "social" to schizophrenic. One recently proposed revision divides the MMPI into a validity scale and a clinical scale. The validity scale has four parameters and measures the individual's willingness to complete the test, ability to read, and psychological defense behavior. The clinical scale has ten parameters and measures various abnormal psychological tendencies (depression, sexual orientation, hypochondriasis, hypomania, hysteria, introversion, paranoia, anxiety, psychopathy, and schizophrenia). See *psychological test.*

Cost $50–$75.

Comments When the MMPI was created in the 1930s, the average United States citizen was 35 years old, married, lived in a small town, had eight years of general schooling, and was employed in a skilled or semiskilled trade. Since that time, developed countries have changed considerably. As an example, discrimination based on race, religion, sex, age, sexual orientation, and presence of mental or physical handicaps, have all but disappeared as part of governmental policy. It is clear that revisions of the MMPI need to reflect societal norms.

mirror image biopsy   A biopsy of the opposite breast when lobular carcinoma-in-situ is found in one breast. This procedure is most often performed as a means of excluding the presence of invasive carcinoma.

Patient preparation The preparation is for that of any biopsy of the external surface of the body. The patient may require a tranquilizer.

Procedure The procedure consists of one or more "passes" of a 14-gauge biopsy needle to obtain tissue that will be examined by a pathologist.

Specimen Tissue.

Reference range No malignancy.

Abnormal values Malignancy or premalignant lesions.

Cost $250–$300.

Comments Lobular carcinoma-in-situ is associated with a ±1% annual risk of malignant degeneration, which requires close follow-up. See *breast biopsy, lumpectomy, mammography.*

mite   See *scabies.*

mitogenic assay   (blastogenesis assay, lymphocyte proliferation assay, lymphocyte proliferation test)   A test of the ability of lymphocytes to respond to nonspecific stimulators of the immune system (mitogens), specific antigens, foreign cells, or microorganisms. Mitogenic assays are usually performed in a research setting. Clinical testing of a person's immune responsiveness is based on the ability to respond to PPD and other antigens, which are injected into the skin surface.

Patient preparation No preparation is required, other than for drawing blood.

Procedure Lymphocytes respond to stimuli (e.g., concanavalin A, phytohemagglutinin, pokeweed mitogen, PPD (the substance used in testing for tuberculosis), *Candida* antigen, and others by dividing. Immune responsiveness can be measured by co-incubating the lymphocytes with radioactively labeled thymidine). The resulting value can be compared to a duplicate "run" of cells that were not stimulated, yielding a stimulation ratio.

Specimen Blood.
Reference range The patient's lymphocytes respond to the immune stimulation by dividing.
Abnormal values The patient's lymphocytes do not respond to the stimulation.
Cost $225–$250.

mixed lymphocyte culture reaction A test of cell-mediated immunity which is used to obtain the closest possible match between a donated organ and the recipient's immune system. The closer the match is to the recipient's immune system, the less likely is the possibility that the donated organ will be rejected after transplantation. The mixed lymphocyte reaction serves to predict the development of the rejection reaction known as graft-versus-host disease.
Patient preparation No preparation is required, other than for drawing blood.
Procedure The donor lymphocytes are "paralyzed" by irradiation, which prevents them from dividing, so that the only cell capable of dividing is the recipient's CD4 (helper) T cell. If the T cell converts to a more primitive form—known as blast transformation—there is a significant immunologic difference between the two cells, which is more intense as the antigenic difference between the individuals increases. The intensity of the blast transformation is measured by the degree to which transformed cells incorporate radiolabeled carbon or hydrogen. MLC is also used to diagnose T-cell immunodeficiency.
Specimen Blood.
Reference range The less the immunologic diffferences between the patient and potential tissue donor, the less cell division (proliferation) will occur.
Abnormal values The greater the immune diffferences between the patient's and potential tissue donor's cells, the more proliferation will occur.
Cost $150–$200.

M-mode echocardiography (unidimensional echocardiography) A technique of ultrasonography that analyzes the heart in motion. The technique provides both high spatial and temporal (time-related) resolution and is used to measure the thickness of the walls of the heart and the volumes of the heart chambers.
Patient preparation No preparation is required.
Procedure The procedure consists of placing a part of the ultrasound device, the transducer, over the region of the heart and registering the echos on a strip recorder, a video recorder, or a printer.
Reference range The normal values on M-mode echocardiography are found in tables used by the cardiologist or clinician.
Abnormal values The type of defect found by M-mode echocardiography is based on comparison of the patient's findings with those of standardized

individuals. M-mode echocardiography is abnormal in left ventricular hypertrophy or dysfunction, intracardiac tumors (most of which are benign), pericardial effusion, and mitral valve stenosis or prolapse.
Cost $175–$250.

MMPI   See *Minnesota Multiphasic Personality Inventory.*

Monospot test   A simple test that detects the presence of heterophil antibodies (antibodies in one species of animal that agglutinate the red blood cells of certain other species of animals), which are typical of Epstein-Barr virus infection.
Patient preparation No preparation is required, other than for drawing blood.
Procedure In the Monospot test, the patient's serum is mixed with red blood cells from a guinea pig (which contain the Forssman antigen), a cow (which contain infectious mononucleosis antigen), and a horse (which contain both).
Specimen Serum.
Reference range Heterophile antibody titers (levels) of less than 1:128.
Abnormal values Heterophile antibody titers (levels) of greater than 1:256. The Monospot test is abnormal in infectious mononucleosis, Epstein-Barr virus infection, chronic fatigue syndrome, Burkitt's lymphoma, and occasionally in hepatitis.
Cost $20–$30.
Comments There are specific ELISA tests for EBV infections, which should be used to confirm a positive Monospot test.

morphine   See *narcotics testing.*

motor development testing   Motor development is the acquisition and coordination of muscle-related activity. Motor development testing consists of a series of measurements used by pediatricians to track an infant or child's physical development. It is based on a child having passed certain so-called developmental milestones, e.g., hopping on one foot without falling by age 4, and others, e.g., Bayley Scale of Infant Development, Gesell Developmental Schedule.

MRI (magnetic resonance imaging)   A noninvasive diagnostic technique that is based on fundamental principles of physics. The hydrogen ions (protons) in the human body are subjected to a highly controlled, high-intensity radiofrequency magnetic field. The person's hydrogen ions respond by emitting a radiofrequency signal that is then processed by computer to produce an image on film or videotape. MRI became widely available for clinical use in the early 1980s, and for many body regions, in particular the brain and musculoskeletal system, has become the diagnostic imaging method of choice.

MRI has the following advantages over computed tomographic imaging:
1. It does not produce ionizing radiation.
2. The difference between normal and pathological tissue is greater.
3. Confusing bone artifacts do not occur.
4. Rapidly moving components appear dark, and blood flow through large vessels can be analyzed as a type of natural contrast.

MRI is well studied and provides diagnostically superior images of the abdomen, blood vessels, bone, brain, chest, extremities, heart, joints, musculoskeletal system, nerve roots, spinal cord, and spinal canal.

Patient preparation The patient must be able to lie quietly, and all metal objects must be removed.

Procedure Images are obtained by passing the patient through a tubular device that generates a powerful electromagnetic field. Radiofrequency waves are transmitted into the patient in a highly controlled manner. The patient's hydrogen ions (protons) emit radiofrequency signals that are processed by the computer to produce the image on film, a method similar to other techniques interpreted by radiologists.

Reference range No structural abnormalties are identified.

Abnormal values MRI is used to identify abnormalties in the form of tumors, malformations, and collections of fluid.

Cost $900–$1200.

Comments MRI is contraindicated in morbid obesity (i.e., weight of over 300 pounds), pregnancy, claustrophobia, clinical unstability (i.e., a patient who requires continued life support and equipment that cannot be used in the MRI suite), presence of any implanted metal (e.g., pacemaker, aneurysmal clips, inner ear implants, scrapnel or bullet fragments) which may dislodge as a projectile and/or cause considerable distortion in the image.

MRI coronary angiography (MRCA)   A form of MRI that is useful in identifying clinically important narrowing of the coronary arteries. With standard MRI techniques, the images of the coronary arteries appear "fuzzy," due to respiratory and cardiac movements, and they are limited to the segments of the coronary arteries nearest to the aorta. In MRCA, the image is obtained while the patient holds his breath, which reduces the respiratory "noise," and the effect on the image caused by the heart's movement is minimized by obtaining the image during mid-diastole. MRCA provides a new approach for evaluating coronary artery patency and may be combined with MR perfusing imaging and anatomic or functional MRI to provide a comprehensive cardiac profile. See *MRI.*

mucin clot test (string test)   A bedside test for determining the viscosity of synovial fluid or "quality" of the mucin clot in synovial fluid.

Patient preparation No preparation is required, other than for aspirating fluid from a joint.

Procedure A few drops of synovial fluid are added to dilute acetic acid

(2%–5%) and the length of the "strand" formed between drops of fluid is measured.

Specimen Synovial fluid.

Reference range The further a drop of synovial fluid falls before separating ("stringing effect"), the greater the fluid's viscosity and the closer it is to normal.

Abnormal values A decrease in the strand length implies deterioration due to inflammatory (e.g., sepsis, gout, rheumatoid arthritis), but not degenerative joint disease.

Cost $35–$50.

Comments The mucin clot test seldom leads to changes in diagnosis, treatment, or patient outcome. Essentially the same information may be obtained from measurement of the synovial fluid viscosity. The mucin clot test is of questionable value and can be eliminated from "routine" synovial fluid analysis. See *synovial fluid analysis.*

MUGA Multiple gated acquisition scan. See *multigated equilibrium heart scan.*

multigated equilibrium heart scan (MUGA) A technique used in cardiology to evaluate the heart's ability to respond to physical stress. A radiopharmaceutical (e.g., 99m-technetium pertechnate) is used to radiolabel either red blood cells or albumin, both of which circulate freely in the bloodstream.

Patient preparation No preparation is required. All laboratory tests that will be performed by radioimmunoassay must be performed before MUGA, because a radioactive agent is injected into the bloodstream that would interfere with the laboratory tests.

Procedure After the red blood cells or albumin are labeled with the radiopharmaceutical, multiple images of the heart are acquired in synchrony with specific intervals of the electrocardiogram. These images can be linked together to produce a "movie" of the movement of the heart wall and to calculate the volume in each pumping stroke (ejection fraction) of the heart.

Reference range MUGA can be used to evaluate the functional status of the heart at rest and in response to exercise.

Abnormal values MUGA can be used to determine the functional impact of coronary artery disease, congestive heart failure, various cardiomyopathies, and cardiotoxic drugs.

Cost $300–$400.

multiphasic screening Any of a number of low-cost tests that identify potentially treatable diseases, most of which can be performed on minimal amounts of blood. The typical multiphasic screen includes a laboratory component, which identifies abnormalities that are specific for common diseases, such as diabetes mellitus (glucose greater than 130 mg/dl), coronary artery disease (cholesterol greater than 200 mg/dl), and prostate cancer (prostate-specific antigen or PSA greater than 4 ng/mL. Multiphasic screening often contains a clinical component, which identifies hypertension by measuring the blood pressure (greater than 160 mm Hg systolic pressure and greater than 90 mm Hg diastolic pressure). Multiphasic screening may be used at health fairs to provide inexpensive tests to large populations that may not regularly visit a physician. There may be a physician available at such fairs to counsel anyone with abnormal results.

Patient preparation No preparation is required, other than for drawing blood.

Procedure The tests are run on any of a number of "bench-top" instruments.

Specimen Blood.

Reference range The normal result for each measured substance is found in this book under the individual test names.

Cost The cost depends on the number of tests being performed. The average is $20 per test.

multiple puncture test A general term for any of a number of tests for sensitivity to tuberculin, in which the test material is introduced with multiple needles or tines, e.g., tine test, Heaf test, and others. Improved reproducibility of the results of a single puncture tuberculin (Mantoux) test has made it the preferred method, and multiple puncture tests have passed into history.

multiple test panel See *profile* in Glossary.

muramidase See *lysozyme*.

muscle biopsy A biopsy obtained from muscle of patients who have symptoms thought to be related to neuromuscular disorders. The muscle biopsy is intended to evaluate primary (e.g., dystrophies, myopathies) or secondary (e.g., drug-related, endocrine, neurologic) muscle disorders or systemic disease (e.g., vasculitis).

Patient preparation Any biopsy is painful, but muscle biopsies may be more painful, as they need to be relatively large (up to one cm in length) to provide adequate diagnostic information. The muscle needs to be rested after the procedure for adequate healing.

Procedure For optimal evaluation, muscle biopies require special handling, which includes stretching the muscle between forceps and transporting it without fixative, usually in physiologic saline, followed by fixation with formalin. It is then processed like other biopsies. A slide of the tissue is made, stained, and then analyzed by a pathologist. A wide range of special studies can be performed on a properly obtained muscle biopsy, including biochemical analysis, electron microscopy, histochemistry, immunohisto-chemistry, and various molecular tests. The site selected for the muscle biopsy is critical; it must be known to be involved, but not so much so that only end-stage changes are seen. The preferred method of obtention is to use a clamp to stretch the biopsied muscle which is then transported on a saline-soaked gauze at "refrigerator" temperatures.

Specimen Muscle.

Reference range A normal "checkerboard" pattern of so-called type 1 and type 2 muscle fibers.

Abnormal values Diseased muscle often loses the normal "checkerboard" pattern and undergoes a "grouping" of muscle fibers. Muscle biopsies are useful in the diagnosis of inflammation (myositis), degenerative disease (Duchenne's muscular dystrophy), or conditions induced by exogenous toxins (e.g., alcohol-induced polymyopathy).

Cost $300–$400.

Comments Most pathologists see very few biopies of muscle tissue in practice, and often send them to other pathologists who are known in the field for their expertise in the diagnosis of muscle pathology.

Mycobacterium The genus *Mycobacterium* contains many species of bacteria, the most well known of which is *M. tuberculosis,* which causes tuberculosis and continues to be a major cause of health problems throughout the world. Another *Mycobacterium* of importance is *M. leprae* which causes leprosy (Hansen's disease). The other species of *Mycobacterium* were thought until recently to be relatively benign. The use of chemotherapeutic (for cancer) and immunosuppressive drugs (for transplantation), along with the appearance of AIDS, have provided the other *Mycobacterium* species with opportunities to cause severe infections in immunocompromised patients.

Patient preparation No preparation is required, other than for obtaining the specimen.

Procedure The specimen is placed in the appropriate culture plate and grown for four to six weeks. In the last few years, major advances have been made in the clinical laboratory, particularly in the ability to detect specific DNA or RNA fragments that can be measured easily, reducing the time for positive identification of *M. tuberculosis* from its former turnaround time of six weeks. In 1996, a new PCR (polymer chain reaction) method became available that can give a positive result for *M. tuberculosis* in 24 hours. Although PCR for diagnosing tuberculosis is more expensive, this cost is more than offset by the public health benefits of rapid diagnosis.

Specimen Sputum, body fluids, urine.

Reference range No growth.

Abnormal values Positive identification of *M. tuberculosis.*

Cost

Culture	$85–$150, depending on the specimen's source.
Polymerase chain reaction	$150–$200.
Antibiotic sensitivity	$85–$100.

Comments Identification of *M. tuberculosis* is made difficult by its slow growth.

Mycoplasma A genus of small infectious organisms that infect epithelial cells and cause "walking pneumonia" (which resolves in four to six weeks) and genitourinary infections. *M. pneumonia* may be identified by hemadsorption and complement fixation. *M. hominis* may cause pelvic inflammatory disease, septicemia, and urogenital infection.

Patient preparation No preparation is required, other than for drawing the appropriate specimen.

Procedure The diagnosis of *Mycoplasma* infection can be made by complement fixation, enzyme immunoassays, and immunofluorescence.

Specimen Serum for antibody detection; two specimens are required—from the acute period and from the recovery (convalescent) period, obtained three weeks apart. For culture, throat, or nasal swabs.

Reference range

    IgG   Less than 1:16 is negative.

    IgM   Less than 1:16 is negative.

Abnormal values In practice, the diagnosis of *Mycoplasma* infection is made based on a four-fold increase in titer when two (or more) specimens have been obtained from the patient on different occasions, or a single titer of greater than 1:256. Culturing is not usually performed to establish the diagnosis of mycoplasma infection because of the long (two- to three-week) incubation period.

Cost

    Culture $95–$105.

    Serology $75–$85 per specimen. See *titer* in Glossary.

myelin-associated glycoprotein antibody (MAG) MAG is a component of the myelin of central and peripheral nervous systems. Antibodies to MAG have been associated with a number of neurologic conditions.

Patient preparation No preparation is required, other than for drawing blood.

Procedure The procedure consists of an immune (antibody-antigen) reaction.

Specimen Serum.

Reference range No antibodies detected.

Abnormal values Antibodies (titers of 1:16 or greater) to MAG are detected in 50% of patients with IgM paraproteinemia, peripheral neuropathy, multiple sclerosis, Guillain-Barre syndrome, chronic polyneuropathy, and myasthenia gravis. The clinical utility of MAG antibody assays is uncertain.

Cost $250–$270.

myelin basic protein A protein that is a major component of myelin, a lipoprotein that develops late in the development of the embryo. In adults, an elevation of myelin basic protein in the serum occurs in multiple sclerosis and indicates active destruction of myelin. Some patients with multiple sclerosis will have normal values, especially during remissions. This test is used to monitor disease activity rather than establish the diagnosis of multiple sclerosis.

Patient preparation No preparation is required, other than for drawing blood.

Procedure Myelin basic protein is measured by radioimmunoassay.

Specimen Cerebrospinal fluid.

Reference range Less than 4 ng/ml is negative; i.e., there is no active demyelination.

Abnormal values Above 6 ng/ml is consistent with active demyelination.

Cost $75–$100.

myelography A radiologic technique for examining the spinal canal, in particular the lumbar region, by the percutaneous injection of a water-soluble radiocontrast material into the subarachnoid space through a lumbar puncture. Myelography is used to evaluate spinal cord defects due to compression of the spinal cord and/or its roots by a herniated disk, degenerative articular lesions, trauma, outline tumors or other masses of the spinal cord or meninges or metastases, multiple sclerosis, or increased intracranial pressure.

Patient preparation Formal written consent is required, as myelography is an invasive procedure. Bleeding defects must be corrected before the procedure. No food should be ingested two to four hours before the procedure.

Procedure The procedure consists of the insertion of a long spinal needle through which a radiocontrast is injected. The images are obtained by fluoroscopy and x rays, using a tilting table.

Reference range Normally, the spinal canal is a narrow space with no zones of widening or constriction.

Abnormal values The spinal canal may be widened or narrowed, depending on the disease.

Cost $200–$300.

Comments Complications include meningitis, infection, hemorrhage, nausea and vomiting, herniation of the brain, seizures, and allergic reaction to the radiocontrast. With the advent of MRI, myelography is performed with decreasing frequency.

myocardial infarction imaging A noninvasive method for identifying the location and extent of a myocardial infarct, which is based on the pooling of a radiopharmaceutical. This pooling results in a "hot spot" in the infarcted region of the heart when an image is captured with a gamma (scintillation) camera.

Patient preparation No preparation is required; any laboratory tests that will be performed by radioimmunoassay must be performed before myocardial infarction scanning because a radioactive agent injected into the bloodstream would interfere with the laboratory tests.

Procedure The patient is injected with the radiopharmaceutical (e.g., ^{99m}Tc pyrophosphate) which localizes to the region of the myocardial infarct (dead heart tissue).

Reference range Normally, the ^{99m}Tc pyrophosphate passes to bone and does not linger in the heart.

Abnormal values If the ^{99m}Tc pyrophosphate is concentrated in the heart, then an infarction has occurred. The amount of tissue death or infarction is determined by visually comparing the intensity of the radioactivity of the heart tissue to that of the ribs, which normally pick up the ^{99m}Tc pyrophosphate.

Cost $200–$300.

Comments Synonyms include acute myocardial infarction scan, infarct-avid scan, (myocardial) infarct imaging, PYP cardiac scan, pyrophosphate cardiac scan.

myocardial perfusion imaging   See *thallium stress test.*

myocardial perfusion scan   See *thallium stress test.*

myoglobin   A protein present in muscle that binds reversibly with oxygen. It makes oxygen available to tissues as needed during exercise or other muscle activity. Myoglobin is increased in muscular dystrophy, inflammation, ischemia, or trauma of the muscle, as well as in myocardial infarction and malignant hyperthermia.

Patient preparation The patient should be well rested; strenuous exercise increases myoglobin in the urine and circulation.

Procedure Myoglobin is measured in the serum and in urine by nephelometry, immunoassay, electrophoresis, and colorimetry. ELISA is the most commonly used methodology.

Specimen Serum, (random) urine.

Reference range 30–70 µg/L in serum; less than 5.0 mg/dL in urine.

Abnormal values

Increased in: connective tissue disease (e.g., polymyositis, dermatomyositis), hereditary (e.g., paroxysmal myoglobinuria, malignant hyperthermia, phosphorylase deficiency [McArdle's disease, a.k.a. glycogen storage disease type V], periodic paralysis), infection (e.g., viral [Epstein-Barr, influenza, herpes] or bacterial [Legionnaire's disease]), toxic (e.g., acute alcohol intoxication, phencyclidine [PCP, a.k.a. angel dust], carbon monoxide, ethylene glycol, insect venom, some diuretics), trauma and/or ischemia (e.g., intense and prolonged exercise, extreme hyperthermia, seizures, infarction due to vascular occlusion, crush injury, heat cramps).

Cost Serum $80–$110; urine $70–$80.

myoglobinuria   The presence of myoglobin in the urine. See *myoglobin.*

myography   See *electromyography.*

Nagler's reaction   A test used in microbiology to identify *Clostridium per-fringens*, in which blood is placed on an agar plate that has zones with and without antitoxin. *C. perfringes* is presumed to be present if precipitation occurs in the zone without the antitoxin.

nailfold capillary microscopy (widefield capillary microscopy)   A technique used to evaluate finger nailfold capillaries, using a wide-angle microscope. Abnormalities such as enlargement, increased tortuosity, or reduction in the number of capillaries are common findings in some of the so-called connective tissue diseases, a family of conditions that are often treated by rheumatologists. Nailfold capillary microscopy is indicated in patients with Raynaud's phenomenon, scleroderma (to evaluate the extent of visceral involvement), mixed connective tissue disease, dermatomyositis, and systemic lupus erythematosus.

narcotics testing   Narcotics are substances that cause euphoria and analgesia at the desired abuse levels, physical dependence, central nervous system depression, stupor, coma, or death when administered in excess. Narcotics may be natural products extracted from the poppy plant—yielding morphine and heroin—or from the coca plant—yielding cocaine and crack; semisynthetic products with opiate activity, such as meperidine and methadone, or synthetics; or from the umbrella grouping of narcotic alkaloids, such as LSD, mescalin, barbiturates, alcohol, marijuana, cocaine, hallucinogens, and stimulants, such as antidepressants. The term *narcotics* also includes completely synthetic products such as fentanyl. Identification of narcotics and other drugs of abuse in a patient takes two completely distinct forms, either as a drug screen for emergencies or for forensic purposes, where a criminal act may be attributed to a substance of abuse. In the former, the physicians need to identify the drug causing a particular reaction in the patient, who may be in an excited state, confused, or requiring treatment. Forensic testing for substances of abuse and narcotics requires considerably more caution, as the specimen must follow a "chain of custody," which means that the specimen should be obtained under direct supervision, and each step in the "chain" from the patient to a verified laboratory result must be documented.

Patient preparation No preparation is required for drug screening, other than for drawing blood or obtaining urine. For forensic testing, the specimens must be handled through a "chain of custody."

Procedure In screening for narcotics, the first specimen is obtained in urine. These substances can be measured by thin-layer chromatography and by enzyme immunoassays. Confirmation of the presence of narcotics, required for medical legal purposes, requires more sophisticated methods, including gas chromatography–mass spectrometry and high-performance liquid chromatography.

Specimen Serum, urine.

Reference range Negative for narcotics.

Abnormal values Any finding of narcotics is abnormal.

Cost $25–$100. The cost depends on the extent of the screening procedure and whether there is a positive finding. See *drug of abuse* in Glossary, *drug screening*.

narcotics screen See *drug screening*.

nasal endoscopy (rhinolaryngoscopy, rhinopharyngoscopy, rhinoscopy) The use of a flexible fiberoptic endoscope to evaluate the upper airways (nasal passages, nasopharynx, oropharynx, and larynx), a procedure that is usually carried out by an ears, nose, and throat specialist or an allergist. Nasal endoscopy is indicated for upper airway disease of unknown cause, chronic or recurring upper airway disease that persists despite adequate therapy, epiglottitis, laryngeal trauma, and to determine the cause of stridor, which in children may be due to foreign objects, and in adults may be due to tumors.

Patient preparation Some physicians require formal (written) consent for the procedure, while others consider nasal endoscopy to be an extension of the normal examination. Aspirin and nonsteroidal anti-inflammatory drugs (e.g., ibuprofen) should be discontinued prior to the procedure, if significant bleeding is anticipated.

Procedure The procedure consists of the insertion of a flexible fiberoptic endoscope, allowing direct examination of the nasal passages, upper airway structures, and throat.

Specimen A biopsy may be obtained, although most changes seen by nasal endoscopy can be diagnosed clinically, i.e., without a tissue diagnosis.

Reference range Negative for any changes.

Abnormal values

Nose	Nasal polyps, vascular defects, inflammation.
Upper pharynx	Ulcers, lymphoid hyperplasia, cysts.
Lower pharynx	Lymphoid hyperplasia, cysts, vocal cord trauma.

Cost $300–$600.

Comments Although nasal endoscopy is a low-risk procedure, complications may rarely occur in the form of bleeding, bronchospasm, laryngospasm, cardiac arrhythmias (due to vasovagal stimulation).

nearsightedness See *vision testing.*

needle aspiration cytology A diagnostic preparation of cells obtained from a clinically or radiologically identified mass, using a thin ("skinny") needle to spread the material on a glass.
Patient preparation The procedure requires informed consent. The patient should not eat anything within four hours of the procedure.
Procedure The procedure consists of the insertion of a long 22-gauge needle, guided by fluoroscopy, ultrasound, or computed tomography, into a previously identified mass. Once material is obtained, the cells and debris are either smeared on a slide or placed in a solution, and a "cell block" is prepared. The cells are then placed on a glass slide, stained, and interpreted by a pathologist under a microscope.
Specimen Cells and debris.
Reference range The cells seen in a normal smear are relatively scant and typical of the site from which the material came.
Abnormal values In well-trained hands, aspiration cytology specimens have a 90% sensitivity and 95% specificity for diagnosing thyroid and breast masses as benign or malignant. The procedure is helpful when positive, but requires further diagnostic procedures when negative.
Cost $100–$200.
Comments Complications include fainting (vasovagal responses), infection, hematomas, and hemorrhage. Rarely, tumor cells may spread along the needle tract.

needle biopsy A diagnostic preparation that in principle is the same as that of aspiration cytology, but because of the larger bore needle (19 gauge), has greater yields of architecturally intact tissue, with a higher diagnostic success rate. CT-guided transthoracic needle biopsies are used for lesions less than 2.0 cm in diameter, while lesions larger than 2.0 cm are best diagnosed by fibroptic bronchoscopy if the mass can be reached by the bronchoscope. Despite the small size of the material obtained, needle biopsies may be analyzed by the techniques of immunohistochemistry, cell culture, electron and immunofluorescence microscopy, receptor analysis, in situ hybridization, and PCR (polymerase chain reaction) and can be cultured for organisms.
Patient preparation The procedure requires informed consent. The patient should not eat anything four hours before the procedure and should undergo coagulation screening with a platelet count, partial thromboplastin time, and prothrombin time to detect any defects in clotting. An intravenous line is placed to allow administration of sedatives, if necessary.
Procedure The procedure consists of the insertion of a long 19-gauge needle, guided by fluoroscopy, ultrasound, or computed tomography, into a

previously identified mass. Once the material is obtained, the tissue is placed in formalin and processed like any biopsy. If the material is extremely scant in nature, a "cell block" of the material is prepared. The cells are then placed on a glass slide, stained, and interpreted by a pathologist under a microscope.
Specimen Tissue.
Reference range Negative.
Abnormal values Inflammation, malignancy, infection.
Cost $100–$200. See *needle aspiration cytology*.

Neisseria gonorrhoeae A bacteria that is a major cause of sexually trans-mitted infections in the United States and Europe. *N. gonorrhoeae* infections may remain undetected in asymptomatic cases and, if untreated, can result in infertility and severe urogenital complications, e.g., obstruction of the fal-lopian tubes. Until recently, culturing of *N. gonorrhoeae* in the microbiolo-gy laboratory was the standard means of identifying gonorrhea. As with most organisms, cultures require several days to become positive, and because *N. gonorrhoeae* is a delicate organism, it may not survive the transit from the patient to the culture plate, resulting in a high false-negative rate due to improper transportation of the specimen. Some immunologic tests may be used for screening, but positive results must be confirmed by cul-ture. Recently, DNA probe technology has been developed that can detect the organism more accurately than culture. The DNA probe methodology has become routine in most clinical laboratories, and both chlamydia and gonorrhea can be detected in the same specimen.

Patient preparation The patient should not have urinated for one hour prior to collection of the specimen.
Procedure For men, the urethra is sampled by rotating the swab 2–3 cm into the urethra. For women, there are two swabs in the kit; the first is used to clean the area. The second swab is inserted 2–3 cm into the endo-cervix and then rotated to collect the epithelial cells from the potentially infected site.
Specimen A swab specimen from the genitourinary region of a male (ure-thral swab) or female (cervical swab) patient. Special transport media is required for either culture (JEMBEC) or DNA probe (GenProbe). Other sites from which *N. gonorrhoeae* can be obtained include the throat and various sites of infection or abscesses. There are now several methods avail-able to detect *N. gonorrhoeae*'s DNA. This makes screening in males much easier. Because of the cost of these newer techniques, they are not yet widely used in clinical laboratories.
Reference range Negative for *N. gonorrhoeae*.
Abnormal values The finding of *N. gonorrhoeae* in any body site is a patho-logic finding that requires therapy.
Cost

Culture	$30–$40.
DNA probe	$45–$55.

Comments *Neisseria gonorrhoeae* is occasionally identified in child abuse cases, a finding that can be confirmed by use of the DNA probe.

neonatal screen Any of a number of low-cost tests performed on newborn infants to identify potentially treatable diseases, most of which can be performed on minimal amounts of blood or urine.

Patient preparation No preparation is required, other than for drawing blood (which can be a difficult exercise in children) or obtaining urine.

Procedure Neonatal screening procedures include the use of reagent strips (e.g., Chemstrip) for infants at increased risk for hypoglycemia; measurement of hematocrit for infants with risk factors for, or symptoms of, various conditions including anemia or polycythemia; serologic test for syphilis; and state board of health mandated tests. Infants of Rh-negative or blood group O mothers should have their blood typed and both a direct and indirect Coombs test on the cord blood. Repeat screening is recommended at one week. The neonatal screen is accompanied by a clinical examination of the infant to identify physical deformities that may require either close attention or therapy (e.g., congenital dislocation of the hip).

Specimen Serum, urine, blood.

Reference range The results of all tests should be within normal limits.

Abnormal values The neonatal screen is designed to identify hypoglycemia, anemia (including sickle cell anemia), polycythemia, syphilis, cystic fibrosis, galactosemia, homocystinuria, hypothyroidism, maple syrup urine disease, and phenylketonuria

Cost $25–$100, depending on the extent of the testing.

neoplasm panel A battery of tests that is considered to be the most cost-efficient means of identifying a malignancy of unknown origin. The panel includes measurement of acid phosphatase, alkaline phosphatase, alpha-fetoprotein (AFP), carcinoembryonic antigen (CEA), chorionic gonadotrophic hormone, and lactate dehydrogenase. Because of the low diagnostic yield of these assays, chemical "cancer screens" have little role in the early diagnosis of malignancy and, when negative, introduce a false sense of security that malignancy is not present. Because of the low diagnostic sensitivity, these panels are not usually used in low-risk situations.

Patient preparation No preparation is required, other than for drawing blood.

Procedure Most of these tests are performed by ELISA.

Specimen Serum.

Reference range Negative.

Abnormal values Any out-of-range laboratory finding when coupled with clinical features, e.g., smoking history, first-degree relative with breast cancer, mammographic findings suggestive of a lesion, should be followed by a more aggressive workup.

Cost $150–$250.

Comments The only test with a proven record in terms of screening for the presence of malignancy is prostate-specific antigen. Some other "markers," such as carcinoembryonic antigen and alphafetoprotein, have proven to be relatively useful.

neostigmine test A clinical test consisting of the administration of neostig-mine methylsulfate, an agent that intensifies the symptoms of myasthenia gravis. The test is performed in individuals who are suspected of suffering from myasthenia gravis but for whom the Tensilon (edrophonium) test is negative.

Patient preparation Because of neostigmine's muscarinic effects (e.g., ven-tricular fibrillation and cardiac arrest), atropine should be adminstered both before, and be available during, performance of this test.

Procedure In myasthenia gravis, neostigmine improves muscle contractility, which is seen in 10 to 15 minutes and peaks at 30 minutes.

Reference range An objective improvement in muscle contractility.

Abnormal values If the patient does not have visible improvement in mus-cle contractility, myasthenia gravis is virtually excluded from diagnostic consideration.

Cost This is a test most often performed in a hospital setting and has a wide range of fees. See *Tensilon test.*

nephrolithiasis See *kidney stone analysis.*

nerve biopsy A biopsy used to evaluate primary or secondary neuropathies or systemic disease (e.g., amyloidosis). A wide range of special studies can be performed on a properly obtained nerve biopsy, including biochemical analysis, electron microscopy, histology, immunohistochemistry, various molecular studies, and virology. The site selected for the nerve biopsy is crit-ical and should come from an area of active disease. Once obtained, the tis-sue must be transported as quickly as possible to the laboratory.

Patient preparation Any biopsy is painful, but nerve biopsies may be par-ticularly painful, as they need to be relatively large (up to one inch in length) to provide adequate diagnostic information. The nerve requires rest after the procedure for adequate healing.

Procedure A section of nerve—the sural nerve is preferred by some neurol-ogists—is excised, sometimes in combination with a muscle biopsy.

Specimen Nerve.

Reference range Negative.

Abnormal values The nerve is often abnormal in chronic asymmetric mononeuropathies, including amyloidosis, angiitis, leprosy, and sarcoido-sis. Except for certain conditions, e.g., metachromatic leukodystrophy and giant axonal neuropathy, nerve biopsy is relatively useless in polyneu-ropathies.

Cost $300–$400.

Comments Most of the changes seen in diseased nerve tissue are inflamma-tory, and relatively straightforward diagnoses. Nonetheless, nerve biopsies are not commonly seen in practice, and a pathologist may prefer to send the tissue to another pathologist known in the field for his expertise.

nerve conduction study A noninvasive method for assessing a nerve's ability to carry a neural impulse and its speed of transmission. In these studies, larger peripheral motor and sensory nerves are electrically stimulated at various intervals along a motor nerve.

Patient preparation No special preparation is required beyond obtaining informed consent. The test is usually well tolerated, although it has the unpleasantness of any test that requires the insertion of a needle.

Procedure Two round metal plates are placed on the skin at a distance from each other. An electrical stimulus passes through one plate and causes the nerve to fire, resulting in a "compound" muscle action potential. The resulting response is displayed on an oscilloscope and may be photographed and/or stored on disk or another magnetic storage medium.

Reference range The maximum (normal) velocity for peripheral nerves requires complete myelination and is between 40 and 80 meters/seconds.

Abnormal values The nerve conduction velocity is often normal in certain neuromuscular diseases, including primary muscle disease, radiculopathies, axonal type neuropathies, anterior horn cell disease, and in early peripheral nerve disease. Nerve conduction may be less than one-half normal in segmental demyelination, as occurs in polyneuropathy, e.g., in Charcot-Marie-Tooth disease, diabetic neuropathy, Guillain-Barré syndrome, diphtheria, and metachromatic leukodystrophy. Entrapment syndromes (e.g., carpal tunnel, tarsal tunnel, and thoracic outlet) result in localized slowing of conduction. Motor nerve conduction studies allow a separation between peripheral nerve or muscle disease and those due to defects of the anterior horn cells by measuring the resulting muscle twitch/action, the so-called M response.

Cost $50–$60. See *electromyography*.

neurologic examination A battery of clinical tests that evaluates a person's neurologic function and mental status. A complete neurologic examination is intended to detect the presence of structural (organic) lesions that may cause changes in neurologic function.

Procedure The clinical tests include:

HISTORY Patient's chief complaint.

MENTAL STATUS Coherency, memory, judgement, comprehension, and other cognitive processes.

CRANIAL NERVES

1. Olfactory (1st cranial nerve) Ability to identify common odors.
2. Optic nerve (2nd cranial nerve) Visual acuity, visual fields, pupil size and response to light, optic examination.
3. Ocular muscles (3rd, 4th, 6th cranial nerves).
4. Trigeminal nerve (5th cranial nerve).
5. Facial nerve (7th cranial nerve).
6. Auditory nerve (Rinne and Weber tests, 8th cranial nerve).
7. Glossopharyngeal (9th cranial nerve) and vagal nerve (10th cranial nerve).

8. Accessory nerve (11th cranial nerve).

9. Hypoglossal nerve (12th cranial nerve).

MOTOR FUNCTION

1. Upper extremities: Finger-to-nose test, extension-flexion of elbow, power of grip, reflexes (e.g., biceps, brachioradialis), sensation (e.g., vibration, pain).

2. Lower extremities: Heel-to-knee test.

Reference range Negative for neurologic abnormalities.

Abnormal values Any abnormality identified by a neurological examination requires further evaluation.

Cost $250–$350. See *psychiatric interview* in Glossary.

neuron-specific enolase (NSE) A form of an enzyme that is produced by neurons and neuroendocrine cells of the central and peripheral nervous systems. NSE is a useful marker for malignancies, as it may be elevated in certain tumors, e.g., medullary carcinoma of the thyroid, neuroblastoma, pheochromocytoma, carcinoid, and small cell carcinomas, especially of the lungs. However, the high rate of false-positive and false-negative results with serum NSE have made it of relatively little use in the diagnosis of tumors.

Patient preparation No preparation is required, other than for drawing blood.

Procedure NSE can be measured by immunohistochemistry.

Specimen Serum.

Reference range Less than 20 ng/ml.

Abnormal values Greater than 20 ng/ml.

Cost $85–$100.

Comments Direct staining of tissues with monoclonal antibodies to neuron-specific enolase has proven useful to pathologists in the evaluation of neuroendocrine tumors.

neutralization test A general term for any test in which a substance (e.g., antiserum, antitoxin, chelator, or other neutralizing agent) is used to block the properties—usually pathogenic—of a microorganism or its products, or of a toxin. An example of a neutralization assay is the Schick test for diphtheria, which is performed on the skin.

neutrophil alkaline phosphatase (leukocyte alkaline phosphatase, LAP, NAP) An enzyme that is concentrated in granules of normal neutrophils. The NAP stain is used most often to differentiate chronic myelogenous leukemia from other disorders that increase the white blood cell count.

Patient preparation No preparation is required, other than for drawing blood.

Procedure The slides must be prepared from the blood and transported to the hematology laboratory as soon as possible. If there is a delay in transport, the slides must be fixed and frozen. Leukocytes are scored (0 to 4) according to the intensity of the staining; 100 cells are counted for a total score ranging from 0 to 400.

Specimen Whole blood collected in a green-top tube.

Reference range The reference range is 20 to 100.

Abnormal values

Increased in: polycythemia vera, myelofibrosis, myeloid metaplasia, corticosteroid therapy, pregnancy, aplastic anemia, chronic myelocytic leukemia in remission, hairy cell leukemia, Hodgkin's disease, leukomoid reactions, trisomy 21 (Down syndrome).

Decreased in: aplastic anemia, chronic myelogenous leukemia, idiopathic thrombocytopenic purpura, infectious mononucleosis, paroxysmal nocturnal hemoglobinuria.

Cost $60–$80.

neutrophils   See *white blood cell* in Glossary.

niacin (nicotinic acid)   A water-soluble "B complex" vitamin that is integrated in the coenzyme nicotinamide adenine dinucleotide (NAD), one of the hydrogen ion acceptors for enzymes known as dehydrogenases. Niacin is formed in the body from trypotophan and is present in high-protein foods (e.g., fish, poultry, meats, yeast). Niacin deficiency (pellagra) is characterized by anorexia, glossitis, headaches, insomnia, rashes, depression, and pseudo-dementia.

Patient preparation No preparation is required, other than for obtaining urine.

Procedure Microbiological methods.

Specimen Urine.

Reference range 0.3–1.5 mg/24 hours.

Abnormal values Less than 0.2 mg/24 hours. Niacin is decreased in states of malnutrition, including chronic alcoholism, cirrhosis of the liver, chronic infections (e.g., tuberculosis), diabetes mellitus, cancer, chronic diarrhea, poor diet, and malabsorption.

Cost $100–$150.

niacin test   Niacin (nicotinic acid) plays a key role in the metabolism of the tuberculosis bacterium, *Mycobacterium tuberculosis*. Although all mycobacteria produce nicotinic acid, *M. tuberculosa, M. simiae,* and *M. szulgai* produce it in the greatest amounts. Differences in nicotinic acid production form the basis of the niacin test, which helps differentiate among the distinct species of mycobacteria. The niacin test is not billed separately but is part of the workup in microbiology when diagnosing tuberculosis.

nitrite reduction test   A test used in clinical microbiology to detect nitrate reductase, an enzyme that is produced by many enteric gram-negative bacteria, especially when their number is greater than 10^6/ml in the bladder. Nitrate reducing bacteria include *Klebsiella, Escherichia coli,* and others, including *Eubacterium lentum, Bacteroides fragilis,* and some strains of *Veillonella.* In the nitrite reduction test, bacteria are cultured in a broth containing nitrates which, in the presence of nitrate reductase (of bacterial origin), are reduced to nitrites. These nitrites appear as a red color when the culture is mixed with sulfanilic acid and alpha-naphthulamine in acetic acid. The nitrate reduction test allows bacteria to be identified with relative certainty and specific therapy to be administered.

Patient preparation No preparation is required, other than for obtaining urine.

Procedure The most common method for detecting nitrite reduction is by reagent strips (dipsticks), in which the paper is dipped in the urine and the color change is evaluated. For proper evaluation, the specimen must be fresh.

Specimen Urine.

Reference range Negative.

Abnormal values A color change indicates a significant amount (greater than 10^6/ml) of bacteria in the urine.

Cost The nitrite reduction is part of the urinalysis procedure, and is not billed separately.

Comments Some bacteria, e.g., enterococcus, do not reduce nitrates to nitrites.

nitroblue tetrazolium test (NBT test)   A test that measures the immune activity of white cells. This conversion indicates that a major immune function, phagocytosis, is intact. NBT reduction is defective in chronic granulomatous disease.

Patient preparation No preparation is required, other than for obtaining blood.

Procedure The test measures the activity of peroxidase, an enzyme in white blood cells, and is based on the conversion by macrophages of NBT into blue-black clumps of reduced NBT, known as formazan.

Specimen Whole blood, anticoagulated with EDTA.

Reference range 3%–10% of cells are positive in adults; a higher percentage is found in newborns.

Abnormal values

Increased in: drugs (e.g., oral contraceptives, indomethacin, typhoid vaccine), infection with viruses, bacteria, fungi, and some parasites lymphomas.

Decreased in: chronic granulomatous disease, drugs (e.g., antibiotics, glucocorticoids, phenylbutazone, salicylates).

Cost $200–$300.

nitrogen washout test   See *pulmonary function test.*

nonspecific urethritis   See *Chlamydia.*

nonstress test   A noninvasive test used in late pregnancy by obstetricians to monitor the well-being of a fetus by measuring the increase of the fetal heart rate (FHR) in response to the fetus' own movement or external movement (e.g., by the obstetrician) of the uterus. The nonstress test evaluates the frequency of fetal movement, the degree of heart rate acceleration, and the beat-to-beat variation of the heart rate, which determines the "health" of the placenta's vessels.

Patient preparation No preparation is required. The mother may experience a minimum amount of anxiety due to the emotional nature of childbirth.

Procedure The procedure consists of recording the fetal heartbeat before and after the fetus moves.

Reference range Normally, the fetal heartbeat should increase by 15 beats or more within a few minutes of after the fetus' kicking or other movement.

Abnormal values If the increase in the FHR is less than 15 beats/minute above the baseline rate (normal rate is 130 bpm) for more than 15 seconds, the patient is a candidate for an oxytocin stress test.

Cost $150–$250. See *fetal monitoring, oxytocin stress test.*

nortriptyline See *tricyclic antidepressants* in Glossary.

NTx See *osteoporosis* in Glossary.

nuclear cardiology An evolving discipline that bridges cardiology and nuclear medicine, the primary reason for which is to determine the functional status of patients with known cardiac and cardiovascular disease. A patient's ability to respond to cardiovascular stress helps to determine the risks for further deterioration of heart muscle and the patient's prognosis. In nuclear cardiology, techniques of nuclear medicine are used to study cardiovascular disease, including myocardial perfusion imaging (either by planar imaging or by SPECT–single photon emission computed tomography), infarction imaging, and evaluation of cardiac perfomance. Nuclear cardiology owes much of its success to the development of radiopharmaceuticals (e.g., ^{201}Thallium and ^{99m}Tc-sestamibi) that have ideal imaging qualities and gamma (scintillation) cameras that capture the image. See *first-pass radionuclide angiocardiography, thallium stress test.*

nuclear scanning (radionuclide imaging) Any of a number of diagnostic procedures (commonly known as scans, as in bone scan, liver scan, thyroid scan) that use a substance containing a radioactive isotope (e.g., 99m-Technetium-^{99m}Tc or 123-iodine-^{123}I). The amount of radioactivity in the isotopes used in diagnostic medicine is minimal and poses no threat to health. The body flushes out or "turns over" the radioactive ions within hours to days after the study's completion. Some nuclear scanning techniques have fallen into disuse and have been replaced by imaging procedures (e.g., CT, MRI, ultrasonography) that provide more precise information on structural abnormalities or defects.

Patient preparation No preparation is required, other than for injecting a radiocontrast into the blood. Blood for analytes that are measured by radioimmunoassay must be drawn before the procedure.

Procedure The radioisotope is linked to a molecule that selectively localizes in a particular tissue. After administration, the compound's distribution in the body is evaluated using a scintillation (gamma) camera.

Reference range No abnormalities in location or degree of uptake of the radioisotope.

Abnormal values Any region that is larger, brighter, or located in different sites than normal is regarded as diagnostic or at least suspicious for a disease process.

Cost $400–$800. See *bone scan, thyroid panel.*

5'-nucleotidase assay 5'-nucleotidase is a liver-related enzyme that is elevated in bile obstruction. Its measurement has not found wide use as a liver function test because the enzyme gamma-glutamyl transferase is thought to be a more reliable indicator of liver disease, and is more easily measured. 5'-NT is not elevated in bone disease.

Patient preparation No preparation is required, other than for drawing blood.

Procedure 5'-NT can be measured by colorimetry or by kinetic (enzyme digestion) studies.

Specimen Serum.

Reference range 0–1.6 U/dL.

Abnormal values

Increased in: metastatic neoplasms of the liver, primary biliary cirrhosis, biliary obstruction, pregnancy (third trimester).

Cost $45–$60.

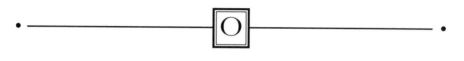

O banding See *oligoclonal bands.*

obstetric hypercoagulability profile A battery of tests performed on a pregnant woman who may be at an increased risk, due to repeated abortions, for clotting disorders. The test results supplement the details provided by an obstetric screening profile and include measurements of proteins C and S, antithrombin III, lupus anticoagulant, fibrinogen, and plasminogen.

Patient preparation No preparation is required, other than for drawing blood.

Procedure This profile is available in most hospitals; however, some of the tests such as protein S and protein C are very specialized and are sent to reference laboratories that concentrate on coagulation testing. Because some of these tests are expensive, they are usually performed only when the PT/PTT or fibrinogen are abnormal.

Specimen Serum.

Reference range All factors are within normal limits.

Abnormal values Any decrease of measured factors warrants further investigation.

Cost $75–$500, depending on the extent of the testing.

obstetric screening profile (obstetric panel) A standard battery of laboratory tests used to evaluate a pregnant woman's baseline health status. The panel is used for women who are not known to have, or to be at risk for, conditions that might complicate labor and delivery. For Medicare or Medicaid reimbursement, the panel must include a CBC (complete blood count) with a differential white cell count, hepatitis B surface antigen, rubella antibody, a quantitative test for syphilis (e.g., VDRL, RPR), an antibody screen, and both ABO and Rh(D) blood typing.

Patient preparation No preparation is required, other than for drawing blood.

Procedure All of the tests in the obstetric profile are available in any secondary care hospital where a woman would go for delivery.

Specimen Blood.

Reference range All factors are within normal limits.

Abnormal values Any abnormality of any measured analyte warrants further investigation.

Cost $100–$150. See *complete blood count, "diff"* in Glossary, *hepatitis B virus, Rh antigen(s), RPR test, rubella, VDRL.*

obstruction series A series of X-ray studies that is obtained from a patient with suspected obstruction or functional paralysis of the intestinal flow.

Patient preparation An obstruction series is by definition not an elective procedure. The standard bowel preparation for a barium enema, in which clear liquid is administered for 24 hours, is not possible.

Procedure The procedure is usually carried out in a two-step fashion. In the first step, plain films (i.e., X rays) are obtained, if possible with the patient erect to detect free air under the diaphragm, which is diagnostic of a ruptured hollow viscus organ. This is followed by a second step in which radiocontrast is instilled in the intestine.

Reference range Normally, the loops of the small and large intestine are not dilated, and radiocontrast material remains within the loops of bowel.

Abnormal values Radiological findings in prolonged obstruction include enlarged (dilated) loops of bowel, which may be filled with air, and loss of the normal markings of the mucosa (internal surface) of the intestine. The series is abnormal in abdominal abscesses, abdominal aortic aneurysm, aortic calcification, bladder distension, bowel obstruction, kidney stones, paralytic ileus, organ perforation, and peritoneal effusion. If the obstruction is prolonged, the imbalance in a person's physiology can be extreme, with a loss of fluid into the intestine. In advanced cases, perforation and ischemia of the bowel with tissue death (necrosis) are possible.

Cost $500–$700.

Comment The indications for performing a radiocontrast obstruction series are controversial. An upper GI series is the most useful study to perform if obstruction of the small intestine is suspected. A barium enema is generally helpful for obstruction of the lower intestine. See *barium enema, upper GI study.*

occult blood testing The testing of stool for the presence of bleeding that is not apparent to the naked eye (usually more than 50 cc per liter is required to visually recognize blood in the stool) to detect possible malignancy.

Patient preparation Patients should not consume vitamin C for one to three days before occult blood testing. A high-fiber, red meat-free diet with restriction of peroxidase-rich vegetables has been recommended for 72 hours before guaiac testing. Alcohol, aspirin, and nonsteroidal anti-inflammatory drugs can cause false-positives with some test methods. Oral iron does not cause false-positive results.

Procedure Fetal blood is detected by:

1. The guaiac method, e.g., Hemoccult II, a low-cost screening technique

that uses a guaiac-impregnated paper to indirectly measure hemo-globin by measuring the activity of an enzyme, pseudoperoxidase. While sensitive, the guaiac method is nonspecific, as peroxidase activity is present in uncooked red meat, fish, uncooked fruits, and certain vegetables, e.g., broccoli and cauliflower. False guaiac positivity occurs in gastrointestinal bleeding at a distance, from the gingiva, stomach, or hemorrhoids. It also occurs with drug therapy, e.g., iron, aspirin, nonsteroidal anti-inflammatory drugs, and topical iodine. False-negative results may be due to improper storage of test slides, intermittent bleeding of the lesion, hypervitaminosis C, and degradation of hemoglobin by colonic bacteria.

2. HemoQuant™ is more specific as it quantifies the conversion of heme to fluorescent porphyrins. It has the advantage of not being affected by peroxidase in the diet, vitamin C, and storage, and it allows an estimation of the amount of blood being lost in the stool.

Specimen Stool in a plastic urine container. Stool collection has been offensive to most patients. New and easier screening tests on cards have been developed for home use. Three specimens should be submitted for the most reliable interpretation.

Reference range Negative.

Abnormal values A positive reaction of any type requires further evaluation.

Cost $15–$25 per specimen when performed in the clinical laboratory. As this test may be performed in a home testing format, the "street" prices may vary.

Comments These tests assume that the carcinoma has produced an ulcer and, therefore, is bleeding. However, 20%–30% of patients with colorectal cancers have a negative fecal occult blood test.

ocular cytology testing Examination of cells from the surface of the eye and conjunctiva using a sterile cotton swab ("Q-tip"). The material obtained is then smeared on a glass slide, stained, and examined by a cytologist or pathologist for the presence of infection by bacteria (*Haemophilus* species), viruses (e.g., herpesvirus, adenovirus), or other microorganisms. Note: Although in theory ocular cytology could be used to identify malignancies, any cancer that is seen in the eyes would be very advanced and evident elsewhere.

ocular plethysmography A noninvasive method for indirectly measuring the flow of blood through the ophthalmic artery and, by extension (since the ophthalmic artery is the first branch of the carotid artery), the flow of blood to the brain. Ocular plethysmography is indicated for patients with symptoms of transient ischemic attacks, carotid bruits, and neurologic defects.

Patient preparation Contact lenses must be removed. The patient must have both eyes, i.e., no ocular prostheses.

Procedure Small photoelectric sensors are attached to the earlobes, which detect blood flow to the ear via the external carotid artery. Ocular pressure is measured through contact lens-like suction cups, which are placed on the eyes and held in place by light suction. Tracings of the pulsations in each eye and the ears are displayed on paper and compared.

Reference range Normally, all pulsations of the eyes and ears should occur simultaneously.

Abnormal values Narrowing (stenosis) of the internal or external carotid artery is manifest by a delay in the pulse tracing of the eye or the ear on the affected side.

Cost $50–$100.

Comments Contraindications include allergy to local anesthetics, cataracts, lens implants, recent eye surgery, and retinal detachment.

ocular ultrasound (orbital ultrasound) A diagnostic technique that uses ultrasound to produce two-dimensional images of the eye and surrounding tissues. Because MRI and CT images are superior, ocular ultrasonography is primarily used in the physician's office to screen suspected masses of the orbital and periorbital region.

O-F test (oxidative-fermentative test) A test that is used in clinical microbiology to detect acid production by fermentative gram-negative bacteria, which cause a wide range of infections of gastrointestinal, respiratory, and urinary tracts. Two tubes are partially filled with different concentrations of fermentable sugars. One tube is overlaid with mineral oil, creating an anaerobic (airless) environment. Oxidative bacteria e.g., *Pseudomonas aeruginosa*, produce acid only in the open tube exposed to atmospheric oxygen. Fermenting bacteria, e.g., *Escherichia coli*, produce acid in both tubes, and nonsaccharolytic bacteria, e.g., *Moraxella,* do not react at all. The results of the test allow the microbiologist to determine the type of bacteria and to guide the physician in treatment of the infection.

oligoclonal bands (O bands) The presence of multiple, distinct bands of immunoglobulins in the γ (gamma) region of cerebrospinal fluid that has been electrophoresed on a gel and stained. The presence of oligoclonal bands supports the diagnosis of multiple sclerosis.

Patient preparation The lumbar puncture—insertion of a long needle into the spinal canal—is a potentially painful procedure and may require sedatives. For drawing blood, no special preparation is required.

Procedure Electrophoresis of cerebrospinal fluid on an agarose gel and stained with Coumassie blue.

Specimen Serum and cerebrospinal fluid obtained at the same times.

Reference range None detected in the cerebrospinal fluid.

Abnormal values While the finding of oligoclonal bands is nonspecific, it occurs in 90%–95% of patients with multiple sclerosis, the diagnosis of which is supported by the presence of an increased myelin basic protein. Oligoclonal bands may also occur in other encephalopathies, including

herpes encephalitis, bacterial or viral meningitis (40%–60% of cases have bands), carcinomatosis, toxoplasmosis, neurosyphilis (60% positive), progressive multifocal leukoencephalopathy, subacute sclerosing panencephalitis (90% have bands), and transiently in Guillain-Barré disease, systemic lupus erythematosus vasculitis, amyotrophic lateral sclerosis, spinal cord compression, diabetes mellitus, and cerebrovascular events including strokes.
Cost $110–$120.
Comments The test is often positive in multiple sclerosis, but is nonspecific. The clinical diagnosis of multiple sclerosis is corroborated by the finding of multiple defects by CT and MRI and an increase in myelin basic protein. Serum protein electrophoresis must be performed concurrently to assure that any cerebrospinal fluid bands detected are not also present in the serum. This could possibly represent another condition, including multiple myeloma.

oncofetal antigen   A general term for any of a number of antigens that are expressed in the fetus but not produced in significant quantities in adults. Oncofetal antigens may re-appear in malignancy, when tumors return to more primitive states (a process known as "de-differentiation"). Oncofetal antigens include alphafetoprotein (AFP), which is elevated in 70% of hepatocellular carcinomas and carcinoembryonic antigen (CEA). CEA is present in the fetal gut, liver, and pancreas. Although it is elevated in many benign or malignant processes in adults, it is commonly used to monitor tumor recurrences in patients who are known to have colonic adenocarcinoma. See *alphafetoprotein, carcinoembryonic antigen.*

open biopsy   A type of biopsy in which a lesion is excised under direct visual examination during an open surgical procedure. See *biopsy.*

ophthalmodynamometry   A technique in which a device (ophthalmodynanometer) is used to exert calibrated amounts of pressure on the eyeball. It was formerly used to approximate central retinal pressure and to screen for atherosclerosis of the carotid artery. Because severe (70%–90%) stenosis is required to detect reduced carotid arterial blood flow, the technique has fallen into disuse and been replaced by other more sensitive techniques, e.g., ocular plethysmography. See *ocular plethysmography.*

ophthalmoscopy   The examination of the back (fundus) of the eye with an ophthalmoscope, which is part of the routine examination of a patient. Ophthalmoscopy allows a magnified evaluation of the blood vessels, nerves, and retina. In absence of a slit lamp, the ophthalmoscope can also be used to evaluate the cornea, iris, and lens.
Patient preparation No preparation is required, other than removal of contact lenses and instillation of drops to dilate the pupils.
Procedure The procedure consists of the use of an ophthalmoscope in a darkened room to shine a beam of light on the fundus for the visualization of various "accessible" structures of the eye.

Reference range Negative for lesions of note.

Abnormal values Abnormalities seen by ophthalmoscopy include retinal hemorrhage, retinal detachment, and clouding of the vitreous fluid. This may be related to intraocular inflammation, optic neuritis, atrophy of the optic nerve, and papilledema, which is due to increased intracranial pressure, vascular occlusion, changes of hypertensive retinopathy, diabetic retinopathy, choroidal tumors, and other lesions.

Cost Ophthalmoscopy is part of a routine physical examination and is not billed separately.

Comment Dilating drops should not be used for patients who have narrow-angle glaucoma or a history of hypersensitivity to dilating agents.

optochin (disk) test (P disc test) Optochin is a quinine derivative that selectively destroys *Staphylococcus pneumoniae* at low concentrations. Typically the zone of lysis around the optochin-impregnated paper disc is 14 mm. The lack of inhibition by optochin implies that the organism on the growth plate is not *S. pneumoniae*. See *minimum inhibitory concentration* in Glossary.

oral lactose tolerance test See *lactose tolerance test.*

orbital ultrasound See *ocular ultrasound.*

orientation test A general term for any part of a neurologic examination that determines whether the patient understands who he or she is and the nature of his/her present situation. Orientation tests include questions about a person's name, address, current location, occupation, marital status, date, how the person arrived to present location, and others.

osmolality Osmolality is the measurement of the number of particles or ions per kilogram of water in a particular body fluid, such as blood or urine. The osmolality of the fluid outside the cells is determined by measuring sodium and chloride in the serum; that of the fluid within the cells is determined by measuring potassium. The kidney normally increases the urine to an osmolality four times that of serum when there is need to conserve fluid, and it dilutes the urine to an osmolality one-fourth that of serum when large volumes of water must be eliminated. Serum and urine osmolality are measured when evaluating electrolyte and water balance, acid-base metabolism, antidiuretic hormone activity, liver disease, and hypersomolar coma, and to determine a person's state of hydration.

Patient preparation No preparation is required, other than for drawing blood and obtaining urine.

Procedure Osmolality is measured by determining the freezing point of a fluid or by vapor depression. Further information is provided by calculating a ratio of the urine to serum osmolality, which should be greater than 3.0 after 12 hours of fluid restriction.

Specimen Urine, serum.
Reference range
  Urine   50–1400 mOsm/kg.
  Serum   275–295 mOsm/kg.
Abnormal values
URINE OSMOLALITY
  Increased in: Addison's disease, azotemia, cirrhosis, congestive heart
    failure, dehydration, diabetes mellitus, hyperglycemia
  Decreased in: diabetes insipidus, high-protein diet, hyponatremia.
SERUM OSMOLALITY
  Increased in: hypernatremia, hyperglycemia, mannitol therapy,
    azotemia, ingestion of ethanol, methanol, ethylene glycol.
  Decreased in: hyponatremia, inappropriate antidiuretic hormone
    secretion which is associated with carcinoma of the lung.
Cost $45–$55.

osmotic fragility test   A test in which red blood cells are tested for their susceptibility to bursting in various salt (sodium chloride or saline) solutions, ranging from the normal concentration of salt in body fluids to greater or lesser amounts of salts. The test is performed to confirm the diagnosis of a rare form of red blood cell disease known as hereditary spherocytosis.

Patient preparation No preparation is required, other than for drawing blood.

Procedure The procedure consists of placing the red blood cells in saline solutions ranging from 0.85%, which is the normal or "physiologic" level of sodium chloride in the body, to 0.2%, which is closer to pure water. The percentage of cells that dissolve, or hemolyze, in each of the tubes after 24 hours at 37°C is plotted on a graph.

Specimen Blood.

Reference range Hemolysis begins at 0.7% sodium chloride concentration and is complete at 0.40% to 0.15%.

Abnormal values Red blood cells in hereditary spherocytosis have a greater osmotic fragility, while those found in iron-deficiency anemia and thalassemia have a decreased osmotic fragility.

Cost $25–$45.

osteoporosis testing   Bone undergoes a continuous cycle of formation (osteogenesis) and resorption (osteoclasis) that is collectively termed remodeling. Substances known as biochemical markers are excreted in the urine and can be used clinically to determine whether bone is being formed or resorbed. The substances excreted during bone resorption include hydroxyproline, deoxypyridinoline, pyridinoline, and the cross-linked N-ends of the protein collagen I (N-telopeptides) which appear to be the most specific indicator of active bone resorption and evolving osteoporosis. Urine markers are being used to reduce the use of bone densitometry and plain films of the vertebrae as a means of evaluating bone integrity and bone loss, as both have the disadvantage of exposing the patient to radiation.

Patient preparation No preparation is required, other than for obtaining urine.

Procedure N-telopeptides, short peptides present in the urine of patients with osteoporosis, can be measured by an enzyme-based test (Osteomark®) that was approved in 1995 for clinical use. This and other tests provide a means for screening for osteoporosis and determining its severity and the need for treatment.

Specimen Urine.

Reference range This is a relatively new test with no clear reference ranges. It is most useful in monitoring changes rather than having definitive ranges.

Abnormal values N-telopeptide is used for monitoring treatment of osteoporosis. If the treatment is effective, the levels decrease.

Cost $65–$85. See *bone densitometry, pyridinium crosslinks.*

ova See *parasite identification.*

oxalate test This test measures any salt or ester of oxalic acid, generally called an oxalate, that is excreted in the urine. An excess of oxalates may result in the accumulation of oxalate crystals in the kidneys, urinary tract, and urine and may, if extreme, cause a blockage of the ureters through the formation of kidney and bladder stones. Oxalates are measured in individuals who have an increased tendency to absorb and excrete a higher-than-normal level of oxalates from the diet. For example, this may occur in malabsorption, which may be found in a person who has had intestinal bypass surgery for extreme ("morbid") obesity.

Patient preparation Vitamin C should be avoided for 24 hours prior to collection of urine. The patient should be ambulatory with normal fluid intake.

Procedure Oxalates can be measured by color changes or by gas-liquid chromatography.

Specimen 24-hour urine.

Reference range 10–41 mg/24 hours.

Abnormal values
   Increased in: cirrhosis, inflammatory bowel disease, diabetes mellitus, kidney stones, overdose of vitamin C, ingestion of antifreeze (ethylene glycol), methoxyflurane anesthesia.
   Decreased in: renal disease.

Cost $70–$80.

oxidative-fermentative test See *O-F test.*

oximetry See *pulse oximetry.*

oxygen saturation (sO_2) Oxygen saturation is a measure of the blood's capacity to transport oxygen and is a normal part of the blood gas profile. It can be estimated from samples obtained from different sites in the heart in cardiac catheterization and, combined with measurements of intracardiac pressures, can be used to detect defects within the heart.

Patient preparation No preparation is required, other than for drawing blood. There is some mild discomfort with the procedure.

Procedure The procedure consists of the insertion of a long, 20- or 18-gauge needle on either side of the navel, from which the arterial blood specimen is obtained.

Specimen The specimen is arterial blood collected anaerobically (without air) in a well-sealed, heparinized (green-top) tube. It is transported on ice to the laboratory for immediate analysis.

Reference range Neonatal period 40%–90%. Otherwise 95%–98% arterial; 60%–80% venous.

Abnormal values

Increased in: high altitude, hypocapnia, hypothermia, increased cardiac output, oxygen therapy, PEEP (positive end-expiratory pressure) ventilation, respiratory alkalosis.

Decreased in: carbon monoxide poisoning, congenital cardiac defects, emphysema, hypercapnia, hypoventilation, hypoxia, respiratory acidosis.

Cost $50–$100.

oxyhemoglobin   See *hemoglobin*.

oxytocin stress test   A clinical test for evaluating the fetus' ability to "weather" labor that uses oxytocin, a hypothalamic polypeptide released into the posterior pituitary (of both mother and fetus), to induce and stimulate uterine contractions and labor.

Patient preparation No preparation is required; the mother may experience anxiety and discomfort at being connected to an infusion pump.

Procedure The procedure consists of recording the fetal heartbeat before and after the fetus moves. Oxytocin infusion is adjusted so that three contractions occur in ten minutes; if three decelerations (slowing down of the fetal heart rate) occur within ten minutes, the fetus is considered to be at risk for labor-related complications and should be delivered as soon as possible. Because uterine contractions cause a decrease in uteroplacental blood flow, a clinically controlled "trial of labor" should be performed in women at high risk for uteroplacental insufficiency. At-risk pregnancies affect women with chronic obstructive lung disease, diabetes mellitus, underlying heart disease, hypertension, narcotic addiction, post-term pregnancy, pre-eclampsia, and sickle cell anemia.

Reference range Normally, the fetal heart rate (FHR) should increase by 15 beats or more within a few minutes of the baby's kicking or other movement. A positive stress test is characterized by consistent late decelerations and ample indication for an expedient delivery.

Abnormal values If the increase in the FHR is less than 15 beats/minute above the baseline rate (the normal rate is 130 beats per minute) for more than 15 seconds, the fetus is at risk and may be a candidate for cesarean section.

Cost $300–$400. See *fetal monitoring*.

P

pancreas sonography   A form of ultrasonography in which the recording probe (transducer) is passed over the abdomen to identify benign or malignant neoplasms, circumscribed inflammation, cysts, or pseudocysts.

Patient preparation The patient should not eat after midnight on the night before the examination. A barium enema should not be performed in the three days before the procedure.

Procedure The procedure consists of the use of a B-mode ultrasonic imager. A gel is applied to the skin, and a transducer is swept across the abdomen to acquire images of the organs of interest, which are recorded on X-ray film.

Reference range No structural abnormalities are seen.

Abnormal values Any mass or fluid accumulation is considered to be abnormal and requires further diagnostic evaluation in the form of an aspiration biopsy or obtention of cells for examination by microscopy.

Cost $300–$400.

pap smear (Papanicolaou test, pap test)   The pap smear is one of the most commonly ordered tests in medicine and consists of a sampling of cells from the uterine cervix and endocervix, which are spread on a glass slide, stained, and interpreted by a cytotechnologist or pathologist. Pap smears were formerly classified by the system devised by Dr. George Papanicolaou, who divided the findings into five groups, from normal (Class I) to malignant (Class V). This classification fell into disfavor with both the cytopathologists (who interpret the smears) and the gynecologists (who base their treatment on the pathologists' interpretation), and has been replaced by the Bethesda system. The Bethesda system provides information on the adequacy of the specimen, the presence of infection and/or inflammation, and the presence of benign, reactive, or malignant processes.

Patient preparation The smear should not be obtained during the woman's menstrual period but ideally at midcycle. Douching and intravaginal medication should not be administered in the 24 hours before the procedure.

Procedure The procedure consists of the insertion of a clamp, known as a speculum, into the vagina, so that it extends to the uterine cervix. Any of a number of elongated swabs are passed through the speculum, and a sampling of material, which includes cells from the cervix and endocervix, is obtained. The swab is withdrawn, and the specimen is spread on a glass slide that is either sprayed with a fixative or, less commonly, dipped in a fixative solution and stained by the pap method.

Specimen A stained smear of cells.

Reference range No significant changes beyond mild inflammation.

Abnormal values The pap smear is the standard method for early detection of HPV (human papillomavirus), herpes, or trichomonad infections, cervical intraepithelial neoplasia (CIN or dysplasia), and carcinoma of the cervix. Less commonly, cells may be sampled from the upper vaginal wall to evaluate the woman's hormonal status, resulting in a value known as a maturation index. The interpretation of a "pap" is highly subjective and less often a science than an art based on the experience of the screening cytotechnologist or pathologist. In the best of laboratories, an error rate of 5% to 15% has been reported in the medical literature.

Cost $35–$55. If the original result is negative, the patient is usually offered the opportunity to have her pap smear slide rescreened, either manually, or by one of the new computerized screening devices, such as Papnet, for which there is an additional $25–$45 fee.

Comments Various factors prevent the pap smear from detecting the theoretical 100% of lesions, including sampling error, insufficient time devoted to screening, and fatigue by the cytotechnologist performing the screening. The pap smear may suffer from lack of clinical information and suboptimal reproducibility. In one study of 481 women with invasive cervical cancer, 33% had not had a pap smear within the previous five years, and 15% of these women did not return for follow-up after an abnormal or inconclusive diagnosis on the pap smear. In 7% of these cases, the laboratory was in error.

paracentesis (peritoneal fluid analysis)   See *abdominal tap.*

parasite identification   Parasites are uncommon in developed nations, which is the combined result of safe water supplies, a high standard of living, and aggressive epidemiologic surveillance of index cases. An individual who acquires parasites is often exposed to unusual circumstances, e.g., uncooked fish (sushi is linked to anisakiasis) or meat (pork is linked to trichinosis) or recent travel to a developing nation (e.g., malaria). Those who have an unremarkable clinical history may suffer from some defect in the immune system (e.g., AIDS, malignancy) that makes them more susceptible to parasite infection. In general, evaluation of a patient for parasites depends on the symptoms and, because of their relative infrequency, may be the last thing that a physician considers when trying to determine the cause of a patient's particular complaint or symptom. The most common parasites reside in the gastrointestinal tract and can be identified in the stool, which may contain parasite body parts or, more commonly, eggs.

Patient preparation Mineral oils, bismuth (e.g., PeptoBismol™), magnesium, antidiarrheals, antibiotics, or barium enemas should not be administered in the seven to ten days before examining the stool.

Procedure Up to three specimens are required, which should be collected in a container and submitted to the laboratory. Once received by the laboratory, the stool is mixed in water, which causes the parasite's eggs (ova) to float. The eggs have specific features that aid in their identification under the microscope. Some roundworms (*Ascaris lumbricoides*) are large enough (up to 35 cm–12 inches in length) that they can be identified based solely on their physical features. For detecting pinworms (*Enterobius*), cellophane (e.g., Scotch tape™) is used with the sticky side out to collect the eggs from the anal region.

Specimen Stool, or the worms themselves.

Reference range Normally no eggs or parasites are present in the stool.

Abnormal values Any finding of eggs or worms is abnormal and requires treatment with the appropriate drugs.

Cost $85–$150.

parathyroid hormone (PTH)   PTH is a hormone that maintains the balance of calcium in the body. It is produced in the parathyroid gland and secreted in response to a decreased serum concentration of calcium. PTH increases intestinal absorption and mobilization of calcium from bone. It also increases the excretion of phosphorus by the kidney. PTH is present in the circulation in one of three different forms—intact PTH and either the N-terminal (the amino end of PTH) or the C-terminal (the carboxyl end of PTH) of the partially metabolized form of PTH, which are cleaved from the PTH molecule in the liver, kidneys, and parathyroid gland. Parathyroid hormone is part of the evaluation of hypercalcemia and in the differential diagnosis of hyperparathyroidism.

Patient preparation No preparation is required, other than for drawing blood.

Procedure PTH is measured by immunoassay, which quantifies either intact N-terminal fragments, the fluctuations of which most accurately reflect an acute change in parathyroid metabolism, or C-terminal fragments, which are of greater use in evaluating chronic diseases of parathyroid metabolism.

Specimen Serum must be separated from the red blood cells and frozen quickly for transportation to the laboratory, because PTH is quickly metabolized to smaller, undetectable fragments. Freezing of the specimen is not required for measuring the C-terminal fragment.

Reference range

Intact PTH	200-300 pg/ml.
C-terminal PTH	400-1700 pg/ml.
N-terminal PTH	250-650 pg/ml.

Abnormal values

Increased in: primary and secondary hyperparathyroidism, hypercalcemia, chronic renal failure, malabsorption, pseudohyperparathyroidism, paraneoplastic syndrome, vitamin D deficiency, osteomalacia.

Decreased in: hypomagnesemia, hypoparathyroidism, nonparathyroid hypercalcemia, Graves' disease, metastases to the bone, sarcoidoisis, vitamin D excess.

Cost

PTH Intact	$170–$180.
PTH, N-Terminal	$190–$210.
PTH, C-terminal	$90–$120.

parathyroid hormone-related protein (PTH-rP) A protein that has a structure similar to PTH and can bind to and stimulate PTH receptors. PTH-rP is produced mainly by solid tumors, but is also found in normal lactating mammary glands, skin surface cells (keratinocytes), placentas, and parathyroid glands. Measurement of PTH-rP may be useful in identifying the cause of hypercalcemia, specifically in separating primary hyperparathyroidism from hypercalcemia related to cancer.

Patient preparation No preparation is required, other than for drawing blood.

Procedure PTH-rP is measured by immunoassay.

Specimen Frozen plasma drawn in a special collection tube.

Reference range Less than 1.5 pmol/L. PTH-rP is not elevated in primary or chronic renal failure.

Abnormal values Elevated in tumor-associated hypercalcemia.

Cost $170–$190.

paroxysmal nocturnal hemoglobinuria See *sucrose hemolysis test.*

partial pressure of carbon dioxide (CO_2) See *arterial blood gas.*

partial pressure of oxygen (O_2) See *arterial blood gas.*

partial thromboplastin time (activated partial thromboplastin time, aPTT) The PTT is a test that evaluates the function of coagulation (clotting) by measuring the time required for plasma to form a fibrin clot after the addition of thromboplastin, a clot-promoting substance. It is commonly ordered before surgery to determine the time required for blood to coagulate.

Patient preparation No preparation is required, other than for drawing blood.

Procedure PTT is a measurement of the time required for plasma to form a clot.

Specimen Plasma obtained from whole blood collected in a citrated collection tube.

Reference range 32–46 seconds.

Abnormal values PTT is prolonged in deficiencies of coagulation factors V, VIII, IX, X, XI, XII, HMW (high-molecular weight) kininogen, lupus

anticoagulants (inhibitors), heparin, prekallikrein, prothrombin, or fibrinogen.
Cost $25–$35.

patch test (contact dermatitis skin test, skin patch test)   The skin is subjected to numerous organic and inorganic chemicals including toxins, carcinogens, irritants, and allergens. The patch test is performed on the skin surface to identify "contact-type" hypersensitive reactions to various allergens in the environment.

Patient preparation The skin should be cleaned with a non-allergenic soap.

Procedure A patch with a minimal amount of a potentially allergenic substance (allergen or antigen) is applied to an unexposed area of the skin, usually the back. The patch is covered with plastic, left in place for two days, and observed one to two days later. The most common sensitizing substances in North America are poison ivy (*Toxicodendron radicans*), nickel, chromate, paraphenylenediamine (a dye constituent), ethylenediamine (a solvent and emulsifier), local anesthetics (e.g., benzocaine), rubber, and neomycin. Patch testing materials have been standardized and are commercially available, either as individual allergens or as batteries of allergens, including those for specific occupations such as hairdressers, printers, and others.

Reference range Normally there is no reaction to the allergens.

Abnormal values The results of patch tests are graded according to the intensity of the reaction, with "+" for a weak positive reaction, characterized by a faint reddening of the skin, "++" for a strong positive reaction with puffiness of the skin and tiny fluid-filled cysts, and "+++" for a very strong positive reaction that spreads and is covered by fluid-filled blisters. Incorrect patch test results are common in the form of false-positives, due to an excessive concentration of allergens in the patches, misinterpretation of the irritant reaction, a nonimmune response to either the "vehicle," a nonallergenic substance in which the allergen is suspended, or the chemicals in the plastic itself, and generalized erythema of the skin-testing site. False-negative results are linked to technical errors and failure to mimic the "real-world" situation in which the person is exposed to the allergen.

Cost The cost depends on the number of patches used, usually $10–$25 each.

Comments Up to 5% of the general population has dermatitis, and 7% or more of a dermatologist's practice is involved in treating allergic contact dermatitis. Up to 50% of occupational absenteeism is related to contact dermatitis. See *prick test, RAST.*

paternity testing   A battery of tests used to identify, with reasonable or absolute certainty, a child's genetic parents. There are a number of maneuvers used to exclude the possibility of one person being the parent of another.

DIRECT EXCLUSION OF PATERNITY

1. The child has a genetic marker that is absent in the mother and not present in the father; in complex systems where a child lacks all paternal antigens, the putative father is excluded.

2. The child is an "amorph," i.e., does not express a gene which is present in both the mother and the father.

INDIRECT EXCLUSION OF PATERNITY

1. A gene is present in the child that can be transmitted only by a male, and which the putative father does not have.

2. The child is homozygous for markers not seen in a parent.

3. The parent is homozygous for a genetic marker that is not seen in the child (paternity is excluded). Indirect exclusions are accepted when they are confirmed by a second method by another laboratory.

Genetic markers are used in "classic" paternity testing, but those of very high or very low frequencies are of limited value in differentiating among individuals, although very low frequency genetic markers are used to determine statistical likelihood of paternity. Genetic markers include red blood cell antigens (M-N, S-s, Rh-C–c, Rh-E-e, K-k, Fy^a-Fy^b, Jk^a-Jk^b), red blood cell enzymes (adenosine deaminase, glucose-6-phosphate dehydrogenase) isomers, HLA antigens, immunoglobulin allotypes, and nonimmunoglobulin serum proteins.

Since the late 1980s, DNA "fingerprinting" has become the legally accepted means of establishing or excluding parentage, using the "Jeffries" probe. Because of the legal implications of this test, relatively few specialized laboratories offer these services. See *chromosome analysis, DNA fingerprinting* in Glossary.

Patrick's test A clinical maneuver performed on a supine patient, in which the hip and knee are flexed, and the external malleolus is placed on the patella of the opposite leg. Pain in the hip resulting from pressure on the knee suggests the presence of sacroiliac disease.

PBI test See *protein-bound iodine test.*

PCP (Phencyclidine) See *drug of abuse* in Glossary.

PCR See *polymerase chain reaction.*

P disc test See *optochin (disk) test.*

pelvic ultrasonography (obstetric ultrasonography) A clinical form of sonography in which a series of real-time images are analyzed to provide information on the fetus or the status of the organs, structures, and masses of the female pelvis.

Patient preparation The patient should drink four 8-ounce glasses of water 45 minutes before the procedure, and not empty the bladder. A barium enema should not be performed within two days of the procedure. The examination itself may last as long as one hour.

Procedure The test is performed using a B-mode, real-time ultrasonography device with a transducer. The abdominal wall is coated with a gel and the transducer is passed on the skin overlying the areas of interest. The images obtained are recorded on X-ray film for permanent records.

Reference range Normal organ size, shape, and placement.

Abnormal values

1. Obstetrics: Pelvic ultrasonography is used in the early diagnosis of pregnancy, including twins (or "higher multiples") and ectopic pregnancy. It is also used to identify placental abnormalties that may adversely affect the outcome of the pregnancy (e.g., placenta previa, abruptio placentae), to differentiate between pregnancy and tumors of the placenta (known as moles and choriocarcinomas), to determine fetal age and position, to determine the placental position prior to amniocentesis, and to monitor the rate of fetal growth

2. Gynecology: Pelvic ultrasonography is used to identify the presence of and difference among lesions (cysts, abcesses, benign or malignant tumors) of the uterus, ovaries, pelvic organs, and tissues. It can also be used to localize intrauterine devices.

Cost $300–$400.

pelvimetry See *radiologic pelvimetry.*

penile blood flow (penile Doppler studies) A clinical test in which the blood circulating through the penis is semiquantified using a Doppler-based ultrasonic device and compared to the circulation in the brachial artery. Penile blood flow is measured in cases of impotence to determine whether it has an organic or psychogenic cause.

Procedure The test is performed using a B-mode, real-time ultrasonography device with a transducer. The penis is coated with a gel, and the transducer is passed on the skin overlying the areas of interest. The images obtained are recorded on X-ray film for permanent records.

Specimen The technique provides information on the adequacy of the blood flow through the major vessels of the penis.

Reference range Adequate blood flow.

Abnormal values The blood flow may be compromised or decreased in primary impotence or in impotence related to vascular insufficiency.

Cost $250–$350.

pentagastrin test A test used to quantify acid secretion by the stomach, which may be used to identify achlorhydria (absence of acid secretion) in patients with gastric cancer.

Patient preparation Because this is a test of the stomach's ability to secrete acid, the patient must be in a fasting state and free from the sight or odor of food. All medications (e.g., antacids) known to alter gastric secretion should be withheld for 24 hours. The patient should be free from environmental situations that are capable of evoking adverse psychological reactions, e.g., fear, anger, or depression, all of which could alter gastric secretion.

Procedure Gastric acid secretion is stimulated by subcutaneous injection of pentagastrin, a synthetic analog of gastrin.

Specimen Gastric juice.

Reference range Increased gastric acid secretion begins within 10 minutes of pentagastrin injection, peaks at 20–30 minutes, and lasts for less than two hours. The peaks in gastric acid secretion are similar to those evoked by histamine, which was formerly used for this same purpose, but which had greater adverse effects. Maximum acid output is 23–28 mEq/hour in males and 15–22 mEq/hour in females.

Abnormal values

Increased in:	DUODENAL ULCER
Men	35 mEq/hour
Women	26 mEq/hour
Decreased in:	GASTRIC ULCER
Men	20 mEq/hour
Women	13 mEq/hour
	GASTRIC CANCER
Men	7 mEq/hour
Women	3 mEq/hour

Cost There is a wide range of fees. The test is rarely performed outside of a university hospital because of the need to ensure that the test is performed under optimal conditions.

pepsinogen A proteolytic enzyme, produced by the acid-secreting regions of the stomach, that closely reflects the test results of maximal acid output.

Patient preparation The patient should be fasting before drawing the specimen. No further preparation is required, other than for drawing blood.

Procedure Pepsinogen is an uncommonly ordered test that is measured by radioimmunoassay.

Specimen Serum transported to a reference laboratory in a frozen state.

Reference range 100–130 ng/ml.

Abnormal values Pepsinogen is increased in states of increased gastrin and gastric output in the presence of increased gastrin-producing cells in the stomach. Pepsinogen is decreased if the increased gastrin is reactive to decreased gastrin-producing cells in the stomach, as occurs in atrophy of the stomach.

Cost $120–$135. See *maximum acid output.*

perceptual-motor integrity test See *psychological test.*

percutaneous transhepatic cholangiography (PTCA) A radiologic technique used to evaluate the gallbladder and intra- and extahepatic bile ducts.

Patient preparation Informed consent is required. Aspirin and nonsteroidal anti-inflammatory drugs should be discontinued, ideally five days before the procedure, in order to minimize the bleeding. Baseline coagulation studies (e.g., platelet count, prothrombin time, and partial thromboplastin time) and renal function tests (e.g., BUN and creatinine) should be performed before the procedure.

Procedure An iodinated radiocontrast dye is injected through the skin, and the contours of the biliary tract are evaluated by fluoroscopy as the radiocontrast fills the biliary tract.

Reference range Normally, no abnormalities are seen.

Abnormal values PCTA can be used to demonstrate biliary obstruction, which may be due to stones, strictures, or malignancy, as well as changes in the pancreaticobiliary tract.

Cost $575–$800.

Comments Complications include allergic reactions, bile peritonitis due to bile spillage after removing the injection needle cannula, and hemorrhage due to the puncture of a blood vessel. PTCA is used less commonly than endoscopic retrograde cholangiopancreatography (ERCP), because it is more prone to complications in the form of allergy to radiocontrast dyes and increased bleeding time.

percutaneous transhepatic portal venography (portal venography)   An imaging technique in which radiocontrast is injected into the portal vein, allowing visualization of the portal vein and of the veins that empty into it. Portal venography can also be used to identify tumors of the pancreas. With a technique known as embolization, it can be used therapeutically to close off varices in the esophagus, which stops esophageal bleeding, a relatively common complication of alcoholic liver cirrhosis.

Patient preparation Informed consent is required. The patient should not eat in the four hours before the procedure. Baseline coagulation studies (e.g., platelet count, prothrombin time, and partial thromboplastin time) and renal function tests (e.g., BUN and creatinine) should be obtained before the procedure.

Procedure The procedure consists of the insertion of a catheter through the skin and the injection of a radiocontrast material. This allows the radiologist to see the major vein of the liver—the portal vein—and all of its branches. Portal venography can also be used to identify tumors of the pancreas by selectively sampling blood at various sites in the portal venous system.

Reference range Normally, no obstruction, varices, or tumors are identified.

Abnormal values Defects in filling of the veins, obstruction, varices, or displacement of vessels. Pancreatic tumors that can be identified include insulinomas, gastrinomas, and the so-called APUDomas (tumors of the neuroendocrine system).

Cost $575–$800.

Comments Portal venography should not be performed in patients with bleeding tendencies, acute renal failure, or marked fluid accumulation (ascites) in advanced cirrhosis.

perfusion lung scan See *ventilation-perfusion scan.*

pericardiocentesis An invasive procedure in which fluid is drawn from the pericardial sac and analyzed for the presence of infection, inflammation, or tumor cells. The indications for performing a pericardiocentesis have been controversial. Some experts believe pericardiocentesis should only be performed in emergencies and advocate an open (surgical) approach which has the advantages of fewer complications, greater ease in obtaining pericardial biopsies, and more complete drainage of the pericardial sac if necessary. Pericardiocentesis is commonly used to detect bacterial or tuberculous pericardial inflammation and malignancy.

Patient preparation Informed consent and hospital admission is required. Before the procedure, oral intake should be limited to clear liquids; baseline coagulation studies, platelet count, potassium level, x ray(s), and an electrocardiogram should be in the chart. Vital signs should be documented. Full emergency equipment (e.g., defibrillator, intubation devices, epinephrine, atropine, antiarrhythmic agents, and oxygen) should be available, and a thoracic surgery team should be notified.

Procedure A long needle is passed through the chest wall, either blindly or guided by ultrasonography or fluoroscopy, to obtain fluids and cells from the pericardial sac. The fluid is then analyzed in the laboratory for the presence of bacterial pericarditis, tuberculous pericarditis, and malignant effusion, i.e., accumulation of abundant malignant cells in the pericardium.

Specimen Pericardial fluid and cells.

Reference range Normally, a few so-called mesothelial cells may be seen in pericardial fluid. See table.

PERICARDIOCENTESIS	REFERENCE RANGE
Appearance	Clear to straw-colored
Red cells	None
White cells	< 300/mm3
Glucose	70–100 g/dL
Protein	< 4.0 g/dL
Volume	Minimal, usually ± 20 mL

Abnormal values Fresh blood and inflamed or malignant cells may be seen, as indicated above.

Cost $250–$350.

Comments Complications include laceration of coronary arteries, lungs, or liver due to puncture, arrhythmias induced by needle-induced irritation, vasovagal arrest, pneumothorax, pneumohemothorax, and infection.

perimetry A clinical test in which a topographic "map" of the visual field is created and used in the diagnosis and evaluation of diseases of optic nerve, retina, and neuro-optic pathways. In the most common form, Goldmann perimetry uses both stationary (static) light sources of increasing intensity and moving light sources to delineate the visual field, defects of which can be either central or peripheral.

Patient preparation The pupils may require dilation.

Procedure The individual being examined stares straight ahead into a device, e.g., a Goldmann perimeter, while points of light of varying intensity are moved inward from the outside until the individual indicates that he or she sees the points.

Reference range The size and shape of the individual's visual perimeter is compared with that of other individuals.

Abnormal values Defects in the visual field are categorized as peripheral (i.e., at the edge) or central (i.e., there are islands of defective sight surrounded by areas of intact vision).

Cost $200–$400.

periodic acid-Schiff stain   See *PAS stain* in Glossary.

peritoneal fluid analysis   See *abdominal tap.*

peritoneoscopy   See *laparoscopy.*

Perl's test   A semiquantitative test, also known as the Prussian blue reaction, for the presence of hemosiderin. A substance of interest is treated with hydrochloric acid and potassium ferrocyanide. The resulting dark blue color is relatively proportional to the amount of hemosiderin. The Prussian blue stain is widely used in hematopathology to determine the amount of iron stored in the tissue, which is information required in evaluating anemia.

permanent section   See *paraffin section* in Glossary.

peroxidase-antiperoxidase technique   A type of immunoperoxidase method used to identify certain substances (antigens) in tissues, using monoclonal antibodies and amplification steps to detect the antigens' "signal."

Patient preparation The preparation is identical to that which precedes a tissue biopsy.

Procedure The tissue is fixed (e.g., with formalin), washed, and incubated with a monoclonal antibody against the antigen to be tested. The monoclonal antibody is coupled to an enzyme (e.g., peroxidase, which is covalently bound to one end of the monoclonal antibody). The tissue is then incubated with a substrate. If the antigen is present in the tissue, the substrate is digested, yielding a color change that can be seen by a microscope or measured by a spectrophotometer.

Specimen Tissue, usually from a biopsy.

Reference range The usual antigens in normal tissue.

Abnormal values Abnormal tissues, in particular malignant tissues, often have antigens that are not normally produced by their benign counterparts from the same body sites.

Cost $100–$200.

personality test Any of a number of psychological tests, including the individual Rorschach ink blot test or the multiple-choice California Psychological Inventory, which are designed to objectively measure certain facets of an individual's personality and possibly predict a person's ability to function in the workplace. Some experts in psychology believe that personality testing is of little benefit and is poorly predictive of future behavior.

Perthes' test (tourniquet test) A clinical test that evaluates the patency (openness) of the deep veins of the legs, and the competency (i.e., whether they close properly) of the valves of the leg veins in the presence of varices of the superficial leg veins.
Patient preparation None required.
Procedure A tourniquet is wrapped around the upper leg of a patient standing erect, which compresses the superficial varices.
Reference range No pain with prolonged testing.
Abnormal values If atherosclerosis is absent, an increase in pain with prolonged testing usually indicates the presence of deep venous obstruction or thrombosis.
Cost The cost of clinical testing may be incorporated into the normal hospital charges.

per umbilical blood sampling (PUBS, cordocentesis) A test that may be used in high-risk obstetrics to identify fetal disease, alloimmunization, metabolic defects, and infection. It can be used to provide the tissues and cells needed for karyotyping. The same technique can be used in reverse to provide a portal of access for fetal therapy, e.g., red blood cell and/or platelet transfusions.
Procedure This "high-risk" procedure consists of the aspiration of umbilical cord blood from a fetus at high risk for a number of diseases that would benefit from therapy before delivery. An ultrasound device is used to guide the needle to the ideal sites of aspiration and away from the fetus' vital structures.
Specimen Blood.
Reference range Negative for infections, immune reactions and chromosomal defects.
Abnormal values PUBS helps identify hemoglobinopathies, hemophilia, autoimmune thrombocytopenia, von Willebrand disease, Rh disease, Kell antigens, alloimmunization with other red cell antigens, alloimmune thrombocytopenia, metabolic disorders, and fetal infection (parvovirus, B19, CMV, rubella, toxoplasmosis, varicella).
Cost $150–$250.
Comments Complications include cord hematoma, bradycardia, and fetal loss in up to 3% of pregnancies.

PET scan See *positron emission tomography.*

pH of blood Living systems function in a "buffered" fluid environment that is usually close to a neutral pH (i.e., neither too acid nor too alkaline), which in the human blood stream is between pH 7.35 and 7.45. The body compensates for changes in pH—which are related to the quantity of carbon dioxide and hydrogen ions in the body—by altering the activity of the lungs and/or kidneys. A decrease in serum pH may be due to an increase in hydrogen ions or to a decrease in compensating carbonate ions and is known as acidosis. An increase in serum pH may be due to a decrease in hydrogen ions or an increase in carbonate ions and is known as alkalosis. Acidosis and alkalosis are categorized according to cause. Those attributed to decreased pulmonary activity with accumulation of carbon dioxide are known as respiratory acidosis, and those attributed to increased pulmonary activity with decreased carbon dioxide are known as respiratory alkalosis. A decrease in excretion of acids by the kidney is termed metabolic acidosis, and an increase of renal excretion of acids is known as metabolic alkalosis. Measuring pH is necessary in diagnosing these conditions.

Patient preparation No preparation is required, other than for drawing arterial blood.

Procedure pH is measured by electrodes.

Specimen Arterial blood drawn in a hepatinized tube, placed in ice, and transported immediately to the laboratory for analysis.

Reference range 7.35–7.45.

Abnormal values Less than 7.35 or greater than 7.45. The body has a complex and interconnected series of mechanisms that compensate for changes in the pH. Therapy is directed at treating the underlying cause, e.g., prolonged vomiting, chronic diarrhea, excess of adrenal steroids, each of which will affect the pH.

Cost The test is usually part of a blood gas panel. The usual cost is $75–$100.

(12–24 hour) pH study A procedure that is used to determine the presence, frequency, and duration of acid reflux and the need for medical or surgical therapy. Studies of pH are indicated for patients with suspected gastroesophageal reflux disease or lung aspiration of gastric contents, which may occur at night. The studies are also used to evaluate the effectiveness of treatment in persons known to have gastroesophageal reflux disease.

Patient preparation Informed consent is required. Coffee, tobacco, and alcohol are not permitted during the study. The patient must follow a bland diet during the study.

Procedure The procedure consists of the placement of an indwelling probe in the distal esophagus (the region where acid refluxes from the stomach) to evaluate acid reflux and the need for medical or surgical therapy.

Reference range Under normal circumstance, the pH in the distal esophagus is 4 or greater. A series of complex calculations was once used to establish the normal values of the pH study. It is now accepted that the length of time that the distal esophagus is exposed to acid and the number of reflux events requiring more than five minutes to clear are sufficiently informative to guide therapy.

Abnormal values Multiple episodes of reflux and increased exposure of the esophagus to acid.

Cost This test has a wide range of fees, ranging up to $1000.

Comments These studies were formerly performed exclusively in a hospital setting, but when performed, are in the form of ambulatory pH monitoring. pH studies are generally used when gastroesophageal reflux cannot be proven by other means. The test is expensive, labor-intensive, and the rates of false-negativity may be high.

pH (urine)   Urinary pH has a wider range than blood pH, because the kidneys (which produce the urine) have a major role in maintaining the pH in the circulation close to neutral (pH 7.35–7.45). If the pH in the blood falls and becomes more acid, the kidneys increase the excretion of hydrogen ions (acids). If the pH in the blood rises and becomes more alkaline, the kidneys increase the excretion of bicarbonate ions (alkalines).

Patient preparation No preparation is required, other than for obtaining urine.

Procedure pH is measured by electrodes.

Specimen Urine.

Normal range 4.6–8.0, usually 6.0.

Abnormal values

  Increased in: alkaline excess, diet (increased ingestion of fruits and vegetables), drugs (e.g., acetazolamide, aldosterone, amphotericin B, cortisone, dichlophenamide, certain diuretics, methazolamide, potassium bicarbonate, potassium citrate, potassium carbonate, potassium gluconate, prolactin, sodium bicarbonate).

  Decreased in: achlorhydria, alkaptonuria, diabetes mellitus chronic obstructive pulmonary disease (COPD), diet, increased proteins, cranberries, drugs (e.g., ascorbic acid, ammonium chloride, certain anesthetics, diazoxide, hippuric acid, methenamine mandelate), methanol intoxication, phenylketonuria, respiratory acidosis, renal tuberculosis, sepsis, starvation.

Cost This test is part of a routine urinalysis, which normally costs $20–$30.

phenobarbital   A barbiturate drug that is used as a sedative, hypnotic, and anticonvulsant. Phenobarbital can affect the metabolism of other drugs, e.g., phenytoin and ethosuximide, and increase the clearance and elimination of chloramphenicol, theophylline, oral anticoagulants, cyclosporine, and oral contraceptives. Use of these drugs in patients who are being treated with phenobarbital should be monitored clinically, and the serum levels of phenobarbital should be measured.

Patient preparation No preparation is required, other than for drawing blood.

Specimen Serum.

Reference range 15–40 µg/ml during therapy.

Abnormal values Greater than 40 μg/ml.
Cost $70–$90.

phenolsulfonphthalein test (PSP test)   A test that evaluates renal tubular function based on the excretion of a dye (PSP) that is eliminated from the circulation as it passes through the kidneys.
Patient preparation 30 minutes after the patient has voided urine and ingested 600 ml of water, 1 ml of phenolsulfonphthalein is injected intravenously.
Procedure The test is based on the excretion of a dye, PSP, which binds to albumin and is eliminated from the circulation as it passes through the kidneys. The dye is measured in the urine by spectrophotometry, therefore colored substance in the urine could interfere with the results. The urine is collected at 15, 30, 60, and 120 minutes, and the amount of dye excreted is measured.
Specimen Urine.
Reference range 25% excretion in 15 minutes, 50% by 30 minutes, 75% by 2 hours.
Abnormal values
   Increased in: hepatic disease, hypoalbuminemia, hypoproteinemia.
   Decreased in: amyloidosis, cirrhosis (compensated), congestive heart failure, drug therapy (e.g., chlorothiazide, penicillin, probenicid, salicylates, sulfonamides), hyperproteinemia, intravenous radiocontrast dyes, primary hypertension, kidney disease (e.g., lower nephron nephrosis, nephrosclerosis, polycystic kidneys, pyelonephritis, renovascular disease), prostatic hypertrophy.
Cost $50–$100.

phenothiazines   A class of drugs that are prescribed as antipsychotic agents, tranquilizers, and antiemetics. The most widely used agent is chlorpromazine (Thorazine®), which is representative of these drugs.
Patient preparation No preparation is required, other than for drawing blood.
Procedure Phenothiazines are measured by immunoassay, gas-liquid chromatography, and high-performance liquid chromatography.
Specimen Serum, urine, gastric juice. Urine is used to screen for the presence of phenothiazine. Serum is used to determine the actual concentration in the body. Gastric content can be used as a source, especially if the patient is in a coma that might be due to a drug overdose.
Reference range
   Chlorpromazine   50–300 ng/ml.
Abnormal values
   Chlorpromazine   Greater than 750 ng/ml.
Cost
   Urine $25–$45.
   Serum $85–$95.
Comments Phenothiazines are not usually monitored because the correlation between serum level and antipsychotic effect is poor.

phentolamine test (Regitine test) A pharmacologic test for pheochromocytoma (a hypertension-causing tumor of the adrenal glands), in which the alpha-adrenergic blocking agent, phentolamine, is administered intravenously.

Patient preparation The patient is recumbent after an overnight fast.

Procedure 5% glucose is administered for 30 minutes. The blood pressure is allowed to stabilize at greater than 160 mm Hg systolic, and between 1 and 5 mg of phentolamine is administered.

Reference range A mild drop in blood pressure is normal.

Abnormal values The diagnosis of pheochromocytoma is suggested by a significant drop (greater than 35/25 mm Hg) in blood pressure but must be confirmed by measuring the catecholamines or their metabolites in the urine.

Cost The fee charged for such "functional" tests is variable and ranges up to $500 or more.

Comments Because of the high rate of false-positive and false-negative results, and because the test may cause severe hypotension, the phentolamine test has waned in popularity. It is a functional test in which the activity of a particular organ or gland is measured based on the activity evoked by the hormone, factor, or other product. See *catecholamines.*

phenylalanine (urine) (PKU) Phenylketonuria is an inherited disease caused by a defect of the enzyme, phenylalanine hydroxylase, resulting in an accumulation of phenylalanine, which, if untreated, causes mental retardation in children. All newborn infants are tested for phenylalanine before being discharged from the hospital. If the screening test is positive, further quantitative and genetic workups are completed. When identified early, defects such as mental retardation and microcephaly and electroencephalographic abnormalities are avoided by dietary restriction of phenylalanine intake.

Patient preparation No preparation is required, other than for drawing blood or obtaining urine.

Procedure The specimen is measured by direct fluorometry or by ion exchange chromatography.

Specimen Whole blood, serum, plasma.

Reference range Less than 4 mg/dL by fluorometry; less than 2 mg/dL by ion exchange chromatography.

Abnormal values Any moderate to marked increase in phenylalanine in the serum is significant and requires that the pediatrician be alerted and the diet changed immediately.

Cost $85–$100.

phenytoin (Dilantin) A drug used to treat generalized tonic-clonic and partial seizures, as well as status epilepticus. Because of its variable absorption, its narrow therapeutic range, and relative toxicity, phenytoin levels in the blood must be monitored. Most phenytoin in the circulation is bound to serum proteins; only the unbound (free) fraction is biologically active. Free phenytoin is not routinely measured as it is not cost-effective. In practice, total phenytoin levels are used to monitor therapy.

Patient preparation No preparation is required, other than for drawing blood.

Procedure Phenytoin can be measured by various immunoassay techniques.

Specimen Serum, plasma. Consistent sampling times are important in patients who are receiving long-term phenytoin therapy.

Reference range

Total phenytoin	10–20 μg/ml.
Free phenytoin	1–2 μg/ml.

Abnormal values

Total phenytoin	Greater than 20 μg/ml.
Free phenytoin	Greater than 2 μg/ml.

Cost

Total phenytoin	$70–$80.
Free phenytoin	$130–$150.

phlebography   See *venography.*

phleborheography   See *plethysmography.*

phlebotomy   The drawing of blood from a patient to be used for diagnostic evaluation. In most hospitals, this task is carried out by individuals (phlebotomists) who are formally trained.

phlegm   See *sputum.*

phonocardiography (echophonocardiography)   A noninvasive technique that amplifies faint, low-frequency sounds of blood flowing through the heart and the great vessels and displays them in a graphic form. Phonocardiography is used to evaluate various types of pulse tracings and to diagnose abnormalities of the cardiac valves, ventricular hypertrophy, and left heart failure. Phonocardiography is usually performed in synchrony with electrocardiography, M-mode echocardiography, or Doppler echocardiography, which allows the changes heard by phonocardiography to be matched with the point at which they occur in the heartbeat.

Patient preparation No preparation is required. Hairy patients may need to be shaved to optimally place the recording devices on the chest wall.

Procedure The procedure consists of the placement of small microphones on the chest wall. Phonocardiography is often performed at the same time as electrocardiography and apexcardiography.

Reference range Normally the baseline phonocardiogram is flat and is punctuated by vibrations from the first (S_1) and second (S_2) heart sounds. The third (S_3) heart sound, or ventricular gallop, occurs after the aortic valve closes and may be normal in children and in adults with an increased cardiac "output," e.g., athletes. The S₃ sound is due to rapid or high-volume early ventricular filling during diastole. The S₄, or atrial gallop, occurs after the onset of the P wave and may be normal.

Abnormal values Increased intensity of the S₁ sound may occur in stenosis (closure) of the mitral or tricuspid valve or tachycardia linked to an increase in contractility of the left ventricle. A decreased S₁ intensity may occur in pericardial effusion, decreased cardiac function related to myocarditis, or in a first-degree heart block. A widened splitting of the S₁ is typical of a right bundle branch block. A widened S₂ splitting during inspiration indicates right ventricular overload and decreased pulmonary vascular resistance. A widened S₂ splitting during expiration may occur in pulmonary thromboembolism and in right bundle branch block. A narrowed S₂ splitting during inspiration occurs in increased pulmonary vascular resistance. An S₃ may occur in ventricular overload due to tricuspid or mitral valve regurgitation. An S₄ may be due to hypertension, aortic stenosis, coronary artery disease, or hypertrophic cardiomyopathy.

Cost $100–$250.

phosphorus (phosphates, PO₄)   Phosphorus is the predominant intracellular anion (negative ion), which is integral to the storage and utilization of energy. It is intimately linked to the regulation of calcium levels, carbohydrate and lipid metabolism, and acid-base balance. Phosphorus is essential to bone formation, and approximately 85% of the body's phosphorous and phosphates are found in bone.

Patient preparation No preparation is required, other than for drawing blood or obtaining urine.

Procedure Phosphorus is measured by automated blood analyzers by colorimetry or enzymatic methods.

Specimen Serum, urine. For best results in urine, a timed or 24-hour collection is recommended. For serum levels, the patient should be fasting.

Reference range

SERUM
  Children   4.0–6.0 mg/dL.
  Adults   2.5–4.5 mg/dL.
URINE
  Adults   0.9–1.3 g/24 hours.

Abnormal values

SERUM
  Increased in: youth, exercise, dehydration, hypoparathyroidism bone metastases, sarcoidoisis.
  Decreased in: antacids, diuretics, diabetic ketoacidosis
URINE
  Increased in: hyperparathyroidism, vitamin D deficiency, renal tubular acidosis, diuretics
  Decreased in: hypoparathyroidism, vitamin D intoxication.

Cost $10–30. Phosphates are usually part of a typical chemistry profile.
Comments Hemolysis of the specimen will cause falsely elevated levels.

photodensitometry See *bone densitometry.*

pilocarpine stimulation See *sweat test.*

pituitary function test A general term for any laboratory test used to evaluate the function of the adenohypophysis (also known as the anterior pituitary gland). Pituitary function tests can be static, i.e., the levels of a pituitary hormone (e.g., ACTH) and linked feedback hormone (cortisol, which is secreted by the adrenal gland in response to ACTH) are measured in the serum; or dynamic, where hormones are administered to evaluate the response of the feedback organs to stimulation by hormones of the anterior pituitary (adenohypophysis). Among the dynamic tests are the combined anterior pituitary test, the insulin tolerance test, and the glucose tolerance test. See *glucose tolerance test.*

placental lactogen See *human placental lactogen.*

plain film See *X ray* in Glossary.

plantar ischemia test A simple clinical test used to evaluate the adequacy of peripheral circulation of the leg, in which the leg is elevated and plantar surface of the foot is examined in flexion and extension. Blanching or loss of the normal pink color on the skin surface often indicates decreased blood flow, which is usually due to severe arteriosclerosis.

plasma renin activity Renin is an enzyme secreted primarily by the kidney, and in lesser amounts by the brain and blood vessels, in response to reduced renal perfusion pressure or decreased kallikrein blood flow to the kidney. It breaks down angiotensinogen to yield angiotensin I, the precursor of angiotensin II, which is a potent vasoconstrictor that stimulates thirst and increases aldosterone production.
Patient preparation No preparation is required, other than for drawing blood.
Procedure Renin is measured indirectly by an assay that measures renin's conversion of angiotensinogen to angiotensin I, the latter of which is measured by radioimmunoassay.
Specimen Plasma with sodium-EDTA anticoagulant. The plasma is placed in ice and centrifuged at 4°C, separated, and frozen until analysis.
Reference range

Children	1.7–11.0 ng/ml.
Adult lying down for 30 minutes	0.2–2.3 ng/ml.
Adult with salt-restricted diet	4.1–7.7 ng/ml.

Abnormal values
Increased in: Addison's disease, chronic obstructive pulmonary disease,

CRF (corticotropin-releasing factor) hypersecretion, eclampsia (and preeclampsia), hyperthyroidism, liver cirrhosis, low-potassium, low-salt diet, malignant hypertension, pregnancy, early, renal failure, renovascular hypertension, functional tumors of the kidney, drugs (e.g., antihypertensives, oral contraceptives, diuretics, furosemide).
Decreased in: Cushing's syndrome, diabetes mellitus, essential hypertension, hypothyroidism, high-salt diet, drugs (e.g., antihypertensives, levodopa, propranol).
Cost $110–$130.

plasma thrombin time   See *thrombin time.*

plasmin (fibrinolysin)   An enzyme formed from plasminogen that is responsible for the removal of blood clots. Plasmin exists in free and bound forms. Free plasmin is destroyed as it is formed by antiplasmins. Bound plasmin acts as an enzyme to solubilize fibrin clots and hydrolyzes lysine and arginine bonds in certain proteins, e.g., fibrinogen and coagulation factors V and VII. There is no direct measurement of plasmin because of its instability. Abnormalities in plasmin activity are inferred from various coagulation factor assays.

plasminogen   A proenzyme present in the circulation, which is synthesized in the liver and produced or stored in eosinophils. It forms complexes with fibrinogen and fibrin. During coagulation, large amounts of plasminogen are incorporated in the fibrin mass or clot. The most common indication for measuring plasminogen is suspected disseminated intravascular coagulation, a serious clinical condition in which it is markedly decreased.
Patient preparation No preparation is required, other than for drawing blood.
Procedure Plasminogen is measured by radial immunodiffusion, spectrophotometry, or fluorometry.
Specimen Plasma in a blue-top tube.
Reference range 20 mg/dL.
Abnormal values
Increased in: deep vein thrombosis, infection, inflammation, malignancy, myocardial infarction, oral contraceptives, pregnancy physical stress (e.g., surgery, trauma).
Decreased in: cirrhosis and other hepatic diseases, disseminated intravascular coagulation, fibrinolysis, hyaline membrane disease, (respiratory distress of the newborn), renal disease, postsurgery (e.g., coronary artery bypass graft).
Cost $145–$165.

platelet   See *platelet count.*

platelet adhesion test   A test that evaluates the ability of platelets to "stick" to surfaces. Platelet adhesion tests are of limited use, given the lack of standardization and the finding that consistently abnormal values only occur in patients with greatly prolonged bleeding time.

Patient preparation No preparation is required, other than for drawing blood.

Procedure Platelet adhesion is measured based on the retention of platelets in a column filled with glass beads.

Specimen Plasma from whole blood drawn into a citrated plastic tube.

Reference range There is a wide range of values seen in normal patients, making platelet adhesion a difficult test to standardize.

Abnormal values

Increased in: aging, atherosclerosis, burns, homocystinuria, hypercoagulability, hyperlipidemia, infection, inflammation, malignancy, myocardial infarction, oral contraceptives, pregnancy, physical stress, surgery, thrombosis, trauma.

Decreased in: afibrinogenemia, anemia, azotemia, Bernard-Soulier disease, Chédiak-Higashi syndrome, cirrhosis and other hepatic diseases, congenital heart disease, disseminated intravascular coagulation, fibrinolysis, Glanzmann's thrombasthenia, glycogen storage disease, hyaline membrane disease (respiratory distress syndrome of the newborn), multiple myeloma, plasma cell dyscrasia, platelet release defects, renal disease, post-surgery (e.g., coronary artery bypass graft), uremia, von Willebrand's disease, Waldenström's macroglobulinemia.

Cost $100–$150. See *platelet aggregation studies.*

platelet aggregation studies A battery of assays that measures the response of platelets to various substances (e.g., ADP, epinephrine, thrombin, collagen, ristocetin, and arachidonic acid) that cause platelets to aggregate. Platelet aggregation studies are used to diagnose abnormalities in the clotting of blood caused by platelet membrane defects.

Patient preparation No preparation is required, other than for drawing blood.

Procedure Platelet aggregation is determined by an increase in optical density of stirred, platelet-rich plasma.

Specimen Plasma from whole blood drawn into a citrated plastic tube.

Reference Range Normal platelets exhibit a primary and secondary (i.e., a second wave) response when exposed to collagen and ADP.

Abnormal values

Increased in: atherosclerosis, diabetes mellitus, hemolysis, nicotine, hypercoagulability, hyperlipidemia, polycythemia vera.

Decreased in: afibrinogenemia, anemia, Bernard-Soulier disease, β-thalassemia, Chédiak-Higashi syndrome, cirrhosis, hepatic disease, Glanzmann's thrombasthenia, idiopathic thrombocytopenic purpura, myeloma, plasma cell dyscrasia, platelet release defects, storage pool disease, uremia, von Willebrand's disease, Waldenström's

macroglobulinemia, and drug therapy (antibiotics, anticoagulants, antihistamines, aspirin, cephalothin, chlordiazepoxide, clofibrate, cocaine, corticosteroids, dextran, diphenhydramine, dipyridamole, furosemide, general anesthetics [e.g., halothane, nitrous oxide], gentamicin, guaifesin, heparin, hydroxychloroquine, ibuprofen, marijuana, meclofenamate, mefanamic acid, naproxen, nitrofurantoin, nonsteroidal anti-inflammatory drugs, penicillin, phenothiazine, phenylbutazone, propranolol, sulfinpyrazone, theophylline, tricyclic antidepressants).
Cost $150–$200.

platelet count A laboratory test consisting of the simple enumeration of circulating platelets, which are a basic component of the blood and, in large part, responsible for the clotting coagulation of blood. Platelets are fragments of megakaryocytes that are produced in the bone marrow and measure about 1 μL in diameter; the platelets' intrinsic properties of adhesion and aggregation provide the first line of defense when blood vessels are torn through trauma.
Patient preparation No preparation is required, other than for drawing blood.
Procedure The platelets are passed through an electronic device that counts particles (i.e., platelets) of a certain size.
Specimen Whole blood collected in a lavender-top tube. In some patients, platelets are affected by EDTA, an anticoagulant, and clump together, causing false low counts. This can be resolved by collecting the whole blood in green-top or blue-top tubes, which contain, respectively, heparin and sodium citrate as anticoagulants.
Reference range 150–400,000/μL (mm³). The "panic values" are less than 20,000/μL and greater than 1,000,000/μL.
Abnormal values
> Increased in: myeloproliferative disorders, polycythemia vera.
> Less commonly in: infections, blood loss, and splenectomy.
> Rarely also: anemia (hemolytic, iron-deficiency, sickle cell), cirrhosis collagen vascular disease, cryoglobulinemia, drugs (e.g., epinephrine, oral contraceptives), exercise, hemorrhage, hypoxia, postpartum, pregnancy, rheumatoid arthritis, tuberculosis.
> Decreased counts (below 20,000/mm³ (μL) are associated with an increased bleeding tendency and occur in: malignancies of bone, gastrointestinal tract, brain, leukemia, kidney or liver disease, aplastic anemia, disseminated intravascular coagulation, idiopathic thrombocytopenic purpura, systemic lupus erythematosus, drugs (aspirin, chemotherapeutic agents, chloromycetin, phenylbutazone, quinidine, thiazide diuretics, tolbutamide).
Cost Platelets are measured as part of a CBC (complete blood count), which costs $20–$30.

plethysmography (venous impedence plethysmography)   A technique that detects the changes in the volume of an organ, limb, or the body itself by measuring the flow of blood through its veins. Impedance plethysmography is used to diagnose acute venous obstruction or vascular insufficiency of an extremity by measuring the change in limb volume with each arterial pulse and during induced (cuff) occlusion of the venous flow from the limb, the manipulation of which allows evaluation of either the arterial or venous flow. Whole body plethysmography measures the volume of gas in the lungs, including that which is trapped in poorly communicating air spaces, a datum of particular use in chronic obstructive pulmonary disease and emphysema.

pleural biopsy A "blind" biopsy of the pleura, the fibrous layer of tissue that covers the lung and the surrounding space, the pleural cavity. A pleural biopsy is obtained through the skin, often in combination with thoracentesis as a means of determining the cause of pleural effusions, which may be due to tuberculosis or other bacterial infection or malignancy, especially adenocarcinomas and mesotheliomas.

Patient preparation Informed consent is required. A sedative may be required, as it is a painful procedure.

Procedure The procedure consists of the insertion of a biopsy needle, e.g., a Vim-Silverman or a Cope needle, in order to remove tissue.

Specimen Fragments of tissue.

Reference range Normal pleural tissue is not inflamed and has only fibrous tissue and a thin covering layer of cells known as mesothelial cells.

Abnormal values The tissue may demonstrate inflammation in rheumatoid arthritis, infection in bacterial or tuberculous pleuritis, or malignancy, due to spread from the lungs, breasts, or elsewhere.

Cost There are two components to a biopsy, the surgical component and the laboratory component. The surgical component involves hospitalization, anesthesia, and physician charges which are variable but are in the range of $2000–$4000. The laboratory component is $50–$200.

Comments Complications include low platelet count, especially if under 20,000/mm^3, and low volume of fluid.

pleural fluid tap See *thoracentesis.*

ploidy analysis A technique in flow cytometry that evaluates the chromosomal content of cells, which is a marker for aggressiveness in malignancy. In general, diploidy (i.e., the presence of two haploid sets of chromosomes), is a normal or near-normal state. In contrast, anaplastic and aggressive tumors are more often aneuploid or hyperdiploid. Ploidy analysis is used to determine the prognosis of cancer of the bone (osteosarcoma), breast, colon, endometrium, lymphoma, and ovary.

Patient preparation No specific preparation is required, as the cells are taken from a portion of tissue obtained during a biopsy.

Procedure The procedure consists of passing cells through a device known as a flow cytometer.

Specimen Cells derived from tissues that have been chopped into small fragments or "minced."

Reference range Diploidy.

Abnormal values Hyperdiploid tumors have a high relapse rate in the early follow-up period and behave aggressively, resulting in a shortened survival for the patient. The same "rule" (diploid, good prognosis; aneuploid, poor prognosis) applies to transitional cell carcinoma of the bladder, lymphoma, and cancer of the bone, breast, colon, endometrium, ovary, and elsewhere.

Cost $175–$250. See *flow cytometry*.

point-of-care testing (POCT)   The analysis of clinical specimens as close as possible to the patient, which can be at the bedside, in the patient's ward (unit), or at "stat" regional response laboratories that service specified areas, including the emergency room or the intensive care unit. While the cost in point-of-care testing are generally much higher than those of similar tests performed in a central laboratory, the total cost may actually be reduced, as labor is performed by personnel, e.g., nurses, physicians' assistants, and others who are already performing different duties at the bedside. While POCT would appear to be clearly useful, no one has proven that improved timeliness of test results improves patient care.

polymerase chain reaction (PCR)   A technique used in molecular biology in which enzymes from high-temperature bacteria are used to rapidly amplify (i.e., increase the number of copies of) a portion of DNA in a sample. Starting from minimal amounts—as little as one copy of a sequence of DNA—the PCR amplifies DNA, synthesizing millions of copies of a DNA segment of interest, and can be used to detect various DNA defects, including gene mutations. PCR has been used to determine fetal sex, diagnose sickle cell anemia, detect HIV-1, and identify gene rearrangements in lymphomas and DNA from suspected criminals. In detecting leukemia in bone marrow, PCR has an accuracy of 99.999%. In addition to human genetic analysis, PCR is being used increasingly in the rapid detection of viruses and bacteria, and PCR tests have been developed for the diagnosis and monitoring of Lyme disease, tuberculosis, and chlamydia (*Chlamydia trachomatis*). While PCR is a costly test, its cost will decrease as it becomes more readily available in clinical laboratories. The major drawback of PCR is the ease with which foreign DNA contaminates the specimens being tested, which may cause false-positive results.

Patient preparation No specific preparation is required, as the DNA is obtained from the cells obtained in a biopsy or from whole blood.

Procedure PCR exponentially "amplifies" DNA, synthesizing millions of copies of a DNA segment of interest within hours. The PCR can be used to detect DNA abnormalities including gene deletions, insertions, translocations, and point mutations. Once a DNA segment has been amplified, it is then evaluated by conventional DNA techniques, including Southern blot hybridization.

Specimen Fragments of tissue or blood samples.
Reference range Negative for the DNA (e.g., HIV-1, sickle cell defects).
Abnormal values Depending on the segment of DNA being amplified, the PCR serves to confirm the presence of an infection or to determine the type of malignancy.
Cost Highly variable, depending on the type of specimen and the type of testing being performed. $200–$500.

polysomnography (cardiopulmonary sleep study, sleep apnea study) A technique for measuring multiple physiologic parameters during sleep. Polysomnography is used to identify nocturnal defects in respiratory control.
Patient preparation The procedure is complex and requires that the patient spend the night at the test site. The patient's hair should be clean and free of oils. All medications should be continued and brought to the test site.
Procedure A complete polysomnography includes electrocardiography, electroencephalography, electromyography, and electrooculography. Noninvasive sensors measure nasal air flow (thermocouple), air flow through the mouth, tracheal sounds (microphone), thoracic and abdominal respiratory effort (inductance plethysmography), and oxyhemoglobin by a finger-pulse oximeter.
Reference range No defects or alterations in physiological parameters.
Abnormal values Polysomnography is abnormal in sleep apnea disorders, chronic obstructive pulmonary disease, and restrictive ventilatory disorders.
Cost $1000–$2000.

porphobilinogen (porphyrin) Porphyrins are breakdown products of hemoglobin, the protein that carries oxygen (O_2), and may be measured in porphyria (a relatively uncommon metabolic disease), liver disease, lead poisoning, and rarely in pellagra.
Patient preparation No preparation is required, other than for obtaining urine.
Procedure Porphyrins are measured in the urine by spectrophotometry.
Specimen Urine, kept in a dark container; quantitative results require a 24-hour urine specimen.
Reference range Because testing procedures vary from laboratory to laboratory, the reference range must be obtained from the laboratory carrying out the analysis. Normally, up to 2.0 mg are excreted in the urine in a 24-hour period.
Abnormal values
  Increased in: congenital erythropoietic porphyria, acute intermittent porphyria, hereditary coproporphyria, liver disease, porphyria cutanea tarda, variegate porphyria.
Cost $40–$60.

porphobilinogen deaminase (uroporphyrinogen synthase) An enzyme that converts porphobilinogen into uroporphyrinogen in the synthesis of heme. Heme is present in red blood cells, lymphocytes, fibroblasts, hepatic cells, and amniotic fluid cells. Porphobilinogen deaminase levels are reduced to 50% normal in acute intermittent porphyria, an inherited condition that may be latent for many years and then triggered by alcohol or drugs (e.g., barbiturates, diphenylhydantoin, estrogens, mephenytoin, meprobamate, sulfonamides, or valproic acid).

Patient preparation No preparation is required, other than for drawing blood.

Procedure The enzyme activity is demonstrated by fluorometry, which measures the rate of conversion of porphobilinogen to uroporphyrinogen.

Specimen Whole blood collected in heparinized (green-top) or EDTA anti-coagulated tubes.

Reference range 1.27–2.01 mU per gram of hemoglobin.

Abnormal values Decreased in acute intermittent porphyria.

Cost $150–$200.

Comments Paradoxically, estrogen-based oral contraceptives have been used to prevent acute attacks of porphyria.

portal venography (portovenography)   See *percutaneous transhepatic portal venography.*

portovenography   See *percutaneous transhepatic portal venography.*

positron emission tomography (PET scan, positron emission transaxial tomography)   A noninvasive imaging used to evaluate blood flow and metabolism in the brain and heart. PET detects positron-emitting radioisotopes, the patterns of which correspond to biochemical and pathologic abnormalities in the body.

Patient preparation None required, other than that for radionuclide imaging, where blood specimens to be analyzed by radioimmunoassay should be drawn before the procedure.

Procedure The technique combines computed tomography with radionuclide scanning, providing a three-dimensional image of the brain and heart.

Reference range No anatomic abnormalities or physical defects are seen.

Abnormal values PET is abnormal in the brain in AIDS-related neuropathology, dementia, epilepsy, malignancy, Parkinson's disease, and psychiatric disorders. PET may also be used in cardiology to detect coronary arteriosclerosis, regional myocardial blood flow, and ischemia.

Cost $700–$1500.

(2-hour) post-prandial blood sugar   See *glucose tolerance test.*

potassium (K+)   The principal positive ion (cation) within living cells. This electrolyte is critical in the synthesis of new molecules within the cell and those involving the transfer of energy. Potassium in the circulation has a narrow range, and both extremely high and low levels may be fatal.

Specimen Serum, plasma, urine. When measuring potassium in plasma, potassium anticoagulants must be avoided, using instead ammonium or lithium heparin anti-coagulants of choice. Urine measurements should be made on timed specimens.

Reference range

Serum, plasma	3.5–5.0 mmol/L.
Urine	26–123 mmol/24 hours.

Abnormal values

Decreased in: crash dieting, Cushing's syndrome, diabetic ketoacidosis, dehydration, drugs (aspirin, corticosteroids, (potassium-wasting), diuretics, estrogen, insulin, laxatives, lithium, sodium polystyrene sulfonate, hyperaldosteronism, licorice (due to aldosterone-like effects of glycyrrhizic acid), malnutrition, metabolic acidosis, nasogastric suction, starvation, stress (burns, surgery, trauma), vomiting.

Increased in: renal insufficiency or failure (anuria, oliguria) tissue injury or destruction, burns, drugs (potassium-sparing diuretics [e.g., spironolactone], epinephrine, histamine, antibiotics [e.g., cephalosporins, isoniazid, penicillin]), excess potassium in intravenous solutions, metabolic acidosis.

Cost $10–$30. Usually performed as part of a chemistry profile.

Comments Because potassium is relatively abundant within red blood cells, hemolysis or lengthy contact between the serum and red blood cells will cause falsely elevated levels. If the test cannot be performed immediately, the serum or plasma should be separated from the red blood cells until analysis is performed.

potential achievement test See *psychological test.*

PPD test A clinical test for detecting exposure to the tuberculosis bacteria, *Mycobacterium tuberculosis.* A small amount of PPD (purified protein derivative, the antigenic material used to detect previous exposure to tuberculosis) is injected intradermally, and the diameter of the reaction is measured after a few days.

Patient preparation No preparation is required. Minimal discomfort is associated with the pinprick of the PPD test.

Procedure A small needle is inserted into the superficial skin, and the response is interpreted between 48 and 72 hours later.

Reference range An indurated zone of less than 10 millimeters is seen after two to three days in normal individuals who have not been exposed to tuberculosis.

Abnormal values An induration of 10 mm or greater after 48 to 72 hours is considered a positive. A negative PPD response may not indicate that the patient has not been exposed to tuberculosis but rather may be due to a

loss of reactivity (anergy), as occurs in immune defects, e.g., AIDS.
Cost $35–$50.

preadmission tests (PAT) A battery of tests required before a patient is admitted to a hospital for elective therapy, e.g., cataract extraction or cholecystectomy. Preadmission tests serve to establish "baseline" values in the patient. In a community hospital setting, a typical PAT battery includes a CBC and leukocyte differential count, PT and PTT, a multichannel analysis of blood chemistries, urinalysis, an electrocardiogram, and a chest film.

Patient preparation No preparation is required, other than for drawing blood, obtaining urine, or passing through the cardiology or radiology services for the appropriate studies.

Procedure The analyses differ according to the parameter being measured.

Specimen Blood, serum, urine, chest X ray, electrocardiogram.

Reference range All parameters should be within normal limits.

Abnormal values Abnormality in the preadmission tests requires physician notification and possibly treatment.

Cost Because each hospital has different requirements for preadmission tests, the charges are highly variable. These tests are generally paid as part of the hospitalization rather than on an outpatient basis.

Comments The usefulness of preadmission testing for ambulatory surgery is limited, as the abnormalities may be ignored and/or extremely expensive for the information they provide.

predictive value of a negative test See *negative predictive value* in Glossary.

predictive value of a positive test See *positive predictive value* in Glossary.

predisposition testing (susceptibility testing) A general term for the screening of a battery of molecular markers in order to identify inherited mutations that have been linked to malignancies, e.g., inherited colon cancer (mutations of MSH2 and MSH1), breast cancer (BRCA1), endocrine tumors (RET), melanoma (p16), and Li-Fraumeni syndrome (p53).

pregnancy test A general term for any of a number of tests used to detect or confirm pregnancy. In the early pregnancy, all of these tests detect the presence of human chorionic gonadotropin (hCG), the principle hormone produced by the developing placenta, which is detectable as early as six days after fertilization of the egg.

Patient preparation No preparation is required, other than for obtaining urine, for home testing kits, or blood for quantifying serum levels in the clinical laboratory.

Procedure Home testing kits operate on the principle of agglutination, in which there is a clumping of antigen-antibody complexes. These tests are very reliable and have less than a 1% error rate. Laboratory testing is more sophisticated. It quantifies the serum hCG levels, and is usually performed by enzyme immunoassay.

Specimen Serum, urine.

Reference range Nonpregnant women and men have less than 3.0 mIU/ml of hCG in the serum.

Pregnancy values

7–10 days	Greater than 3.0 mU/ml.
30 days	100–500 mU/ml.
10 weeks	50,000–140,000 mU/ml.
Above 16 weeks	10,000–50,000 mU/ml.

Abnormal values

Trophoblastic disease	Greater than 100,000 mU/ml.

Cost

Home kit	$25–$50.
Laboratory	$15–$25.

Comments HCG can also be measured in men when testing for particular types of tumors. See *human chorionic gonadotropin.*

pregnanediol Pregnanediol is the principle metabolite of progesterone, which is present in the urine. Progesterone is produced in the ovary during the luteal phase of the menstrual cycle, and by the adrenal glands in both men and women at all times. Pregnanediol is produced by the placenta during pregnancy and is responsible for maintaining an appropriate hormonal balance in women after fertilization.

Patient preparation No preparation is required, other than for obtaining a 24-hour specimen of urine.

Procedure Pregnanediol is measured by gas-liquid chromatography.

Specimen 24-hour urine collected in a preservative, e.g., boric acid.

Reference range

Men	0.1–1.5 mg/24 hours.
Women	0.5–1.5/24 hours.
Pregnancy, less than 20 weeks	5–25 mg/24 hours.

Abnormal values

Decreased in: fetal death, menstrual disorders (e.g., amenorrhea), placental failure, preeclampsia, decreased ovarian function, benign tumors of the ovaries or breast.

Increased in: pregnancy, hyperplasia of the adrenal cortex choriocarcinoma, a malignancy of pregnancy-related tissues.

Cost $110–$130.

pregnanetriol A metabolite of 17-hydroxyprogesterone which is produced in the adrenal gland and excreted in the urine, primarily in women. It is increased in a rare endocrine disorder (congenital adrenal hyperplasia), in certain ovarian tumors, and in Stein-Leventhal syndrome.

Patient preparation No preparation is required, other than for obtaining a 24-hour specimen of urine.

Procedure Pregnanetriol is measured by gas-liquid chromatography.

Specimen 24-hour urine collected in a preservative, e.g., boric acid.

Reference range

Women   Less than 2.0 mg/24 hours.

Abnormal values

Decreased in: decreased ovarian function, hypofunction of the anterior pituitary gland.

Increased in: congenital adrenal hyperplasia, tumors of the adrenal cortex, hyperplasia of the adrenal cortex.

Cost $120–$140.

prenatal tests, fetal   A general term for those laboratory parameters that are used to detect genetic and/or congenital fetal abnormalities that would compromise the infant's well-being and quality of life to such a degree that the parents might choose to have an abortion. These tests include measurement of alphafetoprotein levels in the mother's serum or amniotic fluid, chromosomal analysis, ultrasonography, chorionic villus biopsy (a test that is performed on or after the 8th to 10th week of pregnancy, which carries a 1.0–1.5% risk of spontaneous abortion or miscarriage), amniocentesis (a test that is performed on or after the 16th week of pregnancy, which carries a 0.5% risk of spontaneous abortion or miscarriage), fetoscopy, and embryoscopy. Diseases detected by prenatal tests include thalassemias, defects of sex and autosomal chromosomes, including trisomies, gene deletions, mosaicisms, fragile X syndrome, hemophilia, neural tube defects (anencephaly, spina bifida), polycystic renal disease, and Tay-Sachs disease. See *embryoscopy, fetoscopy.*

prick test (percutaneous allergy test, scratch test)   A clinical test for immediate hypersensitivity, in which the reaction is compared to that obtained with standardized mast cell stimulants (e.g., compound 48/80, codeine, and histamine). In contrast to the intradermal test in which very low concentrations of the allergen are allowed to penetrate below the epidermis, the prick test is more rapid, simpler, causes less discomfort for the patient, can be used to test infants, and produces false-positive results. False-negative results, however, are more common. Both tests evoke increased production of IgE antibodies.

Patient preparation No preparation is required. The patient questionnaire should include all current medications, including the last time antihistamines were administered.

Procedure Diluted allergen is droppered on the skin, and a sterile needle is used to "prick" the skin surface, which is observed 20 minutes later to detect the hypersensitivity reaction, a local welt. Allergens commonly used for prick testing include extracts of trees (e.g., birch, elm, ash, cottonwood, and hickory), weeds (e.g., ragweed), grasses, fungi, molds, and epidermals (e.g., house dust, mites, feathers, dog and cat dander). The materials used to perform prick tests have been standardized and are commer-

cially available, either as individual allergens or as batteries of allergens.
Reference range Normally, the welt that develops in individuals with hypersensitivity to these allergens measures less than 5 mm.
Abnormal values The results of the prick test are graded according to the intensity of the positive reaction. "+" is positive with reddening of the skin measuring less than 2.0 cm; "++" is positive with reddening of the skin measuring greater than 2.0 cm; "+++" is positive with reddening of the skin and welts, but no pseudopods; "++++" is positive with reddening of the skin, welts, and pseudopods. Incorrect prick test results are common in the form of false-positives, due to too high concentration of allergens in the patches, misinterpretation of the irritant reaction (a nonimmune response to either the "vehicle" a nonallergenic substance in which the allergen is suspended), or the chemicals in the plastic, and generalized erythema of the skin-testing site. False-negative results are linked to technical errors and either waning potency or inadequate concentration of the allergen.
Cost $10–$25 per allergen.

proctoscopy (anoscopy)   A clinical test that is most often performed in the physician's office, in which a proctoscope, a rigid tube, is inserted in the rectum and the mucosal surface of the lowermost portion of the colon is examined visually to detect the presence of neoplasms or other lesions. If present, these lesions are biopsied and sent to the pathology laboratory for evaluation, to determine whether the tissue is benign or malignant and whether the patient requires further therapy.
Patient preparation The procedure generally follows a digital rectal examination. Sedatives may be required in some patients.
Procedure The procedure consists of the insertion of a rigid metal or plastic tube measuring 2–5 inches in length, which allows the physician to examine the surface (mucosa) of the lower rectum and, if necessary, obtain a biopsy.
Specimen If the physician or staff performing the proctoscopy deems it appropriate, a biopsy is obtained.
Reference range The normal rectum has no visible lesions.
Abnormal values Common defects in the rectum include polyps, bleeding, and cancer.
Cost $500–$700. See *barium enema, colonoscopy, endoscopy, occult blood testing, sigmoidoscopy.*

progesterone   Progesterone is the principal hormone produced in the ovary by the corpus luteum during the luteal phase of the menstrual cycle. It is also produced by the placenta and adrenal cortex in both men and women and is a critical molecular precursor of corticosteroids, e.g., cortisol. Progesterone is produced by the placenta during pregnancy and prepares the endometrium for the implantation of a fertilized egg. It plays a critical role in maintaining the fetoplacental unit and fetal development during pregnancy, and it is responsible for maintaining appropriate hormone levels in a woman after fertilization. Progesterone levels are high in early pregnancy and continue to rise as pregnancy progresses. Progesterone levels are used to diagnose inadequate luteal phase and to monitor ovulation during fertility studies.

Patient preparation No preparation is required, other than for drawing blood or obtaining urine.

Procedure Progesterone is measured in the serum by various immunoassay methods and in the urine by competitive protein binding.

Specimen Serum, urine.

Reference range

Women

Follicular (proliferative) phase	0.1–1.5 ng/ml (US: 20–150 ng/dL).
Luteal (secretory) phase	2.0–30 ng/ml (US: 250–2800 ng/dL).
Postmenopausal	Less than 1.0 ng/ml (US: 100 ng/dL).
Pregnancy, 1st trimester	9–50 ng/ml.
2nd trimester	20–150 ng/ml.
3rd trimester	60–275 ng/ml.
Men	Less than 0.1 ng/ml.

Abnormal values

Increased in: pregnancy, ovarian cysts, tumors of the adrenal gland or ovary, therapy with ACTH, progestins.

Cost $85–$95.

projective test ("projection test") Any of a number of psychological tests in which a person is presented with external stimuli (often in the form of images, e.g., Rorschach ink blot test, thematic apperception test) that are ambiguous and open to subjective interpretation. Analysis of the person's response to the situations or images in the projective tests provides (in theory) information on the person's unconscious desires, personality traits, and interpersonal dynamics. See *psychological test, Rorschach test* in Glossary.

prolactin (lactogenic hormone) A small polypeptide hormone produced by the anterior pituitary that is critical for the development of the mammary glands and production of breast milk. The serum levels of prolactin are similar in men and women, except during pregnancy or lactation, when they are much higher in women.

Patient preparation No preparation is required, other than for drawing blood or amniotic fluid. See *amniocentesis*.

Procedure Prolactin is measured by immunoassay and radioimmunoassay.

Specimen Serum, amniotic fluid.

Reference ranges

Men: Less than 0.1 ng/ml; diurnal variation peaks 4–5 hours after onset of sleep.

Women: Less than 0.1 ng/ml; diurnal variation peaks 4–5 hours after onset of sleep.

Follicular (proliferative) phase	2–20 ng/ml (US: x ng/dL).
Luteal (secretory) phase	5–40 ng/ml (US: x ng/dL).
Postmenopausal	Less than 12 ng/ml (US: x ng/dL).
Pregnancy, 1st trimester	Less than 80 ng/ml.
2nd trimester	Less than 160 ng/ml.
3rd trimester	Less than 400 ng/ml.

Abnormal values

Increased in: physiologic stimuli (e.g., breastfeeding, exercise, coitus, pregnancy, sleep, stress, hypoglycemia), amenorrhea, cirrhosis, drug therapy (alphamethyldopa, amphetamines, antihistamines, cimetidine, contraceptives, L-dopa, ergot alkaloids, haloperidol, isoniazid, methyldopa, monoamine oxidase inhibitors, phenothiazines, procainamide, reserpine, tricyclic antidepressants, verapamil, hormones [e.g., estrogen, growth hormone, thyroid-releasing hormone], psychotropic drugs), empty sella syndrome, galactorrhea, hypothalamic dysfunction, hypothyroidism, neoplasms (e.g., malignancy with ectopic hormone production, pituitary tumors), renal failure, MEN-I.

Decreased in: postpartum pituitary infarction, drugs (e.g., apomorphine, bromocriptine).

Cost $110–$120.

prostate biopsy (needle biopsy of prostate)   A biopsy of the prostate that is obtained from older men who have either clinical (e.g., increased firmness of the prostate on rectal examination), or laboratory (e.g., increased prostate specific antigen — PSA) findings that are commonly associated with prostate cancer. Prostate biopsies may be obtained from perineal, transurethral, and the most commonly, transrectal approaches. Because of the prostate's anatomy, it is common practice for the urologist to obtain tissue from six different regions, including the base, middle, and apex of the right and left sides. The "needle" biopsies themselves are small. They are sent to a pathologist, who examines the tissue by light microscopy to determine whether the tissue is benign or malignant. If it is malignant, the tissue can be further evaluated to determine prognosis by ploidy analysis.

Patient preparation The procedure requires informed consent. Regional pain and discomfort is normal for this procedure.

Procedure The procedure is most commonly performed on an outpatient basis, consists of the insertion of the biopsy needle transrectally, and does not require local anesthesia.

Specimen "Cores" of whitish tissue that measure 1–2 cm in length by 0.1 cm in diameter.

Reference range No pathologic changes or mild inflammation of tissue.

Abnormal values Benign enlargement (benign prostatic hypertrophy) and

cancer are the findings that lead to therapy in the form of prostate resection.
Cost $350–$500.
Comments Prostate biopsies are difficult to interpret, even for world-renowned experts. See *digital rectal examination*, *Gleason grading system* in Glossary, *ploidy analysis*, *prostate-specific antigen*.

prostate specific antigen (PSA) A small enzyme that is very similar to other enzymes that break down proteins. PSA is secreted exclusively by the prostate and is responsible for lysis of the seminal coagulum. It can be measured in the serum and is slightly increased in patients with benign disease (e.g., acute inflammation and prostatic hypertrophy) and usually markedly increased in cancer of the prostate.
Patient preparation No preparation is required, other than for drawing blood.
Procedure PSA is usually measured by enzyme immunoassay.
Specimen Serum.
Reference range

Men under 60	Less than 4.0 µg/L.
Men over 60	Less than 7.5 µg/L.

Abnormal values Greater than 7.5 µg/L.
Cost $50–$100.
Comments Prostate cancer is present in 22% of those with PSA levels above 4.0 µg/L, and 60% of those with levels above 10 µg/L. Newer and more sensitive test methods are currently being developed. The overlap in serum PSA levels between benign and malignant prostatic disease is considerable and in the past reduced the value of PSA measurement as a screening tool for prostate cancer. Many of the screened individuals fell in a sort of no-man's-land with serum values between 4.1 and 10.0 ng/ml. A small amount of PSA in the circulation is not bound to a carrier protein and is known as free PSA. It has been reported that the free PSA in the circulation is proportionately higher in men with benign prostate conditions than those with prostate cancer. In the future, both free and bound forms may be measured routinely. Although free PSA measurements may be useful in reducing the number of negative biopsies, most laboratorians have not fully endorsed this test.

prostate ultrasonography A noninvasive procedure in which a series of images of the prostate and surrounding tissues are obtained using ultrasonic waves. Prostate ultrasonography is usually combined with measurement of the serum levels of prostate-specific antigen. If a lesion is identified, it is biopsied.
Patient preparation The patient should not void within one hour of the procedure. A cleansing enema should precede the procedure.
Procedure The test is performed using a B-mode, real-time ultrasonography device with a transducer, which is inserted through the rectum.
Reference range Normal size and morphology of the prostate and seminal vesicles.
Abnormal values Any densities or masses require further evaluation.
Cost $300–$400. See *prostate specific antigen*.

protein-bound iodine test (PBI test)   A thyroid function test in which the iodine present in precipitated protein is quantified. This provides a crude indication of thyroid activity. The test has fallen into disuse and has been superseded by more specific tests. See *TSH, T4 uptake.*

protein C   Protein C is a potent vitamin K-dependent anticoagulant that is converted to an active enzyme by thrombin and "accelerated" by protein S. Activated protein C (APC) limits clot formation and enhances the break-down of blood clots.
   Patient preparation No preparation is required, other than for drawing blood.
   Procedure Protein C deficiency can be detected by functional assays that measure either protein C activity or its actual amount.
   Specimen Sodium citrated plasma.
   Reference range
      Functional assay   70%–140% of normal activity of pooled plasma.
      ELISA   0.6–1.13 units/ml.
   Abnormal values Protein C deficiency is a major cause of deep vein throm-bosis and can be inherited or acquired, the latter often due to liver disease.
   Cost
      Functional assay $140–$160.
      ELISA $150–$160.
   Comments Protein C is lower in children than in adults. Protein C assays are generally part of a panel of tests, including protein C, protein S, antithrombin III, lupus anticoagulant, and fibrinogen, which are used to determine the cause of increased blood clotting.

protein electrophoresis (SPEP, serum protein electrophoresis)   Protein electrophoresis is a screening method for detecting significant serum protein abnormalities. When submitted for electrophoresis, the proteins are divided into prealbumin, albumin, $\alpha 1$ and $\alpha 2$, β, and γ zones, indicated in the table below. One or more regions of the protein electrophoresis may be increased or decreased in conditions that affect the production of certain proteins, or variable in the presence of gene polymorphism. The interpretation is com-plex and any abnormality identified should be confirmed by re-running the electrophoresis.
   Patient preparation No preparation is required, other than for drawing blood.
   Procedure The body fluid of interest is placed on a gel, and an electric cur-rent is placed at one end. The proteins migrate to certain points, depend-ing on their electric charges.
   Specimen Serum, cerebrospinal fluid (CSF), urine. Protein electrophoresis of CSF is generally used to detect multiple sclerosis. Protein electrophore-sis of urine is generally performed when the protein electrophoresis sug-gests the presence of abnormal monoclonal proteins in the gamma region.
   Cost $60–$80.

protein fingerprint   A protein fingerprint is a characteristic pattern of spots on a solid support medium, e.g., chromatographic paper, that identifies a protein in a relatively specific fashion. In this technique, an enzyme, e.g., trypsin, digests a relatively pure protein, e.g., hemoglobin, to detect, as an example, the alpha or beta hemoglobin chain of interest. The enzyme cuts the protein after certain amino acids (arginine and lysine). The resulting fragments are electrophoresed. The solid support medium is then turned 90° and electrophoresed a second time under different conditions. This produces a two-dimensional "fingerprint" that is seen by spraying the paper with ninhydrin, which marks the polypeptide fragments as purple spots. See *DNA fingerprinting* in Glossary.

protein S Protein S is a small protein that acts as a cofactor for the activity of protein C, which exists in two forms, free and combined with C4b-binding protein. Protein S is assayed with protein C when investigating patients who have increased clotting tendencies or thrombotic episodes. Both functional and ELISA methods have been developed to measure protein S. Heparin may interfere with these assays.
Patient preparation No preparation is required, other than for drawing blood.
Procedure Protein S is measured by enzyme methods and by functional assays, which measure its activity in blood.
Specimen Sodium citrated plasma.
Reference range
 Functional assay
  Total   78%–103% (males).
            70%–122% (females).
  Free   69%–149% (males).
            50%–130% (females).
  ELISA   0.6–1.13 U/ml.
Cost
 Functional $200–$220.
 ELISA $160–$180.

protein (urine) Normal urine does not usually contain large amounts of protein.
Patient preparation No preparation is required, other than for obtaining urine.
Procedure Protein is most often detected through screening, using a reagent strip (dipstick) coated with certain dyes, e.g., tetrabromophenol blue or tetrachlorophenol-tetrabromosulfophthalein, which is yellow in absence of proteinuria.
Specimen A timed urine specimen is required. Once proteinuria is detected, the amount of protein spilled into the urine is quantified with a 24-hour urine specimen, which contains all the urine the patient produces in a day.
Reference range 30–150 mg/24 hours.
Abnormal values Protein in the urine (proteinuria) in concentrations greater

than 5 mg/dL is abnormal. An increase in normal proteins is usually caused by kidney disease due to glomerular defects and defective renal tubular resorption of albumin. An increase in abnormal proteins (monoclonal proteins) is usually caused by neoplasms (multiple myeloma or lymphomas).

Greater than 1.0 g/dL: glomerulonephritis, nephrotic syndrome, lupus nephritis, amyloidosis.

Greater than 0.2 g/dL: congestive heart failure, drugs (e.g., aminoglycoside antibiotics), infections (acute), multiple myeloma, chemical toxins.

0.05–0.2 g/dL: polycystic kidneys, pyelonephritis, renal tube defects, drugs (e.g., acetazolamide, cephalosporins, contrast media used in radiology, gentamicin, penicillin, sulfonamides, tolbutamide).

Cost $30–$50.

prothrombin time (PT, pro-time)   A coagulation test used to determine the time necessary to form a blood clot, evaluate the blood's clotting capacity, and evaluate the functional activity of certain coagulation factors. PT is most often used to monitor therapy with oral anticoagulants, in particular with warfarin, the intent being to maintain the PT at 2 to 2.5 times greater than the normal control. If it is less than twice the normal control, the thinning of the blood (achieved by the anticoagulant) is inadequate. If it is greater than 2.5 times the normal control, there is an increased bleeding tendency.

Patient preparation No preparation is required, other than for drawing blood.

Procedure In the prothrombin time test, calcium and tissue thromboplastin are added to plasma that has been anticoagulated with citrate or oxalate, and the time needed to form a clot is measured.

Reference range 12–16 seconds. In patients receiving anticoagulants, the intent is to maintain the PT at 2 to 2.5 times the normal reference range.

Abnormal values

Decreased in: drugs (barbiturates, contraceptives, digitalis, diphenhydramine, diuretics, metaproterenol, vitamin K), myocardial infarction, pulmonary thromboembolism, thrombophlebitis.

Increased in: afibrinogenemia, coagulation factor deficiencies, drugs (anticoagulants, antibiotics, chlorpromazine, chlordiazepoxide, methyldopa, reserpine, salicylates, sulfonamides), erythroblastosis fetalis.

Cost $20–$40.

provocation test   Any of a number of tests used to deliberately induce a suspected abnormality, e.g., the provocation of increased intraocular pressure by ingesting excess water. In certain areas of medicine, such tests are potentially dangerous, and the risks may outweigh the benefits of the diagnostic information they provide.

pseudocholinesterase (serum cholinesterase, cholinesterase II)   An enzyme present in the liver and plasma that rapidly metabolizes succinylcholine, a short-acting (5–10 minutes) neuromuscular blocker used in anesthesia. Succinylcholine's duration of action is controlled by its rate of metabolism by pseudocholinesterase. Certain individuals have congenital pseudo-cholinesterase variants with prolonged neuromuscular blockage with "usual" doses of succinylcholine, which can be identified by the "dibucaine" number.

Patient preparation No preparation is required, other than for drawing blood.

Procedure Cholinesterase is measured by colorimetry (kinetic studies in which the enzyme—cholinesterase—consumes a substrate) and fluorometry.

Specimen Serum.

Reference range 5–12 kU/L.

Abnormal values

Decreased in: liver disease (hepatitis, cirrhosis, metastasis), acetylcholinesterase inhibitors (e.g., insecticides), acute infections, anemia, cytotoxic drugs, dermatomyositis, malignancy, malnutrition, myocardial infarction, pregnancy.

Increased in: nephrotic syndrome.

Cost $40–$50.

pseudogout See *synovial fluid analysis.*

PSP test See *phenolsulfonphthalein test.*

psychological test Any of a group of tests used to determine a subject's development, intelligence quotient (IQ), level of "normalcy," occupational aptitude, personality traits, thought processes, and future potential for success. The general format for each broad group of tests is provided below.

PERCEPTUAL-MOTOR INTEGRITY TEST Designed to rule out an organic (structural or physiologic, i.e., treatable) cause for the subject's behavior, including the Bender visual-motor Gestalt test, which can be administered from age 5 to adult, evaluating personality conflicts, ego structure and function, and organic brain disease.

IQ TEST The most commonly used IQ tests in the United States were devised by David Wechsler and include the Wechsler Preschool and Primary Scale of Intelligence (WPPSI, ages 4 to 6), Wechsler Intelligence Scale for Children-Revised (WISC-R, ages 5 to 15) and the Wechsler Adult Intelligence Scale (WAIS-R, age 16 to adult); another commonly used IQ test is the Stanford-Binet test, which evaluates individuals from age 2 to adult.

POTENTIAL ACHIEVEMENT TEST The Vineland Social Maturity Scale evaluates the capacity to function independently and is administered to those up to age 25.

"PROJECTION" TEST Any test that evaluates the sense of reality, e.g., the Rorschach ink-blot test. These tests require considerable skill in administration but yield the greatest insight into personality conflicts, ego structure and function, defensive structure, and affective integration; other projective tests

include the Thematic Apperception Test (TAT), Children's Apperception Test (CAT), the "Draw-a-person" test, and the "Draw-a-family" test.
   Cost $150–$300.

psychometric test   Any of a group of tests used to quantify a particular aspect of a person's mental abilities or mindset, e.g., aptitude, intelligence, mental abilities, and personality.

psychomotor test   Any of a group of tests of the senses or perception that measure the speed and accuracy with which a person can carry out a particular task, e.g., building with blocks or copying a design or picture.

PTH   See *parathyroid hormone.*

PTH-rP   See *parathyroid hormone-related protein.*

pulmonary angiography (pulmonary arteriography)   An imaging technique in which radiocontrast is injected into the pulmonary arteries and its branches to identify obstructions or vascular defects.
   Patient preparation Informed consent is required. The patient should not eat in the four hours before the procedure, although pulmonary angiography is often performed on an emergency basis. Baseline coagulation studies, e.g., platelet count, prothrombin time, and partial thromboplastin time, and renal function tests (e.g., BUN and creatinine) should be obtained before the procedure.
   Procedure The procedure consists of the insertion of a catheter through the skin and into the internal jugular vein or the common femoral vein, followed by injection of a radiocontrast material. This allows the radiologist to see the pulmonary arteries.
   Reference range Normally no abnormalities or other defects are seen within the pulmonary vasculature.
   Abnormal values Pulmonary thromboembolism (a potentially fatal condition that represents a true medical emergency). Pulmonary angiography is less commonly used to identify aneurysms, arteriovenous malformations, and stenosis of the pulmonary artery.
   Cost $1500–$2500.

pulmonary function test (PFT)   A general term for any of a group of techniques and maneuvers that provide information on pulmonary function. These techniques include spirometry, ventilation and perfusion scans, and measurement of lung volumes, airway resistance, carbon monoxide diffusing capacity, and arterial blood gases. Pulmonary function tests may be used in combination with endoscopy (bronchoscopy, mediastinoscopy) and various forms of imaging (chest films, CT, MRI) to provide information on the presence of structural (e.g., abscess or tumor) or functional (e.g., emphysema or heavy smoking, which reduces the exchange of respiratory gases) defects.

Pulmonary function tests are used to measure the volume of air that can be inhaled, the efficiency of the gas exchange, and the strength of exhalation. Below are some of the more common pulmonary function tests.

BRONCHIAL INHALATION CHALLENGE The individual inhales methacholine after having had a battery of tests that establishes a baseline of functional status. Methacholine is a histaminic agent that reduces the values of pulmonary function tests in patients with asthma but has no effect on patients with decreased pulmonary function due to other causes, e.g., heart failure, sinus infections, or intrathoracic tumors. Cold air can be administered as another form of bronchial inhalation challenge with similar reponses in asthmatic patients.

DIFFUSING CAPACITY This test measures the efficiency with which gases in the alveolar space (in particular oxygen) pass into the blood, and the efficiency with which gases in the blood (particularly carbon dioxide) enter the alveoli removal from the body by exhalation.

FORCED EXPIRATORY VOLUME (FEV) This is the maximal amount of air that can be exhaled in a period of time, usually one (FEV_1) or, less commonly, three (FEV_3) seconds. FEV_1 is usually reduced in obstructive airways disease, a general term that encompasses both asthma and chronic obstructive pulmonary disease.

NITROGEN WASHOUT TEST This test measures the time required to eliminate nitrogen gas from the lungs when breathing another gas (usually oxygen). The test is used to identify poorly ventilated regions of the lung.

PEAK EXPIRATORY FLOW (maximum expiratory flow rate) The peak flow is the greatest rate of airflow that can be obtained during forced exhalation. It has a diurnal pattern of fluctuation, which is used to evaluate airway tone. The peak flow can be plotted during the day and used to investigate occupational asthma and detect increases of severity prior to the onset of symptoms. Peak expiratory flow is decreased (and airway tone increased) in various forms of asthma.

PULMONARY COMPLIANCE (pulmonary distensibility) The pressure required to increase the lung's volume, which is decreased in emphysema, pulmonary vascular congestion, and interstitial pulmonary fibrosis.

PULMONARY PANEL (pulmonary profile) A battery of cost-effective tests used to evaluate the functional reserve capacity of the lungs in patients who have a clinical diagnosis of obstructive or restrictive lung disease. The panel measures CO_2 content, $PaCO_2$, PaO_2, pH, O_2 saturation, and a/A ratio.

Cost $250–$500.

Comments In all pulmonary function tests, smoking history is critical to proper evaluation of test results. Based on the information they provide, PFTs can be used for diagnosis, e.g., to determine the cause of clinical symptoms (cough, dyspnea, wheezing) in smokers or asthmatics; monitoring, e.g., to determine the value of therapeutic interventions such as anti-asthmatic therapy; evaluation of disability, e.g., to address issues related to personal injury lawsuits or occupational exposure; and as a tool in public health, e.g., for epidemiological surveys. See *lung volumes, pulmonary panel, spirometry.*

pulmonary panel See *pulmonary function test.*

pulmonary profile See *pulmonary function test.*

pulp vitality test A general term for the use of any technique (e.g., application of extremes of temperature, mechanical pressure, or electrical stimulation) to determine if the tissues of the tooth's root are intact and sensitive.

pulse The rhythmic expansion of a blood vessel, which for certain large arteries can be evaluated clinically using the fingers or stethoscope. The ritual of taking the patient's pulse provides information about the heart rate, and a marked decrease in the strength of the pulse suggests severe atherosclerosis, decreased pumping activity by the heart, or vascular defects in the form of arteriovenous shunts or fistulas.
  Reference range The normal pulse is 60–80 beats per minute. It is decreased in bradycardia, which commonly occurs in athletes, due to the increased size of their hearts. It is increased in tachycardia, which is due to emotional stress, exercise, and various heart arrhythmias.

pulse oximetry (oxygen saturation test) A noninvasive method used to determine the oxygen saturation (SaO_2) of arterial blood in a continuous fashion. A pulse oximeter senses the optical difference between oxyhemoglobin and deoxyhemoglobin and detects the differences as increased or decreased transmission of light as the blood pulses through tissue. The probe is most commonly placed on the earlobe or finger. These optical differences are used to calculate SaO_2. Pulse oximetry is relatively accurate when the SaO_2 is in the 70%–100% range. The accuracy falls when the SaO_2 is below 70% and is less than informative in patients with poor cardiac reserve or abnormal gas exchange. Pulse oximetry detects oxygen desaturation accurately, inexpensively, quickly, and safely, and is used in endoscopy, the recovery room, in intensive care units, and in evaluating obstructive sleep apnea syndrome.
  Patient preparation No preparation is required; if the finger is being used for the test, nail polish must be removed.
  Procedure Pulse oximetry consists of passing light through a capillary bed in the ear or finger. The light at the other side of the capillary bed is measured by spectrophotometry and is proportional to the amount of oxyhemoglobin present relative to the amount of hemoglobin available for binding.
  Reference range Oxyhemoglobin saturation is greater than 95%.
  Abnormal values Any drop of 5% or more in oxyhemoglobin saturation is considered significant for a possible decrease in oxygen saturation.
  Cost $150–$200.

punch biopsy A minor surgical procedure performed in an outpatient setting or dermatology clinic, in which a hollow needle is used to obtain a 3-, 4-, or rarely 6-millimeter in diameter core ("punch") of tissue, almost invariably of skin, which is then evaluated by light microscopy. In practice, punch biopsies are rarely performed on pigmented lesions, as there is always the possibility that the lesion seen may be a type of malignant melanoma. Melanomas must be removed with wide margins at the time of the first procedure, which is virtually impossible with a punch biopsy.

Patient preparation No preparation is required; the procedure may be uncomfortable for the patient. A core of skin and subjacent tissue is removed and cut from the base of the tissue as deeply into the fat as possible. The larger biopsies require one or two stitches to close the wound.

Specimen A cylindrical core of skin.

Reference range Normal tissue, or no changes of significance.

Abnormal values The tissue may have pathological changes ranging from benign (e.g., inflammation, infections, and pigmented or vascular lesions) to malignant (e.g., malignant melanoma and squamous or basal cell cancer).

Cost $300–$400. See *biopsy.*

pupillary reflex A component of a neurological examination in which the ability of the pupils to react to light is evaluated by shining a beam of light in one eye and assessing its response, which under normal circumstances is constriction. Shining a beam of light in one eye results in the constriction of the opposite eye, which is known as the consensual light reflex. See *neurological examination.*

pure tone audiometry A type of hearing test in which the individual is exposed to a series of pure tones over a range of frequencies, the information from which is placed on a graph known as an audiogram. The audiogram is a plot of the tone intensity in decibels (from 0 dB to 80 dB) on the vertical axis and frequency on the horizontal axis (250 to 4000 Hz). The sensation of sound results from the transmission of vibrations at a certain frequency, which occurs both through the air (AC) and through the bones of the head (BC).

Patient preparation A neurologic examination should precede the examination. If the subject is using a hearing aid, it should be brought to the examination.

Procedure In audiometry, the individual's ability to hear sound transmitted through the air (air conduction) is evaluated using special earphones; bone conduction of sound is evaluated using a special bone vibrator.

Reference range In normal individuals the sound threshold through bone is higher than through air, resulting in a normal AC-BC gap. In audiometry, air and bone conduction are analyzed separately but plotted on the same graph.

Abnormal values Hearing loss may be relatively selective, reducing the sensation of one more than the other. As an example, in conductive hearing loss, which may be due to otitis media, eustachian tube dysfunction, or impacted cerumen (earwax), AC is decreased.

Cost $250–$350.

pyridinium crosslinks   Collagen fibers linked together by interchain molecules are refered to as pyridinium collagen crosslinks and are present in all connective tissue except skin. When collagen is broken down by collagenase, small breakdown products are excreted in urine with the attached crosslinks, including pyridinoline (PYD) and deoxypyridinoline (DYPD). Bone collagen is constantly turning over and has a high content of deoxypyridinline and lesser amounts of pyridinoline. Both are excreted in the urine and are useful markers for bone degradation and resorption. They are increased in the urine of patients with osteoporosis.

Patient preparation No preparation is required, other than for obtaining urine.

Procedure Pyridinium crosslinks are measured by immunoassay.

Specimen 24-hour urine, with a dilute acid (hydrochloric or boric) preservative.

Reference range

	DYPD	PYD (NMOL/MMOL CREATININE)
Females	4–21	22–89
Males	4–19	20–61
2–10 years	31–110	160–440
11–17 years	17–100	105–400

Abnormal values

Increased in: osteoporosis, primary hyperparathyroidism paget's disease.

Decreased in: successful treatment of osteoporosis.

Cost $150–$170.

Comments This test is becoming increasingly important in the diagnosis and treatment of osteoporosis. See *bone densitometry, osteoporosis testing.*

pyruvate kinase   An enzyme that participates in the anaerobic metabolism of glucose through the so-called Krebs cycle. Its absence is the most common cause of congenital (nonspherocytic) hemolytic anemia. It is measured in the evaluation of chronic hemolytic anemias.

Patient preparation No preparation is required, other than for drawing blood.

Procedure A lack of pyruvate kinase can be identified by a fluorescence screening assay and confirmed by spectrophotometry.

Specimen Blood, serum.

Reference range 11–19 U/g of hemoglobin.

Abnormal values Pyruvate kinase is decreased in hereditary (nonspherocytic) hemolytic anemia. It is also decreased in acute leukemia and aplastic anemia.

Cost $90–$110.

┌─────┐
│ **R** │
└─────┘

radioactive iodine uptake (RAIU, thyroid scan, thyroid scintigraphy)   A method used to determine the functional status of the thyroid using a radioactive isotope of iodine (iodine-131 or iodine-123). The most commonly performed procedure is that of the 24-hour uptake, in which uptake of iodine is measured approximately 24 hours after its intravenous administration. RAIU is increased in hyperthyroidism, ectopic hormone production, and iodine deficiency in response to thyroid hormone depletion. RAIU is decreased in hypothyroidism, after administration of exogenous thyroid hormone, in defects of hormone storage, and following exposure to excess iodine.

Patient preparation No preparation is required, other than for drawing blood.

Procedure 2 to 15 µCi of iodine-131 is injected intravenously, or 100 to 350 µCi of iodine-123 is administered by mouth.

Specimen Blood drawn at 2-, 6-, and 24-hour intervals.

Reference range

2 hours	Less than 6% uptake.
6 hours	3%–20% uptake.
24 hours	8%–30% uptake.

Abnormal values In hyperthyroidism, the uptake is increased up to 55% in 24 hours. Other cases of increased uptake include hyperactivity of the thyroid without thyrotoxicosis, acromegaly, and acute renal failure. Decreased uptake occurs in hypothyroidism, hypofunction of the pituitary gland, and chronic renal failure.

Cost $100–$150.

Comments Although iodine-131 was more commonly used as a radioactive tracer, iodine-123 is increasingly preferred, as the thyroid's radiation exposure is one-half that delivered by iodine-131. See *T₃ uptake test, thyroxine, thyroid-stimulating hormone.*

radioallergosorbent test   See *RAST.*

radiography (roentgenography, radiographic imaging)   The recording of an image of a body region that is placed in a beam of ionizing radiation. A wide range of instruments are used in radiology, which differ in design depending on the body part being being examined (e.g., mammography), the intensity and type of radiation being delivered (e.g., computed tomography vs. plain films), and whether the image is beng recorded on film or viewed in "real time" as in fluoroscopy. In the United States, radiologic studies, especially in patients with private insurance, are often performed in a free-standing "imaging center." Such centers commonly offer a sophisticated array of radiologic services including computed tomography (CAT scans), magnetic resonance imaging (MRI), mammography, ultrasonography, Doppler imaging, and others, and may have radiography equipment that is better than that available in adjacent hospitals. See *angiography, cholangiography, computed tomography, mammography, MRI, venography.*

radioimmunoprecipitation assay   This laboratory technique, like the Western blot, identifies antibodies to specific viral antigens and requires separation by electrophoresis. Disrupted, purified virus previously grown in culture with a radioactive amino acid is incubated with a test sample which may contain an antibody (immunoglobulin) against the viral antigen. The proteins in the test sample are then subjected to polyacrylamide gel electrophoresis.

radioimmunosorbent test (RIST)   A highly sensitive radioimmunoassay that measures total serum concentrations of immunoglobulin E, the protein that is intimately linked to hypersensitivity reactions, including allergies to house dust and foods. The RIST requires two days to perform and uses anti-IgE antibodies to bind IgE in the serum. Radiolabeled anti-IgE is then used to detect bound IgE. The amount of radiolabeled IgE that binds to a solid support medium is inversely related to the amount of unlabeled IgE in the specimen. IgE levels by RIST are high in patients with atopic dermatitis and hyperimmunoglobulin E syndrome and low in pediatric patients and those with immunodeficiency. See *RAST.*

radiologic pelvimetry (X-ray pelvimetry)   A radiologic study in which the size of the infant and the mother's birth canal are compared to determine whether the bony part of the woman's pelvis is of sufficient diameter to allow a normal vaginal delivery. Because of the radiation exposure, radiologic pelvimetry is confined to highly specific indications, i.e., breech presentation of an infant in a clinical situation where a cesarean section would be difficult, such as a woman with clinical instability who may not withstand the rigors of surgery. X-ray pelvimetry is rarely justified in practice, as it provides little information that is of use in managing the delivery and results in a 1.5-fold increase in the infant's subsequent risk for leukemia.
   Comments Manual "guestimates" of the bony pelvis (manual pelvimetry) are performed, but rarely in a formal fashion, given that in the event of the slightest concern that the birth passage is inadequate, a cesarean section is performed. See *pelvic ultrasonography.*

radionuclide angiocardiography See *equilibrium radionuclide angiocardiography, first-pass radionuclide angiocardiography.*

radionuclide cisternography A rarely performed procedure in which a radiopharmaceutical is injected into the subarachnoid space in the lumbar region, and images of the spinal canal and the cerebrospinal spaces are obtained by a gamma camera that records the radionuclide's scintillations. The technique is used to evaluate hydrocephalus and the patency of implanted ventricular shunts. It is also used to detect the presence of posttraumatic cerebrospinal fluid leakage.

Patient preparation All blood being used to measure substances by radioimmunoassay should be drawn from the patient before performing cisternography. The discomfort associated with the procedure may be considerable and is similar to that of a lumbar puncture.

Procedure The procedure consists of the injection of a water-soluble radiopharmaceutical (e.g., indium-111-DTPA) into the subarachnoid space of the lumbar region. Images of the spinal canal and the CSF spaces are obtained over the ensuing 72 hours using a gamma camera that records the scintillations of the radionuclide.

Specimen The specimen consists of scintigrams that indicate the flow of cerebrospinal fluid.

Reference range Normally, the cerebrospinal fluid flows from the lumbar region to the base of the brain in two to four hours. By 24 hours, the fluid has flowed over the outside of the brain, and by 72 hours, the contrast should have completely cleared. During the test, the patient is ambulatory, but needs to return at specific time intervals to acquire more scintigrams.

Abnormal values Cisternography is abnormal in hydrocephalus and may be used to detect defects in the flow through ventricular shunts or implanted cerebrospinal fluid reservoirs.

Cost $550–$700.

Comments Synonyms include cerebrospinal fluid cisternography, cerebrospinal fluid scan, CSF scan, CSF scintigraphy, emission cisternography, isotope cisternography, radioisotope cisternography.

radionuclide scan of lung See *ventilation-perfusion scan.*

radionuclide venography (radionuclide thrombophlebography) A noninvasive method for detecting thromboembolism, in particular deep vein thrombosis of the lower extremity.

Patient preparation All blood for substances being analyzed by radioimmunoassay should be drawn before performing cisternography.

Procedure A radiopharmaceutical (e.g., technetium–99m) is administered into the dorsal veins of the feet, and images of the legs are captured with a gamma (scintillation) camera.

Specimen Scintigrams of the vascular supply of the legs.

Reference range Symmetrical superficial and deep veins in the legs with no defects in the flow of the radionuclide. The radionuclide does not remain long in the circulation.

Abnormal values Localized venous obstruction is characteristic of deep vein thrombosis.

Cost $500–$750.

rape   See *semen analysis, rape kit* in Glossary.

rapid plasma reagin test   See *RPR test.*

RAST (radioallergosorbent test)   A test used to measure the serum levels of IgE antibodies to certain allergenic substances that are capable of causing rashes, asthma, hay fever, and drug reactions. Although the original form of the test utilized radioactive iodine, this has been phased out with the advent of enzyme immunoassays (e.g., ELISA) and fluorescence immunoassays. RAST correlates reasonably well with bronchial provocation testing. Rare false-positive RAST results from allergies to ragweed/grass. Although RAST is neither more sensitive nor specific than skin testing, it avoids the risk of sensitization and anaphylaxis inherent in testing in living patients. RAST profiles are commercially available for a wide range of allergens, including animal dander (cat and dog), dusts and dust mites, foods (e.g., egg white, grains including barley, oat, and wheat, and shellfish), grasses (e.g., Bermuda grass, perennial rye, Johnson grass, Timothy weed), and mold (e.g., *Aspergillus, Cladosporium, Penicillium*). RAST profiles may also be based on the allergens that are most common in a particular region (e.g., the arid southwestern or the moist southeastern United States). See *patch test, prick test.*

Patient preparation No preparation is required, other than for drawing blood.

Procedure In the RAST, an allergen-antigen complex is bound to a paper disk (an allergosorbent), and the patient's serum is added. Serum that contains the antibodies in question will bind to the "tagged" immunoglobulins, particularly IgE.

Specimen Serum.

Reference range Negative.

Abnormal values Elevated IgE antibodies that react to the antigen of interest.

Cost $10–$20 per allergen tested.

RBC survival study   See *red cell survival (study).*

RDW   See *red blood cell distribution width.*

reagent strip   See *dipstick.*

"real-time" imaging   The visualization of a dynamic process within microseconds after its occurrence, which requires very rapid information processing (i.e., virtually as the process occurs) as in B-mode ultrasonography. Some ultrafast computers in CT allow quasi-real-time imaging. The advantage of real-time imaging is that there is less blurring of the image being acquired, which allows for a more precise interpretation of a mass, if present. Certain imaging modalities, e.g., fluoroscopic angiography and other fluoroscopic procedures, are inherently "real-time" but are not designated as such. These modalities may cause significant radioactive exposure to the user with time. See *ultrasonography.*

red blood cell count (erythrocyte count)   This is the number of red blood cells (RBCs) or erythrocytes per volume of blood, which is measured in microliters (µL) or cubic millimeters (mm^3). RBCs are responsible for carrying oxygen from the lungs to tissues as required for metabolism in an aerobic (oxygen-rich) environment. At birth the RBC count is elevated, followed by a decreased count that levels at about two months of age, then slowly rises to adult levels.

Patient preparation No preparation is required, other than for drawing blood.
Procedure The whole blood is passed through a multichannel analyzer, which is used to evaluate the number, size, and shape of red blood cells, the concentration of hemoglobin, and other paramaters.
Specimen Blood.
Reference range   Males   4.1–5.4 x 10^6/µL.
                       Females   3.8–5.2 x 10^6/µL.
Abnormal values The term polycythemia refers to an increase in RBCs due to any cause. Physiologic or reactive polycythemia (also called erythrocytosis) refers to an increased RBC count that is normal in those who live at high altitudes, in cigarette smokers, in children with certain congenital cardiac defects, and in those with chronic pulmonary disease. When the increase in RBCs is not reactive, but rather neoplastic, it is designated polycythemia vera (true polycythemia) and may itself cause disease. A decreased RBC count is known as anemia, which, like polycythemia, can be physiological (as occurs in those with a high exercise tolerance, e.g., marathon runners) or pathological. Anemias are usually divided into various groups based on the cause, as in iron deficiency anemia, megaloblastic anemia (due to decreased vitamin B$_{12}$ or folic acid), or aplastic anemia (in which the red blood cell precursors in the bone marrow are virtually non-existent).
Cost The red blood cell count is part of the normal CBC (complete blood count), which costs $15 to $30. See *hematocrit, red cell indices.*

red blood cell distribution width (RDW)   An estimation of erythrocyte anisocytosis, a value that is generated by automated red blood cell counters (e.g., Coulter and Cell-Dyne). This parameter is used to detemine the cause of a given anemia (see table); a low RDW in sickle cell anemia indicates milder disease and may be of use in "working up" such patients. In the table, N indicates "normal;" ↑ indicates an increase in the parameter being evaluated, and ↓ indicates a decrease in the parameter being measured.

RED CELL DISTRIBUTION WIDTH

RDW	MCV*	DISEASE STATE
N	↓	α- or β-thalassemia
↑	↓/N	Iron deficiency, hemoglobin H, hemoglobin S
↑	N	Aplastic anemia
↑	↑	Megaloblastic anemia (folate, vitamin B₁₂)
N/↑	↑	Liver disease, myelotoxins, chronic lymphocytic leukemia, chronic myelogenous leukemia, sickle cell anemia, hemoglobin SC, sideroblastic anemia, myelofibrosis, chemotherapy, mixed iron and vitamin B₁₂ deficiency

*MCV = Mean corpuscular volume

red cell indices A group of values obtained from automated blood cell counters (e.g., Coulter and Cell-Dyne) that provide information about the size (i.e., volume) and the concentration of hemoglobin in the red blood cells. Three abbreviations are usually found on the printouts of complete blood counts (CBCs):

MCH (mean corpuscular hemoglobin) A measurement of the hemoglobin in each erythrocyte.

MCHC (mean corpuscular hemoglobin concentration) A value that is derived on automated cell counters from measured parameters.

MCV (mean corpuscular volume) A calculated value for the average volume of peripheral red blood cells.

Patient preparation None required other than that for drawing blood.

Procedure The CBC is performed on automated devices in the clinical laboratory.

Specimen Blood with the EDTA anticoagulant.

Reference range

Mean corpuscular hemoglobin	26–34 pg/red blood cell.
Mean corpuscular hemoglobin concentration	31–36 g/dl.
Mean corpuscular volume	85–100 femtoliter/cell.

Abnormal values RBC indices can be analyzed in a patient with anemia to determine its cause with a fair degree of certainty. In iron deficiency anemia, the cells are small (microcytic), contain less hemoglobin (hypochromic) than normal, and the MCH, MCHC, and MCV are decreased. In megaloblastic anemia, the cells are large (macrocytic), contain the normal amount of hemoglobin (normochromic), and the MCH, MCHC, and MCV are increased.

Comments See *complete blood count.*

red cell survival (study) Rarely performed outside of referral (i.e., university hospital) centers, this highly specialized test is used to determine the length of time that red blood cells survive in the peripheral circulation.

Patient preparation Specimens for any substance being measured by radioimmunoassay should be drawn before performing the red blood cell survival study.

Procedure Red blood cell survival is determined by injecting a radionuclide, chromium-51, into the circulation, which penetrates the red blood cell membrane and binds to hemoglobin. Blood is drawn periodically (over the course of days) from the patient, and the half-life of the RBCs is calculated to determine the amount of remaining RBCs. The patient is also examined periodically with a gamma camera to detect the presence or pooling (sequestration) of chromium-51 in the spleen or other organs.

Specimen Radiolabeled blood.

Reference range The normal red blood cell survival is 120 days.

Abnormal values Reduction of red blood cell survival is indicative of hemolysis, as occurs in chronic lymphocytic leukemia, elliptocytosis, hemoglobin C disease, hemolytic-uremic syndrome, macrocytic anemia, paroxysmal nocturnal hemoglobinuria, sickle cell anemia, and others.

Cost $1000–$1500.

reducing sugar This term refers to any of a number of sugars (e.g., galactose, glucose, fructose, sucrose, and pentose) that cause a "reduction" in copper ions, which results in a change in color. An increase of reducing substances usually translates as an abnormal increase in glucose or galactose in the urine. Copper is also reduced by other sugars (e.g., arabinose, lactose, maltose, ribose, and xylose), as well as other substances.

Patient preparation No preparation is required, other than for obtaining urine.

Procedure Reducing substances are measured by either the Ames' Clinitest reagent tablet, or by the more sensitive Benedict's test.

Specimen Urine.

Reference range Negative. The lower limit of detection of reducing substances for the Clinitest is 250 mg/dl of urine, and for the Benedict's test, 50 mg/dl.

Abnormal values
Increased in: diabetes mellitus, late pregnancy and lactation, galactosemia, excess glucuronic acid, essential pentosuria muscular dystrophy (due to an increase in ribose), drugs (e.g., aminosalicylic acid, cephalosporins, chloraphenicol, corticosteroids, L-dopa, isoniazid, lithium, methenamine, nalidixic acid, nicotinic acid, penicillin G, phenothiazines, probenecid, radiocontrast solutions, streptomycin, sulfonamides, tetracyclines, thyroxine, vitamin C), environmental agents (e.g., bleaches, chloroform, cresol, furazolidine, indican, Lysol, methylprylon, phenols).

Cost $10–$25.

reflex diagnostic testing Reflex testing refers to the performance of a test on a patient specimen only after a particular analyte is abnormal or outside of the reference range. As an example, the finding of hypochromic and microcytic anemia on a CBC suggests the possibility that the patient has iron deficiency anemia. At the ordering physician's request, the laboratory may "reflex" into the more time-consuming and costly tests for iron levels and iron-binding proteins. Reflex testing is a cost-effective way in which a patient can be further evaluated without the need to obtain a second specimen, and reduces to a minimum the inherent delay in beginning appropriate therapy. Reflexes used in clinical laboratories include leukocyte counts greater than 20,000/mm³ which reflexes into a manual differential cell count; a positive sickle cell screen that reflexes to hemoglobin electrophoresis; an albumin/globulin ratio of less than 1.0 that reflexes to serum protein electrophoresis; and serum cholesterol of greater than 240 mg/dL that reflexes to a coronary artery disease risk profile. See *red flag* in Glossary.

Reinsch test A screening test for the presence of heavy (and toxic) metals (antimony, arsenic, bismuth, mercury, selenium, and tellurium) in a fluid of interest (e.g., gastric juice or urine) which is based on the deposition of the metal ions on copper wire.

Patient preparation No preparation is required, as the test may be performed on an emergent basis.

Procedure The procedure consists of dipping a copper strip into the specimen being tested.

Specimen Urine, vomit, gastric fluid from a gastric lavage.

Reference range The test is negative if the concentration of arsenic is less than 25 μg/L, or if the concentration of mercury, selenium, or other metals is less than 50 μg/L.

Abnormal values The Reinsch test results differ according to the metal being tested—antimony is blue-black, arsenic is matte black, bismuth is shiny black, and mercury is silver-gray.

Cost $15–$30.

renal biopsy (kidney biopsy) An invasive procedure in which a long needle is used to obtain tissue from the kidney, which is examined by a pathologist.

Patient preparation Informed consent is required. Baseline coagulation studies (e.g., activated partial thromboplastin time, prothrombin time, platelet count), and certain chemistries (e.g., BUN and creatinine) should be obtained before the procedure. Fluids should be restricted for eight hours before the biopsy.

Procedure A long needle is inserted either blindly or guided by ultrasonography into the kidney to obtain a core of tissue, which is then examined by a pathologist with light, immunofluorescence, and electron microscopy.

Specimen A cylindrical core of kidney tissue.

Reference range Negative for pathological changes.

Abnormal values Nephrotic syndrome, proteinuria, proteinuria with "glomerular" hematuria, acute renal failure, lupus erythematosus-induced nephritis, rapidly progressive glomerulonephritis, transplant rejection, and vasculitis.

Cost $800–$900.

Comments Absolute and relative contraindications include severe clotting disorder (coagulopathy), presence of a single kidney, renal artery aneurysm, or perinephric abscess. Complications include microscopic hematuria (which occurs with virtually all renal biopsies), hematoma, pain, worsening of hypertension, arteriovenous fistula formation, renal laceration or puncture, or laceration of the aorta or arteries, pancreas, spleen, liver, or gastrointestinal tract, and death, which occurs in about 1 of every 3000 patients.

renal scan A study in which a radioactive isotope is administered to evaluate renal blood flow and the risks of renal transplantation.

Patient preparation All blood that will be analyzed by radioimmunoassay should be drawn before the procedure.

Procedure A radiopharmaceutical (e.g., technetium-99m or iodine-123) is administered intravenously, and is chosen based on the region of the kidney where it localizes. Images are acquired for up to one hour after performing the procedure.

Reference range Normally, the radiopharmaceutical flows rapidly to the surface (cortex) of the kidney, then to the collecting system within a few minutes, after which it is excreted into the bladder.

Abnormal values Any delay in the flow of the radiopharmaceutical through the kidneys is abnormal and may correspond to renal obstruction or insufficiency.

Cost $300–$400.

Comments The test is not commonly performed because of the relatively high radiation exposure and low diagnostic yield in the presence of low blood flow or compromised renal function. Commonly used kidney imaging techniques in the current environment include angiography for evaluating blood flow, intravenous pyelogram (IVP) for determining adequacy of urine production, ultrasonography, computed tomography (CT) scans, and MRI for identifying cysts, neoplasms, or other masses. Synonyms include kidney scan, radioactive renogram, radionuclide renal scan, renal scintigraphy, and renogram.

renin (from renal veins) A functional screening test for renovascular hypertension in which peripheral venous blood and blood obtained by catheterization from the renal vein are measured for the ability of the renin to convert angiotensinogen into angiotensin.

Patient preparation Informed consent is required. The following agents should be stopped at least two weeks before measuring renin levels: antihypertensive drugs, corticosteroids, oral contraceptives, estrogens, diuretics, and licorice. A low sodium diet may be ordered for three days only. Upright posture may stimulate renin release.

Procedure A catheter (a thin plastic tube) is advanced to the renal veins, and plasma is obtained from each for the measurement of renin.

Specimen Plasma, drawn in an EDTA tube (lavender top). The specimen should be kept cold until it is analyzed.

Reference range Not sodium-depleted patients 0.6–4.3 ng/ml/hour (mean 1.0–1.9 ng/ml/hour); sodium-depleted patients 2.9–24.0 ng/ml/hour (mean 5.9–10.8 ng/ml/hour).

Abnormal values Increased renin with secondary increase in aldosterone occurs in: severe hypertension, kidney disease, renin-secreting tumors oral contraceptive-induced hypertension.

Cost $110–$130. See *plasma renin activity.*

restriction fragment length polymorphism   See *RFLP* in Glossary.

reticulocyte count   Reticulocytes are immature red blood cells that lack a nucleus and are present in extremely low numbers in the peripheral circulation. The reticulocyte count is a simple way of evaluating the rate of red blood cell production and the response of the bone marrow to anemia.

Patient preparation No preparation is required, other than for drawing blood.

Procedure Reticulocytes have bluish reticulum that corresponds to residual RNA that stains with a supravital dye (e.g., methylene blue and brilliant cresyl blue). The reticulocytes are counted, and the results given in number per 100 or per thousand mature red blood cells.

Specimen Whole blood with an anticoagulant (e.g., EDTA or heparin).

Reference range

Newborn	Less than 6.5% of peripheral red blood cells are reticulocytes.
Children	Less than 2% of peripheral red blood cells are reticulocytes.
Adults	Less than 1% of peripheral red blood cells are reticulocytes.

Abnormal values

Increased in: erythroblastosis fetalis, hemoglobin C, leukemia, blood loss, pregnancy, thalassemia, during treatment of iron and megaloblastic anemia.

Decreased in: adrenocorticol hypoactivity, anterior pituitary hypoactivity, aplastic anemia, cirrhosis of the liver, iron-deficiency anemia, megaloblastic anemia, radiation exposure, renal disease.

Cost $20–$40.

retrograde pyelography (retrograde urography)   A method of diagnostic radiology used to visualize the renal collecting system (i.e., the pelvis and lower urinary tract) based on the excretion of radiocontrast after injection into the renal pelvis or ureter via a ureteral catheter. Retrograde pyelography is used to evaluate suspected kidney disease in the form of inflammation (pyelonephritis), kidney stones (pyelolithiasis), or colicky upper right quadrant pain.

Patient preparation Informed consent is required. The procedure should be performed before barium studies of the gastrointestinal tract. It may be performed at the time of surgery and thus the patient preparation is as for general anesthesia, i.e., nothing by mouth after midnight before the procedure.

Procedure The procedure consists of the injection of a contrast material that is concentrated and excreted by the kidneys and opacifies (makes the system "whiter" to radiologic imaging devices) the ureters and collecting ducts.

Reference range Normally the collecting system and ureters demonstrate bilateral flow into the bladder with no obstruction or stenosis.

Abnormal values Decreased flow of the contrast through the kidneys or anatomic defects of the kidney's collecting system and ureters.

Cost $100–$200.

reverse triiodothyronine (reverse T_3, rT_3)   Reverse triiodothyronine is one of the conversion products of T_4 (thyroxine), the major thyroid hormone. The level of rT_3 reflects the rate of peripheral conversion of thyroid hormones of T_4 to T_3. Most thyroid hormone in the circulation is present as T_4—35% is monodeiodinated to T_3, 15%–20% is metabolized to tetraiodothyroacetic acid, and the remainder is converted to rT_3. Although rT_3 has little or no metabolic activity, an increased rT_3 level in patients with nonthyroidal disease indicates that the patient is not functionally hypothyroid.

Patient preparation No preparation is required, other than for drawing blood; amniotic fluid may be analyzed to identify fetal stress.

Procedure Reverse triiodothyronine is measured by enzyme immunoassay or radioimmunoassay.

Specimen Serum, amniotic fluid.

Reference range Newborn infants, 80–170 ng/dL; adults, 20–80 ng/dL.

Abnormal values

   Increased in: acute surgical stress, glucocorticoids, liver disease, myocardial infarction, old age, oral radiocontrast agents, severe systemic disease, starvation or starvation diet, antithyroid agents, propylthiouracil, methylthiouracil.

   Increased in amniotic fluid in: anemia, diabetes mellitus in the mother, erythroblastosis fetalis, very sick fetuses.

Cost $50–$75. See *thyroxine, thyroxine-binding globulin, triiodothyronine.*

Rh antigen(s)   The Rh system is a complex group of red blood cell antigens present on the surface of RBCs. Rh+ (Rh positive) and Rh- (Rh negative) refer to the presence or absence of the red blood cell-bound antigen D, or Rh-D. Rh "antigen" is actually a group of multiple antigens, which includes Rh-C, Rh-D, Rh-E, and others. The most frequent Rh antigens in whites are Rh-e, 98%; Rh-D, 85%; Rh-c, 80%; Rh-C, 70%; and Rh-E, 30%. Unlike the ABO blood group, antibodies against the D antigen are not formed in the absence of exposure. Thus an Rh- person with anti-D antibodies has been exposed to the Rh antigen by a previous transfusion or pregnancy. Exposure to the D antigen is of concern in obstetrics. RhD-negative mothers who carry Rh-D-positive fetuses often form anti-D antibodies against the infant's Rh-D antigens.

Patient preparation No preparation is required, other than for drawing blood.

Procedure The procedure consists of incubation of test red blood cells that have known Rh group antigens with the serum of a person whose production of anti-Rh antibodies is unknown.

Specimen Blood.

Reference range If the recipient of a blood transfusion is RhD+, the donor can be RhD+ or RhD-, although minor transfusion reactions may occur due to non-RhD antigens of the Rh system. If the recipient is RhD-, he or she will eventually mount an immune response to RhD+ blood, which should not be administered as a transfusion unit. In obstetrics, the same principle applies. If the mother is RhD+, there is little concern that the infant will be affected by an Rh-mediated immune response. If the mother is RhD- and the infant is RhD+, there is risk of sensitization, where the mother mounts an immune response against the infant's RhD antigen, destroying the infants RBCs.

Abnormal values A titer more than 1:16 at the eighth month usually indicates maternal formation of antibodies against the fetal antigens, which is seen in the form of stomatocytes, an altered type of red blood cell present in the mother's blood.

Cost $20–$40.

Comments The mother's anti-D antibodies are immunoglobin G, which are capable of crossing the placental barrier and causing the potentially fatal hemolytic disease of the newborn. With each subsequent pregnancy with an RhD+ child, the mother's anti-D antibody forms earlier in the pregnancy and increases the risk of immune-related complications to the infant. Because of the risk to future fetuses, a preparation of anti-RhD immunoglobulin (RhoGAM) is administered to the mother at the time of delivery. RhoGAM and similar products act to neutralize the infant's RBCs and prevent or reduce immunization of the mother.

rheumatoid factors A group of antibodies directed against a portion of immunoglobulin G and produced by inflammatory cells (neutrophils) in the joints of 80% of patients with rheumatoid arthritis. Rheumatoid factors may result in the formation of immune complexes that activate the complement cascade and release leukocytic enzymes from neutrophils, causing tissue injury.

Patient preparation No preparation is required, other than for drawing blood.

Procedure Detection of rheumatoid factors is not standardized. They can be measured by a wide range of techniques, including erythrocyte agglutination, latex agglutination, nephelometry, fluorescence immunoassay, and enzyme immunoassay (ELISA).

Specimen Serum.

Reference range Negative; titers less than 1:16 are normal.

Abnormal values Rheumatoid factors have a relatively high specificity but low sensitivity for the diagnosis of rheumatoid arthritis. They may occur in infections (bronchitis, kala azar, leprosy, subacute bacterial endocarditis, syphilis, tuberculosis, viral infections), liver disease (biliary obstruction, cirrhosis, fatty liver, granulomas, neoplasms, viral hepatitis), and other conditions (diabetes mellitus, idiopathic pulmonary fibrosis, osteoarthritis, paraproteinemia, Raynaud's disease, sarcoidosis, Sjögren's syndrome), and they occur in 3% of a normal healthy population. Titers of greater than 1:80 are suggestive of rheumatoid arthritis.

Cost $30–50.

RIA (radioimmunoassay)   A method that measures antigens or antibodies based on the principle of competitive inhibition of the binding of radioactively labeled antigens with the binding of unlabeled antigens to specific antibodies. RIA allows measurement of minimal amounts of antigenic substances, including enzymes and hormones, and is widely used in research as it is relatively easy to design an assay to detect a substance of interest. RIAs are being phased out of the clinical laboratory in favor of enzyme, fluorescence, or chemiluminescence assays, which eliminate the waste disposal problems inherent in maintaining radioactive materials on-site.

riboflavin (vitamin B_2)   A water-soluble B vitamin that is widely present in foods of plant and animal origin, which combines with phosphate to form the enzyme cofactors flavin mononucleotide (FMN) and flavin adenine dinucleotide (FAD). Riboflavin is involved in the oxidation-reduction reactions in many metabolic pathways and in energy production in the respiratory chain that occurs in the mitochondria, which are cellular organelles involved in metabolism. Riboflavin deficiency is rare, given the wide distribution of riboflavin in foods, and is almost invariably accompanied by deficiencies of other water-soluble vitamins. Riboflavin is rarely measured in the clinical laboratory, but may be requested in the presence of severe malnutrition and, less commonly, in chronic infections, alcoholism, rapid growth in children, hyperthyroidism, lactation, and pregnancy.

Patient preparation No preparation is required, other than for obtaining urine, which according to the method, may require a 24-hour specimen.

Procedure The methods used to quantify riboflavin include fluorometry, microbiology (based on the growth of *Lactobacillus casei*), and enzymatic (based on FAD-dependent glutathione reductase activity in lysed red blood cells).

Specimen Urine—random, fasting, or 24-hour.

Reference range Infants 500–900 µg/g creatinine; adults 80–270 µg/g creatinine. By the *Lactobacillus casei* assay, greater than 50–120 µg/24-hour urine.

Abnormal values Less than 15 µg/24-hour urine.

Cost $140–$175.

ring test   See *radial immunodiffusion* in Glossary.

Rinne test   A test in which a tuning fork is used to determine whether hearing loss is of the conduction or sensorineural type.

Patient preparation No preparation is required. If the patient has a hearing aid, it should be brought to the test.

Procedure The Rinne test is based on the differences in the sound heard by the individual being examined when a tuning fork (vibrating at 256, 512, 1024, and 2048 Hz) is held close to the ear (air conduction) or placed directly on the mastoid process of the temporal bone (bone conduction).

Reference range For individuals with normal hearing, the sound is heard more clearly and about two-fold longer in the air than when the tuning fork is placed on the bone.

Abnormal values A positive Rinne test is that in which the air conduction is greater than bone conduction, which occurs in normal hearing and in sensorineural hearing defects. A negative Rinne test is that in which the bone conduction is greater than air conduction, which is seen in conductive hearing loss.

Cost $35–$50. See *pure tone audiometry, SISI test, tone decay test.*

RIST   See *radioimmunosorbent test.*

Romberg test   A clinical test used in evaluating dysequilibrium. The Romberg test is used to differentiate central (cerebellar) from peripheral ataxia. In the former, there is no increase in the ataxic (incoordinated) movements with the eyes closed.

Patient preparation No preparation is required; the patient must be able to stand without support.

Procedure The patient stands with the eyes closed and both feet together. Then the patient stands on one or the other foot.

Reference range The patient should not lose his equilibrium with his eyes closed.

Abnormal values Excess swaying implies a severe defect in postural sensation in the lower extremities.

Cost The test is not generally billed separately, as it is a component of more complete neurologic testing. See *vestibular test.*

rosette test (rosetting)   A screening test for detecting significant fetomaternal hemorrhage, where an indicator cell forms easily identified rosettes around individual Rh-D fetal cells that may be present in the Rh-negative mother; this qualitative test can detect a 10 ml or greater fetomaternal hemorrhage, and it should be followed by a quantitative test, e.g., the Kleihauer-Betke test. See *Kleihauer-Betke test.*

Rose-Waaler test   A specialized passive hemagglutination test for detecting rheumatoid factors which uses sheep red blood cells that have been previously sensitized with rabbit anti-sheep red blood cell immunoglobulin G. If rheumatoid factor is present in serum, it combines with the red blood cell membrane-bound IgG, causing agglutination. The Rose-Waaler test is not commonly used as most rheumatoid factor tests use latex particles to establish agglutination, which, while less specific, are much easier to perform. See *rheumatoid factor.*

Rothera test (nitroprusside test)   A method used to semiquantify acetone and acetoacetic acid in urine, which is based on the formation of a purple color that is proportional to the amount of ketones present. The Rothera test is sensitive to 1–5 mg/dL of acetoactic acid and to 10–25 mg/dL of acetone. See *ketone body.*

RPR test (rapid plasma reagin test, reagin test)   A serologic test for syphilis, in which a patient's serum (which may or may not contain syphilis-related antibodies) is incubated with reagin, a fat-rich antigenic complex. Although reagin is not present in or produced by the spirochete (*Treponema pallidum*) that causes syphilis, it is immunologically similar and thus of diagnostic use.
   Patient preparation No preparation is required, other than for drawing blood.
   Procedure The RPR test is performed on a plastic card and measures complement fixation, which appears (in a positive test) as clumps of a modified VDRL antigen, antibody, and charcoal or latex.
   Specimen Serum.
   Reference range Negative.
   Abnormal values 70% of patients with early (primary) syphilis have a positive RPR test; 80% of patients with late (secondary) syphilis have a positive RPR test. The RPR is prone to false-positive results, which are seen in chickenpox, hepatitis, infectious mononucleosis, lupus erythematosus, pneumonia, pregnancy, rheumatoid arthritis, and tuberculosis.
   Cost $25–$50. See *biological false positive* in Glossary, *VDRL.*

rT₃   See *triiodothyronine.*

rubella (German measles)   An acute, usually benign, viral infection that usually occurs in childhood. If a woman is pregnant when first infected, it may cause congenital heart defects, low birth weight, microcephaly, mental retardation, congenital cataracts, or other major defects in the fetus.
   Patient preparation No preparation is required, other than for drawing blood.
   Procedure To determine the patient's immune status (i.e., whether the person has previously had rubella), two specimens are drawn—one in the

acute phase of the infection ("acute" serum) and the second when the patient is clearly recovering from the infection ("convalescent" serum). The levels of antibody (immunoglobulin) are evaluated by serial dilutions (titers) of serum and measured by hemagglutination inhibition, complement fixation, ELISA, and other techniques.

Specimen Serum.

Reference range In the acute phase, the immunoglobulin M (IgM) is increased. As the patient recovers, the immunoglobulin G (IgG) increases.

IgG   Titers of greater than 1:32 indicate previous exposure to rubella and immunity by either natural infection or vaccination

IgM   Titers of less than 1:8 indicate absence of immunity to rubella and the need for vaccination.

Abnormal values A four-fold increase in titers between the acute and convalescent sera indicates that active infection has occurred. A pregnant woman might consider aborting her fetus, which stands a very high risk of suffering congenital malformations.

Cost

IgG	$40-$60.
IgM	$125–$150.

Comments If a woman is pregnant while acutely infected, abortion may be advised, given the frequency of the congenital rubella syndrome. Positive IgG results mean that the patient has been exposed to rubella and is immune to further infection. Positive IgM results mean that there is a current, active infection. See *TORCH antibody panel.*

rubeola   See *measles.*

Sabin-Feldman dye test A serologic test for toxoplasmosis, based on the inability of living toxoplasma (in the presence of specific antibodies) to take up and retain methylene blue. Although it is an excellent procedure, the Sabin-Feldman dye test is cumbersome and rarely performed. Other tests for toxoplasmosis (e.g., indirect immunofluorescence and ELISA) are more easily performed and are equally sensitive to toxoplasma antigens.

salicylic acid (salicylate) The active metabolic product of aspirin, which is used as an analgesic and antipyretic. Salicylates are measured when there is clinical suspicion of acute aspirin intoxication.
  Patient preparation No preparation is required, other than for drawing blood or obtaining urine.
  Procedure Salicylates are measured by colorimetry, fluorometry, gas-liquid chromatography, and high-performance liquid chromatography.
  Specimen Serum, collected in EDTA anticoagulant or 24-hour urine.
  Reference range Less than 100 µg/ml.
  Abnormal values Greater than 100 µg/ml if the patient has gastric intolerance; greater than 150 µg/ml if the patient complains of deafness, dizziness, and tinnitus; and greater than 250 µg/ml if the patient complains of nausea and hyperventilation. Clinical intoxication occurs at levels greater than 500µg/ml.
  Cost $40–$60.

saline wet mount See *wet mount.*

saucerization biopsy (deep shave biopsy) A deep skin biopsy, which has a broad rim of epidermis and dermis. This biopsy is preferred by dermatologists for certain small (less then 1 cm) pigmented lesions, for which the clinical diagnosis is benign although malignant melanoma cannot be ruled out. If melanoma is suspected, a full-thickness excisional biopsy with conservative (i.e., the smallest possible) margins is indicated.

Patient preparation No preparation is necessary. Local anesthesia is required because deep biopsies are painful.

Procedure The procedure consists of the excision of a broad rim of epidermis and dermis and may require sutures.

Specimen Tissue from skin.

Reference range Normally no pathological lesions requiring therapy are seen.

Abnormal values Various benign (e.g., lentigo senilis, seborrheic keratosis), premalignant (e.g., dysplastic nevus), or malignant (e.g., melanoma, squamous cell carcinoma, or basal cell carcinoma) lesions may be identified by the pathologist.

Cost $100–150.

scabies (mite)   A severe form of infestation with the itch mite, *Sarcoptes scabiei*, which spreads by direct physical contact with infected individuals and is thus a disease of families and institutions. Scabies is characterized by intense itching that develops about one month after the first exposure to the mite. While the papules and "tracks" of the burrowing mite are most prominent on the hands and arms, the "scabies rash" is found on the armpits, waist, buttocks, inner thigh, and ankles, sites where *S. scabiei* is rarely found.

Patient preparation A biopsy of tissue may be required.

Procedure The diagnosis is established by dissecting the organisms or the eggs from the mites' tunnels, placing them in 20% potassium hydroxide or mineral oil, and examining them by a microscope.

Specimen Eggs and/or mites from tissue.

Reference range Negative.

Abnormal values Eggs and/or mites from tissue.

Cost $60–$80.

Comments Once scabies is identified, all persons who have had intimate contact with the patient should be examined and, if necessary, treated.

scanning electron microscopy   A type of electron microscope in which the beam of electrons scans the surface of an object, providing a three-dimensional image of the object of interest by analyzing the pattern of deflection of primary and secondary electrons. Scanning electron microscopy has had little use in medicine, given that the image is confined to cell surfaces, although it provides some information in renal pathology. See *electron microscopy* in Glossary, *transmission electron microscope* in Glossary.

Schiller's test   A clinical maneuver used by gynecologists to identify abnormalities on the uterine cervix that need to be biopsied and submitted to a pathologist for histologic examination.

Patient preparation The same as needed for a colposcopic examination of the uterine cervix.

Procedure Schiller's test is performed at the same time as colposcopy and consists of the simple "painting" of the surface of the cervix with a strong iodine solution (Lugol's solution).

Reference range Glycogen-rich areas are brown in color and almost invariably benign.

Abnormal values Areas with reduced glycogen are pale, and when they are viewed by light microscopy often demonstrate histologic changes (e.g., hyperkeratosis and parakeratosis) that have been associated with premalignant (e.g., human papillomavirus infection) or malignant (e.g., cervical intraepithelial neoplasia or carcinoma) lesions.

Cost The cost of Schiller's test is incorporated into a colposcopic biopsy. See *acetowhite lesion, cervical intraepithelial neoplasia, colposcopy.*

Schilling test (vitamin B_{12} absorption test) A clinical test that evaluates the ability to absorb vitamin B_{12}, which is decreased in the absence of intrinsic factor, a glycoprotein produced in the parietal cells of the stomach. Decreased intrinsic factor results in megaloblastic (pernicious) anemia.

Patient preparation No preparation is required, other than for drawing blood.

Procedure A "loading" dose of radioactive (cobalt-57 or cobalt-58) vitamin B_{12} is administered orally, followed by a "flushing" dose of nonradioactive vitamin B_{12}, which is administered intramuscularly. If the renal function is normal, the amount of radioactivity detected in the urine reflects vitamin B_{12} absorption. In another method, the plasma is collected eight hours after oral administration of radiolabeled vitamin B_{12}, which is not followed by a "flushing" dose of unlabeled vitamin B_{12}.

Specimen 24-hour urine.

Reference range At least 7% of the oral dose is excreted in the first 24 hours.

Abnormal values

  Decreased in: chronic pancreatitis, Crohn's disease, cystic fibrosis, giardiasis, gluten-sensitive enteropathy, ileal disease, resection, or bacterial overgrowth, pancreatic insufficiency, pernicious anemia, post-total gastric resection, radiation therapy.

Cost $150–$200.

Comments The Schilling test is being phased out, as it is an indirect means of measuring intrinsic factor, which can now be measured directly by immunoassay. See *vitamin B_{12}.*

Schirmer's test A clinical maneuver used to measure the total tear production by the lacrimal glands under normal (baseline) conditions, as well as response to stimuli, e.g., nasal irritants. It is used to evaluate patients with dry eyes, a relatively common condition of older individuals.

Patient preparation No preparation is required. Contact lenses must be removed.

Procedure A strip of filter paper is placed at the lower eyelid, and the length of filter paper moistened after five minutes is recorded.

Specimen Moistened filter paper.

Reference range Greater than 8 mm of moistening of filter paper is a normal baseline, and greater than 15 mm after nasal stimulation. There is approximately a 15% false-positive and 15% false-negative rate with the Schirmer test.

Abnormal values Any decrease in the length of filter paper moistening is abnormal. Dry eyes may occur as an isolated condition but are more commonly associated with autoimmune diseases, in particular Sjögren syndrome. Dry eyes are also seen in patients with lower motor neuron defects, as may occur in lesions of the geniculate ganglion and the nervus intermedius.

Cost This is a simple clinical test, which is not listed in Medicare price lists. See *autoimmune disease* in Glossary.

Schwabach's test A hearing test used to compare the conduction of sound from tuning forks through the bone of the skull and through the air. The test is used to determine whether hearing loss is due to defects in the conduction of sound or defects in the sensorineural transmission of sound.

Patient preparation None required. If the patient uses a hearing aid, it should be brought to the examining site.

Procedure In Schwabach's test, tuning forks of 256, 512, 1024, and 2048 Hz are placed on the mastoid process of the patient's temporal bone, then on the examiner's temporal bone (whose hearing is presumed to be normal). Each notes the time until the sound disappears.

Reference range In the normal individual, the sound is heard as long by the examinee as by the examiner.

Abnormal values If the sound is heard longer by the patient than by the examiner, the result is termed "Schwabach prolonged" and indicates a conductive-type hearing loss. If the sound is heard for less time by the patient than by the examiner, the result is termed "Schwabach shortened" and indicates sensorineural hearing loss.

Cost $100–$150. See *pure tone audiometry, Rinne test.*

screening test A general term for any evaluation of a person's health status that attempts to identify a disease process not previously known to exist in a patient at the time of evaluation, e.g., hypercholesterolemia, hypertension, or malignancy. Screening tests include measurement of blood pressure (to detect hypertension); sigmoidoscopy (for colorectal cancer); radiologic procedures, e.g., mammography (breast cancer); or laboratory tests, e.g., blood cholesterol (coronary artery disease), guaiac-positive stools (colon cancer), or pap smears of the uterine cervix (cervical cancer). Screening tests generally have high sensitivities and low specificities to allow detection of most of the patients with a morbid condition, while having the acceptable disadvantage of a high rate of false-positivity. Screening strategies are based on whether the population is at high or low risk for a particular disease and whether the course of the disease for which screening is being performed will be affected. Commonly used screening tests include those for:

BREAST CANCER Examination of a woman's breasts by a physician every year after age 40; mammography—every one to two years after age 35, and every year above age 50. Note: Policymakers have recently questioned whether this frequency is justified.

CERVICAL CANCER A pap test from the uterine cervix (cervical cytology) every one to three years, starting at the age of first sexual intercourse.

BLOOD PRESSURE Measurement of blood pressure in normotensive persons every two years, all ages.

CHOLESTEROL Measurement of cholesterol every five years in older individuals. See *cancer screen, diagnostic test* in Glossary, *management test* in Glossary.

Seashore test A battery of recorded sounds used to determine a person's innate musical abilities, in which the individual is evaluated for intensity and pitch discrimination, rhythm, timbre, timing, and tonal memory. Although the test was first used to test musical aptitude, it is believed to be of some use in differentiating between conductive and sensorineural hearing loss. See *pure tone audiometry, Rinne test, Schwabach's test.*

secretin injection test A provocative test used to measure gastrin levels in serum and to evaluate pancreatic function.

Patient preparation Patient should be in fasting state.

Procedure 5 units of nonhuman (e.g., from pigs) secretin is infused for one hour. Blood is drawn at 15-minute intervals, and the gastrin levels are measured by radioimmunoassay.

Specimen Serum, drawn every 15 minutes for one hour.

Reference range The test is used to evaluate exocrine pancreatic function. After secretin injection, the normal pancreas increases its volume of secretion and bicarbonate production.

Abnormal values Gastrin levels are decreased in antral G-cell hyperplasia and duodenal ulcers and markedly increased in gastrinomas and Zollinger-Ellison syndrome. The normal increases in volume of secretion and bicarbonate production, which are stimulated by secretin, do not occur in a pancreas affected by cystic fibrosis, chronic pancreatitis, or carcinoma.

Cost $80–$100 for each specimen drawn. See *gastrin.*

sedimentation rate See *erythrocyte sedimentation rate.*

segmental mastectomy See *lumpectomy.*

Seliwanoff's test A laboratory method measuring fructose in urine, which is increased in several relatively rare diseases of metabolism, including hereditary fructose intolerance and essential fructosuria. In the test, a volume of urine is added to an equal volume of a reagent containing acid and resorcinol. The resulting reaction results in the formation of a red color.

semen analysis A laboratory procedure for evaluating possible causes of male infertility. Sperm counts are decreased in some forms of infertility, chemotherapy, estrogens, and following vasectomy.

Patient preparation The man should abstain from sexual activity for two to five days. The specimen is obtained by masturbation, coitus interruptus, or with a condom and placed in a plastic urine or sputum container with a lid. Specimens from a rape victim require collection by vaginal lavage after the cervix and vaginal wall have been swabbed with an applicator stick and the material obtained therefrom has been placed on a slide for microscopic evaluation. See *rape kit.*

Procedure After the specimen has been delivered to the laboratory, the volume is measured, and several drops are placed on a microscopic slide in order to evaluate the sperm count, morphology, and motility.

Specimen Ejaculate, which should be maintained at room temperature. Analysis should be performed within three hours.

Reference range
Count:	Greater than 20 x 10^6/mL.
Volume	1.0–4.0 mL.
Morphology	More than 75% are mature, without defects.
Mobility	More than 60% of sperm are actively mobile.

Abnormal values Counts of less than 20 x 10^6/mL, volume of less than 1.0 mL, fewer than 60% mature, and fewer than 50% actively mobile.

Cost $80–$100.

Comment The sperm count of the average male appears to have decreased in the twentieth century—113 million/ml in 1940 to 66 million in 1990, a decline believed by some to be related to environmental pollutants that have estrogenic activity. In the event of suspected rape, the specimens must follow a "chain of custody," which ensures that the information such specimens provide is acceptable from a medicolegal standpoint.

serial sevens test A neurologic test that consists of the patient subtracting 7 from 100, from 93, from 86, and so on, as a test of the patient's level of consciousness. It is of use in administering anesthesia in preparation for general surgery.

serologic test A general term for any test performed in the clinical laboratory that measures the components (e.g., antibodies, complement) and reactions (e.g., complement fixation, hemagglutination, hemagglutination inhibition precipitation) that reflect the immune status, especially antibody titers. The term has undergone subtle changes and is now widely understood to mean those tests that measure the immune responses to pathogens, particularly viruses. See *acute serum* in Glossary, *adenovirus, convalescent serum* in Glossary, *RPR test, rubella.*

serum neutralization test (protection test) A test in which a patient's serum (which is presumed to contain a neutralizing antibody) and a microorganism of interest (e.g., an adenovirus or enterovirus) are either placed in a cell culture or injected into a host organism to measure the levels of antibodies that are protective against the pathogen of interest.

Patient preparation No preparation is required, other than for drawing blood.

Procedure The patient's serum is mixed with a sample containing the suspected organism.

Specimen Serum.

Reference range Negative.

Abnormal values Neutralization of the microorganism's activity is seen.

Cost $100–$150.

sex chromatin test See *chromosome analysis.*

sex hormone-binding β-globulin (steroid-binding β-globulin) A protein produced in the liver that is the principal carrier of testosterone. The protein has a weaker affinity for estrogen.

Patient preparation No preparation is required, other than for drawing blood.

Procedure The specimen is measured by electroimmunodiffusion or radioimmunodiffusion.

Specimen Serum.

Reference range

Males	0.1–1.2 mg/dL.
Females	0.3–1.5 mg/dL.

Abnormal values

Increased in: liver disease, hyperthyroidism, increased estrogens, oral contraceptives.

Decreased in: advanced age, androgens, growth hormone, hypothyroidism.

Cost $80–$100.

SGOT (serum glutamic-oxaloacetic transaminase) See *asparate aminotransferase.*

SGPT (serum glutamic-pyruvic transaminase) See *alanine aminotransferase.*

shake test See *foam stability index.*

shell vial assay A rapid culture technique based on the immunofluorescence seen in the early growth of viruses. The shell vial assay can be used to detect the growth of some viruses (e.g., CMV, herpesvirus 1, herpesvirus 2, varicella) within 16 hours of inoculation. This short turnaround time contrasts with that of conventional methods for identifying viruses, which are based on the effects on cells in culture that are caused by the viruses and may require up to 14 days for evaluation. See *cytopathologic effect* in Glossary.

Patient preparation None required other than that for obtaining the specimen from the relevant body site.

Procedure The specimen is placed in the receptacle (shell vial) which contains a coverslip from a microscopic slip. After incubation of the specimen for up to 24 hours, the coverslip is stained with the appropriate antibody and examined by an immunofluorescence microscope.
Specimen Throat swab, vesicles from herpetic lesions of the skin, and others.
Reference range Negative.
Abnormal values Specific changes are seen on the cells attached to the coverslip that are typical of each virus.
Cost $150–$250.

sialography A method of diagnostic radiology for visualizing the salivary glands and ducts after instillation of radiocontrast. Sialography is of use for evaluating suspected salivary gland disease (e.g., dilatation of ducts or ectasia, cysts, calculi, strictures, fistulas) and dry mouth.
Patient preparation None is required. It should not be performed in patients with acute inflammation.
Procedure A 22-gauge polyethylene tube is used to inject 0.5 to 1.0 ml of radiocontrast material.
Specimen Films obtained by the radiologist.
Reference range Negative for anatomic abnormalities, masses, or stones.
Abnormal values Salivary duct ectasia, fistulas, strictures, stones, or calculi.
Cost $250–$400.
Comments For evaluating suspected salivary gland neoplasms, sialography has been largely replaced by regional computed tomography.

sickle cell test (hemoglobin S test, sickling test) Sickle cells are erythrocytes (red blood cells) that have a "sickled" shape due to a mutation in the genes that encode the beta chain of hemoglobin. The sickle cell test is used to screen for the presence of sickling hemoglobins, in particular hemoglobin S, the most common cause of sickle cell anemia.
Patient preparation No preparation is required, other than for drawing blood.
Procedure In the sickle cell test, certain agents (sodium metabisulfite or sodium dithionate) are used to desolubilize hemoglobin S to the crystallized deoxygenated form, which causes the abnormal red blood cells to undergo the sickling change.
Specimen Whole blood, EDTA anticoagulant, stored at 4°C for up to 20 days.
Reference range Negative.
Cost $20–$30.
Comments 0.2% of black persons born in the United States have the sickle cell trait, in which the red blood cells are not normally sickled. Far fewer blacks have sickle cell anemia, in which sickled cells are usually seen in a simple peripheral blood smear.

sigmoidoscopy A clinical test that is most often performed in the physician's office, in which a flexible endoscope is inserted via the rectum, and the surface of the rectum, sigmoid colon, and proximal colon are examined. Sigmoidoscopy is used to detect the presence of neoplasms or other lesions. The lesions are biopsied and sent to a pathology laboratory for evaluation to determine whether the tissue is benign or malignant and whether the patient requires further therapy. Sigmoidoscopy is indicated for screening healthy, asymptomatic older individuals for colorectal cancer and for evaluating patients with suspected disease in the lower gastrointestinal tract based on clinical signs, e.g., blood in stool, diarrhea, colicky lower abdominal pain, and recent loss of weight.

Patient preparation A phosphosoda (Fleet®) enema administered a few minutes before the procedure usually is sufficient to allow adequate visualization of the mucosal surface of the colon.

Procedure A flexible endoscope measuring 35 or 60 cm (depending on the model) is inserted via the rectum, and the mucosal surface of the rectum, sigmoid colon, and proximal colon are examined directly.

Specimen Tissue biopsy of abnormal findings.

Reference range The normal sigmoid colon has no visible lesions.

Abnormal values Sigmoidoscopy may reveal bleeding, benign or malignant tumors, submucosal air, or diverticuli.

Comments Although there are few contraindications for sigmoidoscopy, the procedure should not be performed in patients with acute diverticulitis, acute peritonitis and/or abdominal perforation, toxic megacolon, severe or decompensated cardiac or pulmonary disease, or massive gastrointestinal hemorrhage.

Cost $700–$900. See *barium enema, colonoscopy, endoscopy, occult blood testing, proctoscopy.*

signal averaged electrocardiography A technique that amplifies late electrical potentials in the heart, which are thought to be due to fragmented and delayed conduction through the borders of a myocardial scar. The delayed conduction of late potentials allows reentry of electrical impulses and increases ventricular arrhythmias. Signal averaged electrocardiography is a useful noninvasive test for identifying increased risk of ventricular tachycardia, but it is of little use for patients with conduction defects. See *electrocardiography.*

single fiber electromyography (SF-EMG) A test used in neurology to evaluate the activity of single fibers of selected muscles (e.g., the common extensor of the fingers) which is displayed as an action potential on a cathode-ray oscilloscope. SF-EMG may detect early defects in neuromuscular junction diseases (e.g., myasthenia gravis, Eaton-Lambert syndrome, and botulism) even before clinically obvious neurologic changes occur.

Patient preparation No preparation is required. The procedure may be performed at the same time as conventional electromyography.

Procedure The procedure consists of the insertion of a small (25 μm in diameter) wire into a superficial muscle to evaluate muscle jitter and muscle fiber density.

Reference range Action potentials of single fibers appear as fibrillation potentials. The fiber density for the common extensor muscle of the fingers is 1.3 to 1.8, and its "jitter" is approximately 55 msec.

Abnormal values Jitter is markedly increased in neuropathic conditions (e.g., myasthenia gravis) that are accompanied by denervation and reinnervation but are normal or near-normal in myopathic disease. Fiber density is increased in those conditions in which there is regrowth of nerves in the early stages of disease. Since this may occur in both neural and muscle disease, fiber density lacks specificity.

Cost $250–$350.

SISI test (short increment sensitivity index test) A hearing test used to determine differential sensitivity to changes in loudness.

Patient preparation None is required. If the patient uses a hearing aid, it should be brought to the site of examination.

Procedure The individual is exposed to a pure tone of 1000 Hz, the intensity of which is increased in 1–5 dB intervals. The person being tested indicates to the examiner each time he/she hears an increase in intensity.

Reference range A low (less then 60%) detection percentage of changes in intensity is normal.

Abnormal values A damaged cochlear system results in an increased detection rate (greater than 60%), as there is an increased sensitivity to changes in sound.

Cost $150–$250. See *pure tone audiometry, Rinne test, Schwabach's test, tone decay test.*

skeletal survey The radiologic examination of the entire skeleton, which is of use in suspected cases of child abuse and to detect metastases to the bone (metastatic series) from primary malignancies, e.g., prostate or breast cancer. For detection of malignancy, the skeletal survey has been replaced by radionuclide imaging ("scans") of the skeleton because bone scans detect lesions about three months earlier than plain radiographs of the same region.

Cost $600–$1000.

skin biopsy Any of a number of procedures (e.g., shave, punch, excisional biopsy) in which tissue is obtained from the skin in order to establish a diagnosis on which therapy is to be based. Skin biopsies for possible malignancy must take into account location—adjacency to vital facial structures (e.g., the eyelids, cosmetically sensitive zones) and inadequate margins (e.g., those involved by tumor) which will force the surgeon to obtain more tissue and biology. Malignancies in the skin have a wide range of expression and may be primary or secondary. Primary malignancies arise in the skin itself. The most common primary skin cancer is basal cell carcinoma, which is indolent, slow-growing, and evokes little panic on the part of the managing physician, even if the margins are involved with tumor. This contrasts with malignant melanoma, a malignancy for which the prognosis is based on the depth of invasion. Secondary skin cancers arise elsewhere (e.g., breast, gastrointestinal tract), metastasize to the skin, and almost invariably indicate a poor prognosis.

Patient preparation No preparation is required. The biopsy itself may cause some anxiety, especially if stitches are needed to close the wound.

Procedure The procedure consists of the excision of various amounts of skin. The shave biopsy is used for surface lesions, the punch biopsy for deep lesions, and the excisional biopsy for complete removal of a lesion with margins of normal-in-appearance tissue.

Specimen Tissue from skin.

Reference range Normal tissue or no changes of significance.

Abnormal values The tissue may have pathological changes ranging from benign (e.g., inflammation, infection, pigmented, or vascular) to malignant (e.g., malignant melanoma, squamous cell carcinoma, and basal cell carcinoma).

Cost $75–$150.

"skinny" needle biopsy A 22-gauge needle used for obtaining percutaneous, often radiologically or fluoroscopically guided biopsies or aspiration cytology specimens from masses of the breast, lungs, and sites difficult to access. When positive, skinny needle biopsies circumvent the need for open biopsies. Negative results, however, may result from sampling errors and should be followed by open biopsy if the lesion is suspected as potentially malignant.

Patient preparation Informed consent is required. Baseline coagulation studies (e.g., activated partial thromboplastin time, prothrombin time, platelet count), and certain chemistries (e.g., BUN and creatinine) should be obtained before the procedure.

Procedure The procedure consists of the insertion of a long 22-gauge needle into various sites of the body. It may be performed in the radiology suite.

Specimen Cells and small fragments of tissue.

Reference range Negative for significant pathological changes.

Abnormal values Inflammation, malignancy.

Cost $100–$200.

sleep study See *polysomnography.*

slit lamp This microscope, fitted with a specialized illuminating system for generating collimated light, is used to examine the anterior portion of the eye. The slit lamp allows the ophthalmologist to examine the conjunctiva, sclera, cornea, iris, lens, anterior chamber, and ocular fluids.

Patient preparation No preparation is required, other than removal of contact lenses. Dilation of the pupils by mydriatic agents is often required.

Procedure In the examination the patient sits in front of the slit lamp, the room is darkened, and the eyes are examined by a low-power binocular microscope.

Reference range Negative for abnormalities.
Abnormal values The slit lamp is of particular use in detecting dendritic keratitis, foreign bodies of the cornea, and tumors of the iris.
Cost $25–$50.

small intestinal biopsy (small bowel biopsy)   A biopsy that may be performed with an upper GI endoscope from the duodenum or upper jejunum in an ambulatory or outpatient setting (e.g., physician's office), often as part of an evaluation for nonmalignant conditions.

Patient preparation Informed consent is required. Food and fluids should be restricted for eight hours before the procedure. Baseline coagulation studies (e.g., activated partial thromboplastin time, prothrombin time, platelet count) and certain chemistries (e.g., BUN and creatinine) should be obtained before the procedure. Local anesthesia is required for the insertion of the endoscope.

Procedure The procedure consists of the insertion of an endoscope past the stomach into the small intestine. A biopsy forceps is passed through a channel in the endoscope, and tissue is obtained from areas that appear abnormal. As with other biopsies, once the specimen is obtained, it is sent for microscopic examination to a pathologist. The biopsy may require special stains (e.g., Congo red for amyloidosis or PAS for Whipple's disease) for optimal evaluation. This may result in a delay in issuing a final report.

Specimen A rounded fragment of tissue, which is usually placed in formalin.

Reference range Negative for significant pathological changes.

Abnormal values Pathological lesions occur in: abetalipoproteinemia, agammaglobulinemia, amyloidosis, Eosinophilic gastroenteritis, immunoproliferative small intestinal disease (which may precede or accompany regional lymphoma), radiation enteropathy, scleroderma, sprue (either celiac or tropical sprue), systemic mastocytosis, vitamin B_{12} malabsorption, Whipple's disease.

Cost $900–$1000.

sodium (Na^+)   A critical electrolyte that is the main positive ion (cation) in extracellular fluids, including the blood circulation. Sodium is critical in homeostasis of body fluids, conductance of neuromuscular impulses, and enzyme activity.

Patient preparation No preparation is required, other than for drawing blood or obtaining urine.

Procedure Sodium is measured by any of a number of techniques, including emission photometry and atomic absorption spectrophotometry.

Specimen Serum, heparinized plasma, or urine.

Reference range

Serum	135–145 mEq/L.
Urine	40–220 mEq/24 hours.

Abnormal values
> Serum increased in: adrenal hyperfunction, congestive heart failure, dehydration, drugs, e.g., some antibiotics, corticosteroids, cough medicines, estrogens, laxatives, licorice, methyldopa, phenylbutazone, reserpine, sodium bicarbonate, hepatic failure, high-sodium diet.
> Serum decreased in: burns, drugs (e.g., acetazolamide, cyclophosphamide, ethacrynic acid, mannitol, salt-wasting diuretics, [furosemide], spironolactone, thiazides, triamterene, vasopressin, vincristine), prolonged parenteral nutrition, low-sodium diet, nasogastic suctioning, salt-wasting renal disease, tissue injury, syndrome of inappropriate secretion of ADH (SIADH), vomiting.
> Urine decreased in: adrenal hyperfunction, congestive heart failure, hepatic failure, low-sodium diet, renal failure.
> Urine increased in: adrenal hypofunction, anterior pituitary (adenohypophysis) hypofunction, essential hypertension, high-sodium diet.

Cost $10–20. Sodium is measured as part of a routine chemistry profile.

solubility test (turbidity test)   A test for sickle cell anemia, which is based on the decreased solubility of hemoglobin S in dithionate. It is less accurate than the sodium metabisulfate or sickle cell test, and requires additional testing to confirm sickle cell anemia. See *sickle cell test*.

somatotropin   See *growth hormone*.

specific gravity   A measure of the solutes in a fluid, which is the ratio of the density of a substance (e.g., urine) to the density of water. In laboratory testing this value reflects the kidney's ability to concentrate urine in order to conserve water. If a random urine specimen has specific gravity greater than 1.023, the kidney's ability to concentrate is assumed to be normal.

Patient preparation No preparation is required, other than for obtaining urine.

Procedure Specific gravity is tested by refractometry, which measures the ratio of the velocity of light in air to the velocity of light in a solution.

Specimen Urine.

Reference range 1.016–1.022

Abnormal values
> Decreased in: renal tubular damage, chronic renal insufficiency, diabetes insipidus, malignant hypertension.
> Increased in: syndrome of inappropriate secretion of antidiuretic hormone, uncontrolled diabetes mellitus, proteinuria, eclampsia, obstructive uropathy.

Cost $25–$50. Specific gravity is measured as part of a routine urinalysis.

speech threshold audiometry   A type of hearing test in which the individual's ability to discriminate recorded speech transmitted through earphones. Speech threshold audiometry is used to determine the lowest hearing level necessary to detect and comprehend human speech, to screen for hearing impairment, and to confirm thresholds obtained by pure tone audiometry. See *pure tone audiometry.*

sperm antibody   See *anti-sperm antibodies.*

sperm-binding assay (Mannose-binding assay)   A highly specific test for infertility that evaluates the ability of an enzyme on the sperm's surface to bind with mannose receptors on the ovum. See *semen analysis.*

sperm penetration assay   A type of fertility test that evaluates the ability of sperm to penetrate hamster eggs. The test sperm are compared to those from a male known to be fertile. The assay is highly predictive for normal fertility in a man who has a positive test. In the presence of unfavorable sperm parameters, the correlation of the test results with the ability to fertilize human eggs in vitro is less clear.
   Patient preparation The man should abstain from sexual activity for two to five days. The specimen is obtained by masturbation, coitus interruptus, or with a condom, and placed in a plastic urine or sputum container with a lid.
   Procedure After the specimen has been delivered to the laboratory and the sperm parameters are documented, the specimen is incubated with zona-free hamster eggs.
   Specimen Ejaculate, which should be maintained at room temperature. Analysis should be performed within three hours.
   Reference range Positive, i.e., greater than 10% penetration of the hamster eggs.
   Abnormal values Negative, i.e., less than 10% penetration of the hamster eggs, which may indicate a male factor in infertility.
   Cost $100–$200.

S phase analysis   Analysis of the fraction of the cells in a tissue or fluid that are actively synthesizing DNA, which provides useful information on a tumor's rate of proliferation. The S phase fraction is most easily measured by flow cytometry and is a parameter often measured when evaluating certain malignancies. See *flow cytometry* in Glossary, *ploidy analysis.*
   Patient preparation None required beyond that needed for obtaining the specimen, e.g., blood or a biopsy of tissue.
   Procedure A specimen containing the cells in the appropriate fluid is aspirated and processed through a flow cytometer.
   Specimen The specimens that can be analyzed for cells in the S phase include cells from the peripheral blood, sputum, and body fluids, as well as tissues that have been minced into small pieces in order to "harvest" the cells.
   Reference range Less than 10% of the cells in the specimen should be in the S phase of the cell's reproductive cycle.

Abnormal values The finding of more than 10% of the cells in the S phase of the cell's reproductive cycle is suggestive of an aggressive malignancy. *Cost* $150–$300.

Comments S phase analysis provides information on the prognosis of a lesion or tumor, not on whether it is benign or malignant.

spinal fluid cell content See *cerebrospinal fluid* in Glossary.

spinal tap See *lumbar puncture.*

spiral computed tomography (helical scanning) A type of computer tomography, in which a large image volume is acquired at a relatively high speed by continuous rotation of the detector. This method allows the acquisition of a 10–inch, three–dimensional block of "gapless" radiologic information in a single breath. The information obtained with spiral CT scanning is markedly superior to the single "slice" images from the current generation of CT imagers, and improves the images obtained from the heart and lungs, as the image acquisition time is shorter, which results in less blurring of organs that are constantly in motion. See *computed tomography.*

spirometry The measurement of the movement of air in and out of the lungs during various breathing maneuvers, as a means of preoperative evaluation of pulmonary function. Spirometry is the most important of the pulmonary function tests.

Patient preparation Heavy meals should be avoided before testing. Smoking history, time of last cigarette, and information about current medications, particularly corticosteroids and bronchodilators, should be obtained.

Procedure The patient breathes into a plastic tube attached to a spirometer, which measures either volume displacement or the flow of air over time.

Specimen The "specimen" consists of either exhaled volume or rates of flow.

Reference range The values in spirometry should be within 20% (i.e., 80% of predicted values) of normal for the person's age, height, and sex.

Abnormal values The spirometric values are decreased in patients with obstructive lung disease (e.g., asthma, chronic bronchitis, emphysema), restrictive lung disease (e.g., respiratory distress syndrome and interstitial fibrosis), and in neuromuscular disease (e.g., myasthenia gravis). 70%–79% of predicted values are regarded as minimal impairment of pulmonary function; 55%–69% as moderate impairment; 45%–54% as severe impairment, and less than 45% as very severe impairment. *Cost* $50–$75.

sputum A semiliquid diagnostic material that is obtained by deep coughing from the lungs, bronchi, and trachea and is most commonly analyzed in the laboratory in one of two fashions. In cytologic examination, the sputum is smeared on a glass slide, stained with one of several dyes, and examined by light microscopy. The only cells seen in a normal sputum are those that line the tracheobronchial tree and the lungs. In culture and sensitivity, the sputum is swabbed on a culture plate in the microbiology laboratory to detect the growth of potentially harmful bacteria or fungi.

Patient preparation No preparation is required.

Procedure Sputum is obtained by a variety of methods, usually expectoration. If the sputum is especially thick, it may require hydration, physiotherapy (e.g., clapping on the chest wall), or drainage by changing position. Sputum can also be "harvested" by tracheal suction or bronchoscopy.

Specimen Sputum, as above indicated.

Reference range The normal sputum has many white blood cells and relatively few squames or epithelial cells, which would imply that the specimen is from the mouth rather than from the lower respiratory tract.

Abnormal values Sputum can be cultured to demonstrate infection with various bacteria, e.g., *Streptococcus pneumoniae* and *Haemophilus influenzae*, both of which cause acute bacterial pneumonia, as well as *Mycobacteria tuberculosis,* which causes tuberculosis. Sputum is also used to detect cancer, as it may contain malignant cells, which are analyzed by light microscopy by a cytopathologist.

Cost The cost depends on the procedure needed to obtain the specimen. The laboratory component costs $75–$200. The bronchoscopy per se costs $1000 to $1500. See *cytology.*

standard acid reflux test (Tuttle test)   A clinical test used to evaluate the intensity and duration of the regurgitation (reflux) of acid from the stomach into the esophagus, which is similar to the Bernstein test in format and information provided. See *Bernstein test, maximum acid output, stimulated acid output* in Glossary, *upper gastrointestinal endoscopy.*

Stenger test   A functional test used to differentiate between feigned and true unilateral hearing loss, in which sounds below the normal threshold of hearing are presented to either ear in succession. See *pure tone audiometry, Rinne test, Schwabach's test.*

steroid-binding β-globulin   See *sex-hormone binding β-globulin.*

stimulation test   A general term for any clinical test that evaluates the synthetic reserve capacity of a substance of interest, providing information on whether the production of the hormone is at its maximum. Stimulation tests include the metapyrone test for adrenal hypofunction and the maximum acid output assay in Zollinger-Ellison syndrome. See *maximum acid output, provocative test, suppression test.*

stool   See *parasite identification.*

stress test A general term for any of a number of clinical maneuvers used to evaluate the body's ability to respond to cardiac, mental, pharmacologic, physical, or supraphysiologic stress that are performed under monitored conditions. In practice, the term "stress test" is usually understood to mean cardiac stress test. See *exercise tolerance test, thallium stress test.*

string test A bedside test for determining the viscosity or "stickiness" of synovial fluid. This is a measure of the "quality" of the synovial fluid, which reflects the ability of proteins to bind to each other.
  Patient preparation No preparation is required, other than for obtaining synovial fluid, which requires aspiration from a joint, usually from the knee.
  Procedure A few drops of synovial fluid are added to 10 ml of diluted (2%–5%) acetic acid, and the length of the "strand" formed between drops of fluid is measured.
  Specimen Synovial fluid.
  Reference range The further a drop of synovial fluid falls before separating ("stringing effect"), the greater is the fluid's viscosity and the more normal it is.
  Abnormal values A decrease in the strand length implies chemical deterioration due to inflammatory joint disease (sepsis, gout, rheumatoid arthritis) but not to degenerative joint disease.
  Cost This is a test that is performed at the bedside or in conjunction with synovial fluid analysis, which usually costs between $100 and $200. See *synovial fluid analysis.*

Stypven time test A type of one-stage prothrombin time for clotting disorders that uses the venom from the Russell viper.
  Patient preparation No preparation is required, other than for drawing blood.
  Procedure The procedure is a variation of the one-stage prothrombin time, in which Stypven is added to plasma to accelerate the clotting reaction.
  Specimen Plasma, which should be removed and frozen until analysis.
  Reference range 11 to 15 seconds.
  Abnormal values The Stypven time is prolonged in deficiencies of prothrombin, coagulation factor V, some defects of coagulation factor X, and when the platelets are decreased (thrombocytopenia). It is abnormally shortened in the presence of lipemia (increased fat in the blood) and when the platelets are increased (thrombocytosis).
  Cost $25–$50. See *partial thromboplastin time, prothrombin time.*

sucrose hemolysis test A test used to screen for the presence of paroxysmal nocturnal hemoglobinuria, which is based on the increased binding of complement protein to red blood cell membranes.
  Patient preparation No preparation is required, other than for drawing blood.

Procedure In the sucrose hemolysis test, red blood cells from the patient are incubated in an isotonic saline solution mixed with sucrose.

Specimen Blood anticoagulated with citrate or oxalate, but not with EDTA.

Reference range Normally, less than 5% of red blood cells are lysed (broken apart).

Abnormal values Lysis of more than 10% of the red blood cells being tested is strongly suggestive, but not diagnostic, of paroxysmal nocturnal hemoglobinuria.

Cost $25–$50.

suppression test   A general term for any clinical test or assay, e.g., dexamethasone suppression test, that is used to evaluate a substance (hormone or protein) being produced in excess. If the substance of interest is under the control of a regulating or releasing factor, it will respond to a feedback loop that will eventually "down-regulate" its activity. If the excess production is not being controlled by the feedback loop, it is said to be autonomous, a finding that is typical of tumors of the endocrine system. See *stimulation test*.

susceptibility test   See *predisposition testing, antibiotic sensitivity and identification.*

Swan-Ganz catheterization   An invasive procedure in which a Swan-Ganz catheter is used to monitor blood circulation in critically ill patients. Swan-Ganz catheterization is most often performed in an intensive care unit and requires continuous electrocardiographic and blood pressure monitoring.

Patient preparation Because Swan-Ganz catheterization is often performed on a patient who is comatose, the appropriate guardians or caretakers must be contacted for consent. Baseline coagulation studies (e.g., activated partial thromboplastin time, prothrombin time, platelet count) and certain chemistries (e.g., BUN and creatinine) should be obtained before the procedure. If possible, aspirin and nonsteroidal anti-inflammatory agents should be discontinued before the procedure. The effects of the anticoagulants warfarin and heparin should be reversed.

Procedure The procedure consists of the insertion of a Swan-Ganz catheter through a large vein (e.g., the internal jugular or subclavian) into the pulmonary artery in order to monitor the blood flow (hemodynamics) in critically ill patients. At the same time the catheter is being inserted, the electrocardiogram and the blood pressure are monitored on a continuous basis.

Reference range Swan-Ganz catheterization provides information on the blood pressure in the right atrium, right ventricle, and the pulmonary artery. The "wedge" pressure, which is obtained when the catheter is "jammed" into the smaller pulmonary arteries, is the difference in oxygen saturation between the right atrium and ventricle. Swan-Ganz catheterization can also be used to measure cardiac output and pulmonary and systemic vascular resistance.

Abnormal values Indications for Swan-Ganz catheterization include acute myocardial infarction in the presence of hemodynamic instability, adult respiratory distress syndrome, suspected cardiac tamponade, congestive heart failure that responds poorly to diuretics, rupture of papillary muscle(s) of the mitral valves, severe hypotension, and septic shock. It is also used to monitor the hemodynamic status during cardiac surgery, e.g., coronary artery bypass surgery.

Cost $1500–$2500.

Comments Contraindications include severe coagulopathy, left bundle branch block, severe hypothermia, and inadequate monitoring equipment. Complications include thrombosis, embolism (e.g., pulmonary embolism), infection, infarction, arrhythmias, perforation of pulmonary artery, hemothorax, pneumothorax, and heart valve trauma. The interpretation of normal and abnormal values for hemodynamic studies is highly specialized.

sweat test (sweat chloride test)   A diagnostic test for cystic fibrosis, which measures the chloride present in sweat and is ideally performed after the age of two months. Normal subjects have less then 50 mEq/L (mean, 18 mEq/L) and those with cystic fibrosis have more than 60 mEq/L (average, 100 mEq/L) of chloride in the sweat.

Patient preparation Most patients being tested are children or infants who need to be told that they will feel no more than a slight tickling sensation.

Procedure The procedure consists of iontophoresis, in which a gauze pad saturated with a predetermined amount of pilocarpine (a sweat inducer) is "driven" into the skin by a low amount of electricity (4 milliamperes in 15 to 20 second intervals for 5 minutes). After 5 minutes, a dry weighed gauze pad is taped in place on the site where the pilocarpine was driven into the skin, and after 30 to 40 minutes, the gauze pad is removed, weighed, and the sodium and the chloride concentration are analyzed in the laboratory by rehydrating in distilled water.

Specimen Gauze pad with chloride and sodium.

Reference range

Chloride	10–30 mEq/L.
Sodium	10–35 mEq/L.

Abnormal values

Chloride	50–110 mEq/L.
Sodium	50–130 mEq/L.

Chloride is increased in: Addison's disease, adrenogenital syndrome cystic fibrosis, ectodermal dysplasia, fucosidosis, glucose-6-phosphatase deficiency, hypothyroidism, malnutrition, mucopolysaccharidosis, nephrogenic diabetes insipidus, nephrotic syndrome, renal insufficiency, tjechnical errors in performing the sweat test.

Cost $25–$45.

Comments The sweat test is notoriously difficult to perform, even in the hands of experts. An error rate of 43% was recorded in one referral center. When the sweat test is performed properly in duplicate, it has a sensitivity of 90%–99%. See *cystic fibrosis* in Glossary.

swinging flashlight test   A clinical test for comparing "direct" and "consensual" (the eye that is not being stimulated) reactions of each pupil, which is used to identify pupillary defects of the afferent cortical pathways.

Patient preparation None required.

Procedure A flashlight (or penlight) is swung back and forth between the two pupils.

Reference range Usually the direct reaction (i.e., that which is seen when the light is shone directly into the eye) is stronger than the consensual reaction (i.e., that which is seen in response to the light being shone in the opposite eye).

Abnormal values If the afferent pathway is impaired by disease, the direct response will be weakened and the consensual efferent response unchanged. As light shines on the eye with the affected afferent defect, the pupil will paradoxically dilate, a phenomenon known as the Marcus Gunn pupil or the afferent pupillary defect.

Cost This test is performed as part of a complete neurological examination, and there is not a separate diagnostic fee.

synovial fluid analysis   A laboratory test that evaluates synovial fluid, a pale yellow viscid liquid found in the joint that serves as a lubricant. Synovial fluid analysis is most commonly performed in younger patients to detect infection (e.g., with staphylococcus or tuberculosis) and in older patients to categorize the type of inflammation (e.g., rheumatoid arthritis, pseudogout) and exclude the possibility that the patient's joint complaints are caused by gout.

Patient preparation No preparation is required, other than for obtaining synovial fluid from a joint.

Procedure For nonspecific (e.g., "arthritic") complaints, synovial fluid is usually aspirated from the knee, which has the greatest fluid volume. Other synovial joints include the shoulder, hip, and elbow. After obtaining the fluid, it is submitted to the laboratory for analysis of gross (macroscopic) and microscopic appearance, detection of crystals, bacterial culture, chemical analysis, and, rarely, performance of serologic testing, which is more commonly performed on serum.

Specimen Synovial fluid.

Reference range See table.

Abnormal values See table.

Cost $100–$200.

SYNOVIAL FLUID ANALYSIS*

TYPE	NORMAL	NONINFLAMMATORY	INFLAMMATORY		
			MILD	SEVERE	SEPTIC
Appearance	Clear yellow	Clear yellow	Slightly turbid	Turbid	Turbid to purulent
GLUCOSE‡	<10 mg/dL	<10 mg/dL	<20 mg/dL	<40 mg/dL	20mg/dL
WBCs/mL	<200/μL	<2000/μL	<5000/μL	<50 000/μL	50000/μL
(% PMNs)	<25%	<25%	<50%	50%–90%	90%
Viscosity	↑	↑	↓	↓	↓

‡Synovial fluid and blood difference.

*JB Henry, Ed, Clinical Diagnosis & Management by Laboratory Methods, 18th edition, WB Saunders, Philadelphia, 1991.

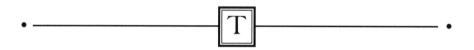

T₃ suppression test   See *thyroid suppression test* in Glossary.

T₃ uptake test (triiodothyronine uptake assay)   A test that indirectly measures free thyroxine (T₄) as a reflection of thyroid function that is based on the amount of T₃ (triiodothyronine) that can be bound to carrier proteins, in particular to thyroxine-binding globulin (TBG). In the T₃ uptake test, a known amount of radioactive T₃, which is in excess of the normal binding capacity of thyroxine-binding globulin (TBG), and a binding resin are added to the serum. The radioactive T₃ that remains after occupying the TBG's binding sites then binds to the resin, which can then be measured by radioimmunoassay. The test has fallen into disfavor as TSH, freeT₃, and freeT₄ can be measured directly by less cumbersome methods. See *reverse triiodothyronine, thyroxine, thyroxine-binding globulin, triiodothyronine*.

T₄   See *thyroxine*.

TAT (Thematic Apperception Test)   A projection-type psychological test that evaluates a child's sense of reality and personality traits and gives insight into his fantasies. In the TAT, the individual being tested is shown a standard series of pictures with human figures in an ambiguous or "neutral" context and then asked to construct a story of the events leading to the image seen in the picture, and its outcome. The stories created by the individual are then analyzed to identify the individual's needs, internal and external conflicts, and emotions. See *psychological test*.

Tc-labeled red blood cell scintigraphy   See *Technetium-labeled red blood cell scintigraphy*.

Technetium-labeled red blood cell scintigraphy   A noninvasive method used to identify the site of slow or intermittent gastrointestinal hemorrhage.
   Patient preparation No preparation is required, other than for drawing

blood. All blood work performed by radioimmunoassay should be drawn before the study. Barium studies should be performed at least two days before the study.

Procedure In this test, red blood cells that have been labeled with technitium are injected and images are obtained from the patient with a gamma camera, which detects scintillation and identifies areas of increased radioactivity.

Reference range Negative study.

Abnormal values Any focal area of increased radioactivity is suggestive of abnormal bleeding. which may correspond to extravasation of radiolabeled cells from the large or (less commonly) the small intestine.

Cost $500–$750.

Comments Synonyms include blood loss localization study, gastrointestinal bleed localization study, gastrointestinal blood loss scan, GI bleeding scintigraphy, and lower GI blood loss scan.

Tensilon® test (edrophonium test) A clinical test used in patients with known myasthenia gravis to distinguish between a myasthenic and cholinergic crisis.

Patient preparation No preparation is required. The test requires intravenous administration of Tensilon.

Procedure The short-acting cholinesterase inhibitor, Tensilon (edrophonium chloride), is administered with a syringe containing 10 mg. If there is no change in muscle strength one minute after 2 mg has been injected, then the remainder is injected. The physician may wish to have the patient exercise the muscle being examined, before injecting the Tensilon, in order to fatigue it.

Reference range Normal muscle usually undergoes fasciculation (quivering) in response to Tensilon.

Abnormal values The muscle strength in patients with myasthenia gravis usually improves dramatically after Tensilon injection. In a cholinergic crisis, the weakness will worsen and be accompanied by colicky pain and fasciculation of the eyelids.

Cost $45–$75.

test of healing A therapeutic trial of H_2-blockers, e.g., cimetidine, ranitidine, that is used in patients with a gastric ulcer, in whom a decrease in ulcer-type of pain is equated with therapeutic success. Nonresolution of symptoms after three to six weeks of H_2-blocking therapy is considered an indication for endoscopy and endoscopic biopsy because the possibility of a gastric carcinoma must be excluded. The test of healing is not commonly performed in clinical practice.

testosterone The principal and most potent androgenic (male) hormone, which is produced by the testis and also (in far smaller amounts) by the ovary and adrenal cortex. Testosterone is responsible for nitrogen retention, which results in a net buildup of protein and muscle, and the induction and maintenance of the secondary male characteristics (e.g., facial hair). Testosterone secretion is regulated by luteinizing hormone, which is produced by the anterior pituitary gland. Most of the testosterone in circulation is bound to the sex hormone-binding globulin. The remainder is "free" (i.e., unbound) and is the active form of testosterone that is measured in functional disorders.

Patient preparation No preparation is required, other than for drawing blood.

Procedure Testosterone is measured by radioimmunoassay.

Specimen Serum.

Reference range
    Men   0.3–1.0 µg/dL.
    Women   0.03–0.1 µg/dL.
Note: The units reported for the reference range depend on the reagent manufacturer and can vary from laboratory to laboratory.

Abnormal values
    Decreased in: alcoholism, anterior pituitary gland hypofunction,
      estrogen therapy, Klinefelter's syndrome, testicular hypofunction.
    Increased in: male sexual precocity, hyperplasia of the adrenal cortex
      adrenogenital syndrome, polycystic ovary syndrome.

Cost $135–$190.

testosterone-estrogen-binding globulin See *sex hormone-binding globulin*.

thallium stress test (pharmacologic stress imaging, myocardial perfusion scan) A technique used to evaluate the regional blood flow (perfusion) through the heart muscle (myocardium). By determining the distribution of blood and oxygen, the thallium stress test provides information on the heart's ability to withstand a reduction in blood flow in the form of a blood clot or stenosis. In the TST, the radionuclide thallium-201 (^{201}Tl) is injected as a diagnostic adjunct to cardiac stress tests, with the purpose of detecting regional ischemia or infarcts. The TST is an increasingly popular alternative to the exercise stress test. It is used to evaluate patients with coronary artery disease who cannot perform an exercise stress test, and it allows the physician to determine a person's risk of angina or a heart attack.

Patient preparation Alcohol and tobacco should be restricted 24 hours before the test. Food should be restricted for three hours before the test. All blood work that will be analyzed by radioimmunoassay should be drawn before the test.

Procedure A radiopharmaceutical (e.g., thallium-201-^{201}Tl or, more recently, technetium-99m-^{99m}Tc) is injected intravenously (in the arm) and images are captured with a gamma (scintillation) camera. Dipyridamole is infused intravenously, producing marked coronary arteriolar vasodilation, leaving the peripheral arterioles relatively intact. In the myocardial regions perfused by coronary arteries of normal diameter, the blood flow increases in the endocardium and epicardium, indicating normal coronary artery reserve.

Reference range Negative for anatomic abnormalities.

Abnormal values In coronary artery stenosis, there is diminished uptake and clearance of intravenously administered ^{201}Tl, resulting in an initial ^{201}Tl defect that is followed by a delayed redistribution in images viewed two to four hours after injection; the side effects induced by dipyridamole are immediately reversible with aminophylline.

Cost $600–$1200.

Comments Synonyms include stress thallium scan, thallium-201 scan, thallium stress test.

thematic apperception test See *TAT.*

theophylline A drug that relaxes smooth muscle of the bronchi and bronchioles, gastrointestinal tract, and blood vessels, resulting in an increased blood flow to the lungs and kidneys with increased diuresis. Theophylline is also a central nervous system and myocardial stimulant.

Patient preparation No preparation is required, other than for drawing blood.

Procedure Theophylline can be measured by enzyme immunoassays, high-performance liquid chromatography, and radioimmunoassay.

Specimen Serum. For best results, specimens should be drawn just before the last dose, when monitoring treatment levels.

Reference range 8–20 µg/ml.

Abnormal values Above 20 µg/ml.

Cost $65–$75. See *therapeutic index* in Glossary.

therapeutic drug monitoring (TDM) The periodic measurement of the serum levels of drugs (common drugs monitored include carbamazepine, digoxin, gentamycin, procainamide, phenobarbital, phenytoin, theophylline, tobramycin, valproic acid, vancomycin) that require close "titration" of doses in order to ensure that there are sufficient levels in the blood to be therapeutically effective, while avoiding potentially toxic excess. The concentration of a particular prescribed drug is a function of multiple factors. These factors include patient compliance (i.e., whether the patient is actually taking the drug); how tightly it is bound to proteins or other carrier molecules in the circulation; interaction with foods; degree of absorption from the gastrointestinal tract; fat-solubility; whether it is broken down as it passes through the liver, or eliminated as it passes through the kidneys; age and sex; presence of other conditons; and genetic factors, which may affect a person's ability to metabolize certain drugs, or which may be due to a lack of enzymes.

Therapeutic drug monitoring requires that:

1. The method measures what it is designed to measure, and not bioinactive metabolites, and has a turn-around time short enough to allow adjustment of doses.

2. The method has a well-defined therapeutic range, the toxic and therapeutic ranges are close enough to require monitoring, and tolerance to
the drug does not develop.

3. The concentration of the drug in the serum is proportional to the concentration at the site of action (i.e., at the receptor), and there is a correlation between the concentration in the serum and the therapeutic
effect. See *therapeutic index* in Glossary.

thiamin (vitamin B₁)   A water-soluble vitamin that is present in many foods,
including grains, yeast, and milk. It is a necessary cofactor in decarboxyla-
tion, which is linked to the metabolism of glucose, the main source of energy in animals; it is also involved in the production of so-called "high energy" phosphates.

Patient preparation No preparation is required, other than for drawing
blood or obtaining urine.

Procedure Thiamin is quantified by spectrophotometry, based on the activity of transketolase from lysed red blood cells, in which a colored substrate
is consumed or another compound converted or formed.

Specimen Serum, urine.

Reference range 0–2.0 μg/dL; 0%–15% substrate conversion is normal.

Abnormal values Less than 27 μg/g creatinine. Alternatively, greater than
25% conversion occurs in severe clinical deficiency (beri-beri), which is
uncommon in developed countries.

   Increased in: Hodgkin's disease, leukemia, polycythemia vera.

   Decreased in: deficiency states (e.g., alcoholism, dietary insufficiency,
   malnutrition), congestive heart failure, diarrhea (prolonged),
   hyperthyroidism, lactation, pregnancy, strenuous exercise.

Cost $130–$150.

thin-layer chromatography (TLC)   A technique in which a thin layer of
alumina, polyacrylamide gel, silica gel, or starch gel is bonded to a glass
or plastic plate, then bathed for 30–90 minutes in a solvent containing a
substance of interest (e.g., acetaminophen, diazepam, morphine, nicotine) which allows the substance to migrate by capillary action. If further
identification of the substance is required, the "spot" of drug may be
scraped off for further analysis by gas-liquid chromatography. TLC
is often used to "screen" for the presence of drugs of abuse. See *drug
screening*.

thoracentesis (pleural fluid "tap," pleurocentesis)   The drainage of fluid for
therapeutic or diagnostic purposes from the pleural space using a long needle. Once obtained, the fluid is analyzed for chemical composition, and the
cells are examined by a pathologist. Thoracentesis is used in determining the
nature, i.e., benign or malignant, of a collection of fluid (effusion) in the
pleural space that has been identified clinically or radiologically.

Patient preparation Informed consent is required. Baseline coagulation studies (e.g., activated partial thromboplastin time, prothrombin time, platelet count), and certain chemistries (e.g., BUN and creatinine) should be obtained before the procedure.

Procedure The procedure consists of the insertion of a 18- or 20-gauge needle through the chest wall after the injection of a local anesthetic. Fifty to 100 ml of fluid is collected in sterile tubes and is sent to the laboratory for cytologic and chemical analysis, and culture.

Specimen Pleural fluid and cells.

Reference range Normally, a few mesothelial cells may be seen in the fluid obtained from an abdominal tap.

Abnormal values Fresh blood and inflammatory or malignant cells may be seen, as indicated above.

Cost $100–$200.

Comments Complications include pneumothorax, hemothorax, laceration of intercostal arteries, puncture of liver or spleen, infection, air embolism, and subcutaneous emphysema. See *pericardiocentesis.*

throat culture The obtention of material from the posterior pharynx (throat) which is submitted to the laboratory for identification of bacteria. The throat may also be cultured for viruses, although most laboratories do not perform this specialized procedure. They send it to a reference laboratory.

Patient preparation No preparation is required. The patient should be warned about the uncomfortable gag reflex caused by aggressive swabbing of the back of the throat.

Procedure The procedure consists of the swabbing of the back of the throat with a sterile applicator.

Specimen Applicator with material for bacterial or viral culture.

Reference range Negative for growth of pathogenic organisms.

Abnormal values Growth of bacteria, e.g., group A β-hemolytic streptococci (*Streptococcus pyogenes*), the most common cause of "strep throat," *Bordetella pertussis* ("whooping cough" agent), and *Corynebacterium diphtheriae.*

Cost $50–$75. A positive culture incurs additional costs due to the requirement that the bacteria be identified and sensitivity to antibiotics determined.

thrombin time (thrombin clotting time)   A laboratory test used to evaluate the clotting of blood, specifically at the final stage of the coagulation cascade, where fibrinogen is converted to fibrin. The TT is used clinically to determine the adequacy of the dosage of thrombolytic therapy, which is optimal when maintained at 1.5 to 3 times normal.

Patient preparation No preparation is required, other than for drawing blood.

Procedure The test is performed by adding thrombin to plasma that has been anticoagulated with sodium citrate and by measuring the time it takes to form a clot.

Specimen Blood drawn in sodium citrate anticoagulant; plasma.
Reference range 10–16 seconds.
Abnormal values The thrombin time is increased in deficiency or defects of fibrinogen in the presence of fibrin degradation products or heparin-coagulation products.
Cost $35–$45.
Comments The thrombin time test is of some use in monitoring the bleeding complications of therapeutic thrombolysis, which also requires the determination of fibrinogen levels, tests for fibrin degradation products, and euglobulin lysis time.

thromboplastin generation test An elaborate laboratory test used to detect defects in the formation of thromboplastin and defects in the relevant coagulation factors. The test is used to differentiate between hemophilia A and hemophilia B, and is helpful in the diagnosis of lupus inhibitors.
Patient preparation No preparation is required, other than for drawing blood.
Procedure In the first stage of the test, prothrombinase formation is initiated by the addition of calcium to a mixture of serum, adsorbed plasma, and a source of platelet factor 3. In the second stage, the prothrombinase formed is measured by adding some of the reaction mixture to normal plasma, which should contain normal amounts of prothrombin and fibrinogen.
Specimen Blood collected in three tubes—one without anticoagulant, one with citrate or oxalate anticoagulant, and one with citrate anticoagulant for platelets. If commercial phospholipid is used, the last tube is not needed.
Reference range 8–15 seconds, substrate clotting time.
Abnormal values Decreased with heparin therapy.
Cost $50–$75.

thyrocalcitonin See *calcitonin.*

thyroid antibodies See *antimicrosomal antibodies, antithyroglobulin antibodies.*

thyroid aspiration and biopsy The obtention of cells and tissue fragments from a thyroid gland that is clinically enlarged or hyperactive. An enlarged thyroid may cause difficulties in breathing and swallowing, vocal cord paralysis, increased neck size, and bleeding. Thyroid hyperfunction causes weight loss due to increased thyroid hormone production, which increases metabolism.
Patient preparation Informed consent is required. Baseline coagulation studies (e.g., activated partial thromboplastin time, prothrombin time, platelet count) should be obtained before the procedure.
Procedure A needle is inserted in the anterior neck, and cells and tissue fragments from the thyroid are aspirated into a syringe. The material may

be scant or bloody and can be spread directly onto glass slides for microscopic examination. The syringe may be washed into a container with fixative, so that the remaining cells and tissue can be processed by pathology and further evaluated by microscopy.

Specimen Fragments of cells and tissue cores from the thyroid.

Reference range Negative for pathological changes.

Abnormal values By far, the most common lesions of the thyroid are benign and include nontoxic goiters, Hashimoto's thyroiditis, and subacute granulomatous thyroiditis. Malignant tumors of the thyroid are relatively uncommon and include papillary and follicular carcinomas.

Cost $85–$125.

thyroid panel A standard panel (or battery) of laboratory tests used to evaluate the baseline thyroid status. For Medicare or Medicaid reimbursement, the thyroid panel includes total thyroxine (T_4), total T_3 resin uptake, and TSH. With the advent of more sensitive TSH tests and the availability of free T_3 and free T_4, many physicians are using ultrasensitive TSH tests as the screening tests of choice. See *thyroid-stimulating hormone, thyroxine.*

thyroid-stimulating hormone (thyrotropin, TSH) A glycopeptide hormone produced by the pituitary gland in response to thyroid-releasing hormone, which is released by the hypothalamus. TSH controls thyroid growth, development, and secretion. Its production is regulated by thyroid-releasing hormone. A low serum level in older (over age 60) people is associated with certain manifestations of subclinical hyperthyroidism, e.g., atrial fibrillation.

Patient preparation No preparation is required, other than for drawing blood.

Procedure TSH is measured by enzyme assay; radioimmunoassay has been phased out.

Specimen Serum, heparized plasma.

Reference range

Adults	2–10 µIU/ml.
Infants	Less then 25 µIU/ml.

Abnormal values

Increased in: primary hypothyroidism, chronic (Hashimoto's) thyroiditis, antithyroid therapy for hyperthyroidism, therapy with lithium, potassium iodide.

Decreased in: secondary hypothyroidism, hyperthyroidism (Graves' disease), hypofunction of adenohypophysis (anterior pituitary gland), drugs (e.g., aspirin, corticosteroids, L-dopa, heparin).

Cost $90–$100.

thyroid-stimulating hormone receptor antibodies (TRAb, TSH receptor antibodies) Antibodies that are pathogenically linked to Graves' disease, which may be quantified by **1.)** Bioassays that measure the ability of a patient's immunoglobulins to stimulate thyroid activity, which are less sensitive than **2.**) Radioreceptor assays that measure inhibition of binding of labelled TSH to its receptor. Both assays confirm the diagnosis of euthyroid Graves' disease with ophthalmopathy and hyperthyroid Graves' disease. See *antithyroglobulin antibodies, antithyroid antibodies.*

thyrotropin-releasing hormone stimulation test (TRH stimulation test)   A clinical test used to determine the point in the endocrine system, which is regulated by long and short feedback loops, that is responsible for decreased secretion of TSH (thyroid-stimulating hormone, thyrotropin) by the pituitary gland.

Patient preparation No preparation is required, other than for drawing blood.

Procedure TRH is administered and blood is drawn at periodic intervals, usually at 30 and 60 minutes.

Specimen Serum drawn before the test, and at 30- and 60-minute intervals.

Reference range

	Baseline	5–60 pg/ml.
Less than age 40	30 minutes	Greater than 6 μU/ml.
Over age 40	30 minutes	Greater than 2 μU/ml.

Abnormal values If the hypothyroidism is due to a defect in the hypothalamus, TSH levels in the blood will increase; if the defect is at the level of the hypophysis, the TSH levels do not increase.

Cost $90–$110.

thyroxine (T$_4$, 3,5,3',5'-tetraiodothyronine)   A hormone that stimulates metabolism and oxygen consumption, which is secreted by the thyroid gland in response to TSH (thyrotropin) produced in the anterior pituitary gland. TSH in turn is produced in response to TRH (thyrotropin-releasing hormone), which is produced and secreted by the hypothalamus, which is located in the base of the brain.

Patient preparation No preparation is required, other than for drawing blood.

Procedure Thyroxine is measured by enzyme immunoassay.

Specimen Serum.

Reference range

	TOTAL THYROXINE	FREE THYROXINE
Adults	5–10 μg/dL	0.7–2.4 ng/dL
Infants	12–24 μg/dL	

Abnormal values

Increased in: acute thyroiditis, drugs (e.g., clofibrate, oral contraceptives, estrogens, perphenazine), hyperthyroidism, myasthenia gravis, preeclampsia, pregnancy, viral hepatitis.

Decreased in: drugs (e.g., corticosteroids, chlorpromazine, heparin, lithium, phenytoin, propranolol, reserpine, salicylates, sulfonamides, testosterone, tolbutamide), hypofunction of anterior pituitary gland, hypothyroidism, malnutrition, renal failure, vigorous exercise.

Cost
 Thyroxine $30–$50.
 Free thyroxine $100–$120. See *reverse triiodothyronine,*
thyroxine-binding globulin, triiodothyronine.

thyroxine-binding globulin (TBG)   A protein that is the main carrrier protein for thyroxine (T_4) and triiodothryonine (T_3). TBG measurements are based on the assumption that there is no underlying abnormality in the protein itself. TBG is measured to determine the ability to bind thyroxine in patients with hyperthyroidism, and to detect patients with hereditary TBG deficiency.
 Patient preparation No preparation is required, other than for drawing blood.
 Procedure Thyroxine-binding globulin is measured directly by radioimmunoassay or indirectly by either electrophoresis or ion exchange, which provides information on the functional ability of thyroxine-binding globulin to transport (or bind) T_3 and/or T_4.
 Specimen Serum.
 Reference range
  Adults   21–52 µg/dL.
  Infants
   0–1 week   21–90 µg/dL.
   1–12 months   21–76 µg/dL.
 Abnormal values TBG's thyroid hormone-binding capacity is
  Increased in: acute intermittent porphyria, drugs (e.g., estrogens, methadone, oral contraceptives, perphenazine, phenothiazines), hereditary defects, hepatic disease, hypothyroidism, neonates, pregnancy.
  Decreased in: acromegaly, drugs (e.g., androgens, cortiosteroids, corticotropin, phenytoin, prednisone), hereditary defects, hepatic disease, nephrotic syndrome, ovarian hypofunction, protein-losing enteropathy, underlying disease, following surgery, thyrotoxicosis.
 Cost $90–$110.

tick identification   The formal exercise of identifying a tick, a hematophagous arthropod. Ticks are classified as either hard ticks (family Ixodidae) or soft ticks (family Argasidae). Ticks are common carriers of bacterial and viral infections. The tick that causes most human diseases is *Ixodes dammini*, the Northern deer tick, which is the vector of the Lyme disease agent, *Borrelia burgdorferi. Dermacentor andersoni* is the North American vector for Rocky Mountain spotted fever, Colorado tick fever, tularemia, and tick paralysis. Size is a critical factor in identifying ticks. The Lyme disease tick is about the size of a pencil point, which contrasts to the dog tick, which is nearly the size of a lentil. See *Lyme disease.*

tine test   See *tuberculin test.*

tissue pathology (surgical pathology)   A general term for the evaluation of tissues obtained by biopsy or other surgical procedure.

Patient preparation The preparation required depends on the site from which the tissue is obtained. For small biopsies from the skin, no preparation is required. For tissues taken from relatively inaccessible sites, e.g., the lungs, liver, and elsewhere, the preparation may be that of a surgical procedure, for which baseline coagulation studies and assessment of renal function are necessary.

Procedure The procedure is also a function of the site of the biopsy. For superficial skin biopsies, the tissue may be "shaved," punched, or excised, requiring a Band-Aid™ or one or two sutures. For inaccessible sites, e.g., the kidney, the biopsy needle may be guided by fluoroscopy, and the patient may need observation after the procedure, should bleeding or other complication occur.

After the tissue is removed from a patient, it is placed in a fixative (usually formalin), transported to a pathology laboratory, placed in paraffin, sliced into very thin sections, stained with various dyes, and then examined by light microscopy. A wide range of further tests can be performed on the tissue, ranging from the relatively primitive (various stains) to those cutting-edge techniques of immunohistologic stains and techniques of DNA ploidy analysis, in situ hybridization, and the PCR (polymerase chain reaction).

Specimen A piece of tissue.

Reference range No significant pathological changes.

Abnormal values Tissues may demonstrate a wide range of change, including inflammation, infection, vascular lesions, and benign and malignant tumors. In the case of malignancy, critical questions asked of the pathologist are whether the margins are free of tumor involvement and, for larger specimens, whether lymph nodes are involved by tumor, both of which impact on the tumor's prognosis.

Cost The fee charged is in part a function of the complexity of the tissue, the need for special stains, the difficulty in establishing the diagnosis, and whether a second opinion is being sought by the pathologist. The cost ranges from $50 to $300.

tobramycin A broad-spectrum antibiotic that is effective against many gram-negative bacteria. It is of particular use in *Pseudomonas* infections of the lungs, urinary tract, and surgical wounds, which have failed to respond to penicillins or cephalosporins. Because of its narrow therapeutic index and adverse effects on hearing and balance, tobramycin should not be administered to patients with renal failure (as it is excreted by the kidneys) and should not be used in combination with other neurotoxic or nephrotoxic antibiotics, e.g., amikacin, cephaloridine, colistin, gentamicin, kanamycin, neomycin, polymyxin B, streptomycin, or vancomycin. See *therapeutic drug monitoring, therapeutic index* in Glossary.

Patient preparation No preparation is required, other than for drawing blood.

Procedure Tobramycin can be measured by any of a number of methods, including enzyme immunoassay, radioimmunoassay, and gas-liquid chromatography.

Specimen Serum. Two specimens should be submitted—one taken 30 minutes after intravenous administration of tobramycin, commonly known as the "peak," and the second, taken just before the next dose, the "trough."

Reference range

| Peak | 4–10 µg/dL. |
| Trough | Less than 2 µg/dL. |

Abnormal values

| Peak | Greater than 12 µg/dL. |
| Trough | Greater than 2 µg/dL. |

Cost $130–$160 for two specimens.

tocainide An antiarrhythmic agent that is used to reduce the incidence of premature ventricular complexes.

Patient preparation No preparation is required, other than for drawing blood.

Procedure Tocainide is measured by gas-liquid chromatography or by high-performance liquid chromatography.

Specimen Serum.

Reference range 4–10 µg/ml.

Abnormal values Greater than 12 µg/ml.

Cost $100–$120.

Comments Side effects include nausea, vomiting, anorexia, tremor, rashes, memory loss, vertigo, anxiety, tinnitus, pulmonary fibrosis, and bone marrow depression with agranulocytosis, which may occur in up to 18% of patients, seriously limiting its usefulness.

tolbutamide An oral hypoglycemic agent used to treat mild adult-onset diabetes mellitus.

Patient preparation No preparation is required, other than for drawing blood.

Procedure Tolbutamide can be measured by gas-liquid chromatography and colorimetric methods.

Specimen Serum.

Reference range 80–240 µg/dL.

Abnormal values Greater than 640 µg/dL.

Cost $50–$75.

tone decay test A type of hearing test that evaluates defects in adaptation to sounds, formally known as auditory fatigue (tone decay), which indicates a defect in retrocochlear transmission of nerve impulses from the ear that may be caused by pressure or damage to the eighth cranial nerve. In the tone decay test, an auditory threshold near 4000 Hz is established in the person being tested. The intensity of the sound is increased by 5 dB increments, and the individual signals when the perception of the sound disappears. The test is stopped when the perception of the sound does not disappear after one minute. The amount of tone decay is determined by adding the number of 5 dB increments, which is 10–15 dB or more in a person with an eighth nerve defect. See *pure tone audiometry, Rinne test, Schwabach test, SISI test.*

tonography   A technique that indirectly measures, based on the softening of the eyeball as fluid decreases, the outflow of fluid from the eye in response to external pressure placed on the eye, which is related to intraocular pressure. Tonography is used to evaluate open angle versus angle closure glaucoma. See *tonometry.*
   Patient preparation Nothing should be taken by mouth for eight hours before testing, including liquids.
   Procedure The procedure consists of the measurement of the flow of aqueous fluid from the eye in relation to the intraocular pressure, which may incorporate a water provocation test. A water provocation test consists of the drinking of a predetermined amount of water to evaluate the rate of flow.
   Reference range The coefficient of outflow is greater than 0.18 in most normal individuals.
   Abnormal values The outflow of fluid from the aqueous humor is markedly reduced in angle closure glaucoma and is also decreased in inflammation and myasthenia gravis.
   Cost $25–$50.

tonometry   A technique that measures intraocular pressure (in mm Hg) by contact (indentation of or applanation on) or noncontact (by a puff of air) on the eyeball. Tonometry is used to diagnose and manage glaucoma and ocular hypertension, and in routine ocular examination. See *tonography.*
   Patient preparation No preparation is required, other than removal of contact lenses.
   Procedure After administration of a local anesthetic, a tonometer is placed directly on the cornea with an initial weight of 5.5 g. A rhythmic pulse should be detected that exceeds 4 on the calibrated scale. The weight is increased up to 15 grams or until the reading exceeds 4.
   Reference range Normal intraocular pressure ranges from 15 to 20 mm Hg.
   Abnormal values The finding of increased intraocular pressure is suggestive of glaucoma, which must be confirmed by further testing in the form of visual field testing and ophthalmoscopy.
   Cost $25–$50.

TORCH antibody panel   A standard battery of laboratory tests used to evaluate the possible presence of prenatal infection in a newborn. The TORCH agents—toxoplasma, rubella, CMV, and herpes simplex—can cause in utero infections resulting in major malformation and prominent neurologic defects, e.g., seizures, hydrocephalus or microcephaly, and others. Many obstetricians order a TORCH antibody panel, or permutation thereof, to ensure that the woman or newborn infant has not been infected with one of the TORCH agents during pregnancy.

The TORCH antibody panel measures antibody titers for immunoglobulins IgG and IgM. The finding of increased IgM in the newborn infant implies an in utero infection by one of these agents, which should be further characterized by measuring the IgM levels for specific organisms.

TORCH AGENTS

TOXOPLASMOSIS may cause obstruction of cerebral foramina resulting in hydrocephalus. With prolonged survival, the infant suffers intracranial calcification; necrosis of the liver, adrenal glands, lungs, and heart; and extramedullary hematopoiesis.

RUBELLA often causes low birth weight, hepatosplenomegaly, petechiae, purpura, congenital heart disease, cataracts, micro-ophthalmia, and microcephaly. The central nervous system symptoms caused by rubella include lethargy, irritability, hydrocephaly, and seizures.

CYTOMEGALOVIRUS may cause hepatosplenomegaly, hyperbilirubinemia, neonatal thrombocytopenia, microcephaly, and a mortality of 20%–30%. After birth, other manifestations may become evident, including mental retardation, deafness, psychomotor delays, defective teeth, chorioretinitis, and learning disabilities. CMV infection is very common—an estimated 30,000 cases of congenital cytomegalovirus cases are believed to occur each year in the U.S., of which only 10% are symptomatic.

HERPES SIMPLEX may cause prematurity, and becomes symptomatic after the first week of life. Central nervous system symptoms include irritability, seizures, chorioretinitis, hydrocephalus, flaccid or spastic paralysis, decerebrate rigidity, and coma. In neonatal HSV infection, no deaths occur in those with localized disease; 15% die if encephalitis is present and 57% die if HSV is disseminated, which may evoke disseminated intravascular coagulation.

SYPHILIS is regarded by some neonatologists as an "optional TORCH" agent. Congenital syphilis has increased to epidemic rates in certain urban areas of the U.S. since the mid-1980s. The clinical findings are nonspecific and include fever, lethargy, failure to thrive, and irritability.

Patient Preparation No special preparation, other than that for drawing blood.

Specimen Serum.

Procedure All of the above tests use immunoassay techniques to detect the presence of specific antibodies.

Cost $150–$175.

Comments The quantitative TORCH screen has a high rate of false-positive and false-negative results. See *toxoplasmosis, rubella, cytomegalovirus,* and *herpesvirus* for a complete discussion of reference ranges and abnormal values.

total catecholamine test This is a test used to identify the presence of catecholamine-producing tumors, e.g., pheochromocytoma and neuroblastoma. Catecholamines are excreted in the urine in both free (unconjugated) and bound (conjugated to glucuronide and sulfate) forms. The total cate-cholamine test measures both. In the clinical laboratory, measurement of urinary free catecholamines is preferred to measurement of total cate-cholamines.

Patient preparation No preparation is required, other than for obtaining urine.

Procedure Total catecholamines are measured by removing the glucuronide and sulfate groups from the conjugated catecholamines before the analysis and measuring by ultraviolet spectrophotometry.

Specimen 24-hour urine.

Reference range

Infants   10–50 µg/m²/day.

Adults   Less than 280 µg/day.

Abnormal values

Increased in: pheochromocytoma, neuroblastoma, paraganglioma multiple endocrine adenomatosis syndrome.

Cost $150–$170.

Comments The total catecholamine test has a wide range of "normalcy," which may obscure the presence of a tumor that produces low amounts of catecholamines. It also measures catecholamines in the diet. Total cate-cholamines are prone to false positivity due to interference from therapy with epinephrine, antihypertensive agents, quinidine, tetracycline, and other drugs, or from vigorous exercise, burns, or progressive muscular dys-trophy, which can cause nontumor-related increases of catecholamines. See *catecholamines, vanillylmandelic acid.*

total hemoglobin   See *hemoglobin.*

total iron-binding capacity   See *transferrin.*

toxoplasmosis   An infection by *Toxoplasma gondii* which is seen in two dis-tinct clinical situations. The first, congenital toxoplasmosis, affects newborn infants, is acquired transplacentally, and is often accompanied by major neu-rological defects. The second, acquired toxoplasmosis, is commonly linked to ingestion of undercooked meats with cysts or to exposure to infected feline feces. In the normal host, the infection is benign with transient swelling of lymph nodes. In an immunocompromised host (for example, a person who has AIDS), toxoplasmosis may be accompanied by myocarditis, pneumonitis, and, in more than 50% of cases, central nervous system involvement, often in the form of necrotizing encephalitis, a condition that may cause considerable destruction of brain tissue.

Patient preparation No preparation is required, other than for drawing blood at two intervals—at the time of acute infection and 2 to 3 weeks later.

Procedure Toxoplasmosis is detected by indirect fluorescent antibody test-ing. An increase in IgM anti-*Toxoplasma gondii* antibodies indicates an acute (current) infection; increased IgG antibodies indicate past infection.

Specimen Serum.
Reference range
  IgG-negative   Indicates no prior exposure.
  IgM-negative   Indicates no active infection.
Abnormal values Indirect fluorescent antibody titers of 1:16 are considered positive for previous exposure of *Toxoplasma*. Titers from 1:32 to 1:256 are typical of chronic infection, and titers of 1:1024 are typical of an acute infection.
Cost
  IgG $60–$80.
  IgM $80–$100.
Comments Most laboratories automatically test for IgM if the IgG antibody is positive.

TPHA test See *Treponema pallidum hemagglutination test.*

TPI test See *Treponema pallidum immobilization test* in Glossary.

TRAb See *thyroid-stimulating hormone.*

transbronchial lung biopsy A biopsy taken from the lung by forceps guided through a fiberoptic endoscope. The tissue obtained is used to diagnose both benign (e.g., interstitial fibrosis, sarcoidosis) and malignant (e.g., cancer, lymphoma) lung disease. The diagnostic yield from a transbronchial biopsy ranges from 60%–80%, depending on the size of the lesion and whether it is visible and accessible to the bronchoscope.
Patient preparation Informed consent is required. Baseline coagulation studies (e.g., activated partial thromboplastin time, prothrombin time, platelet count), certain chemistries (e.g., BUN and creatinine), and a chest X ray should be obtained before the procedure. Fluids should be restricted for eight hours before the biopsy. A transbronchial biopsy is recommended after performing computed tomography and bronchoscopy.
Procedure The procedure consists of the insertion of a forceps through the channel of a fiberoptic endoscope. If a lesion is identified, multiple tissue fragments are obtained, which are placed in formalin, processed like any other tissue in pathology, and interpreted by a pathologist.
Specimen Tissue fragments from the lung.
Reference range Negative for significant pathological changes.
Abnormal values Benign lesions identified by transbronchial biopsy include interstitial fibrosis and sarcoidosis. Malignant lung lesions include cancer arising in the lung or other sites, e.g., breast, stomach, and lymphoma.
Cost $300–$400.
Comments Complications include bleeding (1%–2%) and pneumothorax (up to 5%), neither of which are often important clinically.

transbronchial needle aspiration biopsy An endoscopic technique used to obtain a specimen from a lesion underlying the bronchial mucosa or an otherwise inaccessible lung mass, which may be compressing the bronchi from outside. This method is used to diagnose carcinomas, bronchogenic cysts, lymphoma, sarcoid, pneumonia, and abscesses.

Patient preparation Informed consent is required. Baseline coagulation studies (e.g., activated partial thromboplastin time, prothrombin time, platelet count), certain chemistries (e.g., BUN and creatinine), and a chest X ray should be obtained before the procedure.

Procedure A fine (22-gauge) needle is passed through the chest wall or bronchial wall into a mass identified by fluoroscopy, computed tomography, or bronchoscopy. The aspirated material is then evaluted by a pathologist under a microscope.

Specimen Cells and tissue fragments from the lung.

Reference range Negative for significant pathological changes.

Abnormal values Benign lesions identified by transbronchial biopsy include interstitial fibrosis and sarcoidosis. Malignant lesions include cancer arising in the lung or other sites, e.g., breast, stomach, and lymphoma.

Cost $175–$200.

Comments Complications include pneumothorax, hemomediastinum, hemorrhage, bacteremia, and rarely, false-positive diagnosis of malignancy. The diagnostic "yield" of fine needle aspiration biopsies has been reported to be 56%, which contrasts with 35% for sputum and 70% for forceps biopsies. See *bronchial washings, transbronchial lung biopsy, "skinny needle" biopsy.*

transcranial Doppler ultrasonography   A noninvasive technique used to produce images of the intracranial circulation at bedside in critically ill hospitalized patients or outpatients. The procedure is used to diagnose vasospasm, assess collateral circulation and stenoses, confirm brain death, and monitor the vascular circulation in neurosurgical patients.

Patient preparation No specific patient preparation is required.

Procedure A gel is placed on the head at the site being imaged, and the ultrasonographic device's transducer (a type of imaging "wand") is swept across the region of the skull that is of interest.

Reference range Negative for abnormalities.

Abnormal values The images seen in the intracranial vasculature are abnormal in the presence of stenosis, occlusion, spasms, and vascular shunting.

Cost $200–$300.

transesophageal echocardiography   (two-dimensional transesophageal color-flow Doppler echocardiography)   An ultrasonographic imaging technique used to evaluate cardiac structures (valves, chambers, and inflow and outflow tracts) and function, in which a transducer—the portion of the instrument used to acquire the image—is placed immediately behind the heart in the esophagus and stomach. Because there are no interfering air spaces or bone, the image is superior to that obtained by transthoracic echocardiography (TEE) and is of particular use in evaluating the status of the endocardium, e.g., to identify cardiac valve lesions.

TEE is a noninvasive imaging technique for analyzing abnormalities of regional fluid distribution or blood flow patterns, and is as sensitive (97.7%) as MRI (98.3%), but less specific (77%) than CT (87%) or MRI (98%) for identifying thoracic aortic aneurysms. Although aortography is the current "gold standard" in the diagnosis of traumatic rupture of the thoracic aorta, it may be displaced by transesophageal echocardiography as the modality of first choice.

Patient preparation Six to eight hours of fasting is recommended before the procedure because of the risk of aspiration. The procedure should be fully described to the patient; the transducer is passed into the esophagus, which is uncomfortable.

Procedure The procedure consists of the insertion of a modified gastroscope with an echo transducer into the esophagus to capture the images in various echo (ultrasound) formats, e.g., two-dimensional echocardiography, pulsed Doppler, and color flow images.

Reference range Negative for significant alterations in the heart physiology.

Abnormal values TEE is used to evaluate prosthetic valve (especially the mitral valve) dysfunction, left atrial thrombosis and masses, bacterial endocarditis, and intracardiac shunts.

Cost $175–$200. See *echocardiography, two-dimensional echocardiography.*

transferrin (siderophilin)   A beta globulin (protein) that is the major carrier of iron (it binds two atoms of iron) in the circulation. Transferrin levels correspond to the maximum amount of iron that can be bound to the protein, a value that is designated "total iron-binding capacity" (TIBC). Transferrin levels may be requested in the presence of suspected iron-deficiency anemia, or in those with chronic liver disease, renal failure, malnutrition, lead poisoning, and other conditions.

Patient preparation No preparation is required, other than for drawing blood.

Procedure TIBC was formerly measured by filling all of the sites that transferrin has available for binding iron, which is more cumbersome than the current method which measures transferrin directly by enzyme immunoassay. Other methods for measuring transferrin include radial immunodiffusion, electroimmunodiffusion, and nephelometry.

Specimen Serum.

Reference range Two values are given—the amount of iron in the blood, most of which is bound to transferrin, normally 65–170 mg/dL, and the theoretical amount of iron that could be bound to the transferrin, which is 220–400 mg/dL. Under normal conditions, the transferrin in the circulation is 20%–50% saturated with ironis bound to iron.

Abnormal values

Increased in: estrogens, oral contraceptives, pregnancy, severe iron deficiency anemia.

Decreased in: burns, severe, cancer, chronic infection, corticosteroids,

protein loss by kidneys, protein-losing enteropathy, decreased protein production due to liver damage, inflammation, acute and chronic, iron overload, liver disease (e.g., alcoholic cirrhosis, biliary cirrhosis, subacute hepatitis, congenital liver disease), malignancy, starvation, testosterone.
Cost $50–$75.

treadmill exercise test (exercise electrocardiography) A test that is the most commonly used clinical maneuver for assessing a person's risk of death from cardiovascular disease. It is designed to test the heart's ability to respond to an increased demand for oxygen, by increasing its rate without causing pain, discomfort, or fatigue.

Patient preparation No preparation is required. A baseline electrocardiogram is normally performed. The patient should be well-rested before the test.

Procedure In the treadmill exercise test the patient walks on a treadmill with leads attached to an electrocardiograph, and a line for monitoring blood pressure. The results are scored based on the duration of the exercise, the changes seen in the electrocardiogram (termed ST-segment deviations) and the severity of the pain experienced during the test. For specific details on scoring the test, see the formula below.

TREADMILL EXERCISE TEST (FORMULA FOR CALCULATION)
Duration of exercise in minutes
  – 5 times the maximal ST-segment deviation (on the EKG in millimeters during or after exercise)
  – 4 times the treadmill angina index, defined as no angina during exercise = 0, nonlimiting angina = 1, exercise-limiting angina = 2

Reference range Based on the above formula, a score of 15 is normal for a person at no known increased risk of death from cardiovascular disease.

Abnormal values A score of minus 25 is given to those who are at highest risk of death from cardiovascular disease and whose ST-segment depression is greater than 1 mm, and who must stop the test before the allotted time.
Cost $250–$400. See *thallium stress test*.

Treponema pallidum darkfield examination A test for the early diagnosis of syphilis, in which the *Treponema pallidum* spirochetes are demonstrated by "darkfield" microscopy.

Patient preparation No preparation is required, other than that needed to obtain scapings from the earliest lesion of syphilis, known as a chancre.

Procedure After cleaning the chancre, the scrapings are placed on a glass slide, which is transported immediately to the laboratory and viewed under a darkfield microscope.

Specimen Serum.

Reference range Negative.

Abnormal values Spirochetes with the morphology *Treponema pallidum*.
Cost $50–$75.

Comments Darkfield examination of lesions of the oral cavity are of limited value, given that the mouth contains other (nonpathogenic) spirochetes.

Treponema pallidum hemagglutination test (TPHA test)   A specific serologic test for the diagnosis of syphilis, which is caused by the spirochete *Treponema pallidum*, a bacterium.
Patient preparation No preparation is required, other than for drawing blood.
Procedure In the TPHA test, the patient's serum is incubated (i.e., placed in solution) with tanned (tannin-treated) red blood cells from sheep, which have been coated with *Treponema pallidum* antigens.
Specimen Serum.
Reference range Negative.
Abnormal values If syphilis is present, the tanned red blood cells will clump together.
Cost $60–$80.
Comment Darkfield examination for spirochetes is regarded as the definitive test for syphilis, when spirochetes are found in the appropriate clinical setting. However, spirochetes may be absent as manifestations of later stages of syphilis develop. In syphilis that has advanced beyond the primary (chancre) stage of disease, the serologic tests—e.g., the *Treponema pallidum* hemagglutination test and the VDRL—are of greatest diagnostic importance.

trichophytin test   A skin sensitivity test for the presence of allergy to extract of dermatophytes (*Trichophyton*) that is used to measure cell-mediated immunity, which is compromised or lost in acquired immunodeficiency states such as AIDS. See *patch test*.

triglyceride test (triacylglycerol)   A laboratory test that measures the serum levels of triglyceride, a fatty acid that constitutes 95% of adipose tissue by weight, which is the major form of lipid stored in the body. Triglycerides are believed to be associated with an increased risk of cardiovascular disease. Increased triglyceride levels warrant further laboratory investigation in those with a family history of premature cardiovascular disease, high cholesterol levels, hypertension, cigarette smoking, obesity, and secondary causes of increased triglyceride levels.
Patient preparation The patient should fast for 12 hours before the blood is collected.
Procedure Triglycerides are measured by enzymatic methods in autoanalyzers.
Specimen Serum or plasma collected from a fasting patient in an EDTA anticoagulated tube.
Reference range 50–250 mg/dL.
Abnormal values
   Increased in: acute myocardial infarction, alcoholic cirrhosis, diabetes mellitus (untreated), high carbohydrate diet, hyperlipoproteinemia (some forms), hypertension, hypothyroidism,

nephrotic syndrome, pregnancy, therapy (e.g., oral contraceptives, estrogens).

Decreased in: congenital β-lipoproteinemia, hyperthyroidism, malnutrition, vigorous exercise, therapy (e.g., ascorbic acid, clofibrate, metformin, phenformin).

Cost $25–$35. Because triglycerides are measured as part of a chemistry or lipid profile, they are not billed separately.

Comments Serum triglyceride levels do not appear to play an independent role in predicting coronary artery disease mortality.

triiodothyronine (T_3 3,5,3',-triiodothyronine) A hormone derived from the parent compound thyroxine (T_4), which occurs in the liver and kidney. Although the T_3 and T_4 serum levels rise and fall together, there are exceptions, in particular T_3 thyrotoxicosis, in which T_4 and free T_4 values are in the normal range. Unlike T_4, most T_3 is not bound to a carrier molecule in the circulation. Patients with T_3 thyrotoxicosis are clinically "heterogeneous" and lack distinctive signs and symptoms, They represent about 4% of those with hyperthyroidism caused by Graves' disease, toxic nodular goiter, thyroid adenoma, and hyperthyroidism seen in geographic regions with low iodine levels.

Specimen Serum.

Reference range
　　Free T_3　　Usually 3% of circulating T_3 is in the free form.
　　Total T_3　　60–160 ng/dL.

Abnormal values
　　Increased in: drugs (e.g., clofibrate, oral contraceptives [progestins], estrogens, methadone, perphenazine), hyperthyroidism (T_3 thyrotoxicosis), pregnancy.
　　Decreased in: drugs (e.g., corticosteroids, ethionamide, heparin, iodides, lithium, methimazole, phenylbutazone, phenytoin, propranolol, propylthiouracil, reserpine, salicylates, sulfonamides, testosterone, tolbutamide), euthyroid sick syndrome, hypothyroidism, increased free fatty acids, malnutrition.

Cost
　　Free T_3　　$170–$190.
　　Total T_3　　$80–$90. See *thyroxine, thyroxine-binding globulin.*

triiodothyronine (resin uptake) test See *T_3 uptake test.*

triple marker screen A term for the measurement of three specific substances—alphafetoprotein, human chorionic gonadotropin (HCG), and unconjugated estriol—that are increased in Down's syndrome. The screen has been reported to increase the rate of detection of Down's syndrome and to decrease the false-positive rate (which may cause the parents to opt for abortion) from 6.6% to 3.8%. The triple screen is not a definitive battery of tests and must be followed with ultrasound, and possibly amniocentesis with chromosome studies.

Patient preparation No preparation is required, other than for drawing blood.
Procedure The markers are measured as indicated elsewhere in this book.
Specimen Serum.
Reference range There is no reference value for this group of tests. The results are given by statistical analysis of the age of the mother, number of pregnancies, and the combined results of the three tests. The result is presented in terms of probability of the presence of defects in the fetus. If the probability is high, follow-up testing using sonography and amniocentesis is recommended.
Abnormal values See reference range.
Cost $175–$225.
Comments Because up to one thousand women must be screened to detect a single case of Down's syndrome, the cost to the health care system per case of Down's syndrome detected is $150,000–$200,000, which some view as an acceptable price to pay for preventing this condition. See *alphafetoprotein, human chorionic gonadotropin, unconjugated estriol.*

triple test A colloquial term for the use of three diagnostic modalities (e.g., clinical, radiographic, and cytopathologic data) to arrive at a diagnosis. A positive triple test is critical in those areas where each method being used is significantly less than 100% specific. As an example, in breast cancer, each component of the triple test may be suggestive of malignancy, but is not, on its own, enough to make a definitive diagnosis of malignancy.

tryptophan loading test An indirect test that detects the relative deficiency of vitamin B_6. The test is ordered in a person who is suspected of vitamin B_6 deficiency, which occurs in chronic alcoholism, malnutrition, normal pregnancy, renal failure, neonatal seizures, and industrial exposure to hydrazine compounds.
Patient preparation No preparation is required, other than for obtaining urine.
Procedure A 2–5 gram load of tryptophan is administered orally at breakfast, after which the patient collects his/her urine for 24 hours. Tryptophan's main metabolite, xanthurenic acid, is measured in the urine.
Specimen 24-hour urine.
Reference range Less than 25–50 mg of xanthurenic acid.
Abnormal values In vitamin B_6 deficiency, xanthurenic acid is markedly increased, to 100 or more mg/day.
Cost $125–$150.

TSH See *thyroid-stimulating hormone.*

TSH stimulation test (thyroid-stimulating hormone stimulation test) A test formerly used to determine whether hypothyroidism was due to intrinsic defects of the thyroid gland or to a lack of thyroid-stimulating hormone. This use of the TSH stimulation test has been replaced by the direct measurement of TSH levels in serum and measurement of TSH response to thyroid-releasing hormone. The TSH stimulation test is still used in the following rare situations: to determine if the thyroid is capable of functioning in a patient taking full replacement doses of thyroid hormone and detect thyroprivic hypothyroidism without withdrawing hormone therapy; to determine if nonfunctioning regions of the thyroid are capable of functioning; to determine if the absence of radioactive thyroid hormone accumulation is due to partial agenesis of the thyroid; or to determine if the remaining thyroid tissue is capable of resuming function after the removal of a hyperactive tumor nodule. See *reverse triiodothyronine, thyroxine, thyroxine-binding globulin, triiodothyronine.*

tuberculin test A general term for any superficial skin (intracutaneous) test used to diagnose tuberculosis. The test is based on hypersensitivity to tuberculin, a concentrated preparation of tuberculosis antigen, the standard preparation of which is PPD (purified protein derivative). In the most commonly performed test, the Mantoux test, a short needle is used to inject PPD, which is interpreted at 48–72 hours. An induration of the area at the site of injection of less then 10 millimeters (less than 5 millimeters if they have AIDS, active tuberculosis, or have had contact with those with tuberculosis) is read as negative, and of more than 15 millimeters as positive. True-negatives mean that the individual does not have tuberculosis. False-negative results may occur in patients with sarcoidosis, intercurrent viral infection, corticosteroid therapy, and defects in the reticuloendothelial system. The tine tuberculin skin test, which injects the test material more superficially than the Mantoux test, has been largely relegated to a secondary role in the diagnosis of tuberculosis and is now rarely performed. See *Mantoux test.*

tuberculosis test Any of a number of tests used to detect exposure to, or current infection, by the bacterium, *Mycobacterium tuberculosis,* that causes tuberculosis. In practice, tuberculosis tests are of the following two types:
1. Those that identify current infection, either by a direct smear of sputum, or by culturing a specimen (e.g., sputum, lymph node, or lung biopsy). The causative organism, *M. tuberculosis,* is notoriously slow to grow, and requires up to three weeks for definitive identification when cultured in the traditional fashion. More recently, molecular techniques have been used to shorten the turnaround time for test results. See *acid-fast stain.*
2. Those that evaluate the immune response. See *Mantoux test, tuberculin test.*

tuberculosis skin testing See *Mantoux test, tuberculin test.*

tularemia testing Tularemia is an infectious disease of small animals (e.g., rabbits and rats) caused by *Francisella tularensis,* an aerobic bacterium, which can be transmitted to man by bites or via arthropod vectors (e.g., ticks). Tularemia should be suspected in anyone with an unusual pattern of fever who has had contact with wild animals and livestock, has ingested unpurified water, or has been exposed to microbiology cultures or laboratory animals.

Patient preparation No preparation is required, other than for drawing blood.

Procedure The diagnosis can be established "directly" by fluorescent examination of cultured specimen, or serologically by agglutination.

Specimen Serum.

Reference range Negative.

Abnormal values Agglutination titers as low as 1:40 are regarded as positive.

Cost $70–$80.

turbidity test   See *solubility test.*

two-dimensional echocardiography (cross-sectional echocardiography)   A procedure that is the most common ultrasound-based diagnostic method in cardiology, which provides high-resolution, real-time (i.e., obtained as they occur) images of the heart and great blood vessels.

Patient preparation No preparation is required.

Procedure Ultrasonographic images are obtained using a specific echocardiography device while monitoring the electrocardiogram.

Reference range Negative for significant alterations in the heart physiology.

Abnormal values Because of the clarity of the images, two-dimensional echocardiography is the noninvasive method of choice for the diagnosis and management of congenital, pericardial, myocardial, and cardiac valve disease and is used to evaluate heart volumes, ventricular wall thickness, and depressed cardiac function.

Cost $175–$275. See *echocardiography, transesophageal echocardiography.*

two-dimensional transesophageal color-flow Doppler echocardiography See *transesophageal echocardiography.*

two-step prothrombin time test   A timed clotting test that measures the adequacy of the extrinsic pathway of coagulation. The two-step prothrombin time is not commonly used in practice, as it is more complicated and not performed on an automated instrument.

Patient preparation No preparation is required, other than for drawing blood.

Procedure The test is performed by mixing tissue extract (e.g., from brain or lung), excess calcium, and measuring the time for clot formation.

Specimen Whole blood, anticoagulated with sodium citrate.

Reference range 11 to 22 seconds.

Abnormal values The two-step prothrombin time test is prolonged in the presence of a coagulation inhibitor or one or more deficiencies of coagulation factors II, V, VII, X, and fibrinogen. It is decreased in the presence of increased antithrombin III.

Cost $75–$100. See *prothrombin time*.

Tzanck test A rapid method for determining the nature of cells in blistering diseases of the skin (e.g., herpesvirus lesions, pemphigus vulgaris).

Patient preparation No preparation is required.

Procedure The procedure is performed by scraping the base of a "virgin" blister or vesicle, spreading the adherent cells on a glass slide, staining the cells with Giemsa or Wright's stain, and examining the cells under a microscope.

Specimen Cells from a blister.

Reference range Negative.

Abnormal values Cytologic evidence for herpes simplex virus and varicella-zoster virus include atypical keratinized epithelial cells with large nuclei, "ground-glass" cytoplasm, multinucleated giant cells, nuclear molding, and peripheral margination of chromatin.

Cost $25–$75.

Comments In practice, the Tzanck test is rarely obtained in an adequate fashion, and thus does not offer clinically useful information.

ultrasonography A diagnostic method that generates images based on the differences in the ability of tissues of various densities to slow (ultra)sound waves. Electricity applied to a piezoelectric crystal or ceramic in a "transducer" causes a high-frequency (2.25–5.0 MHz/s) mechanical vibration, which emits ultrasound in the form of "pressure waves." These waves are transferred into tissues and organs, and at each tissue interface, a portion of the ultrasound wave is reflected, generating echoes. As the echoes return in the direction of the transducer, there is a slight distortion or deformity of a piezoelectric crystal in the transducer, which produces minute voltage pulses that are then amplified and displayed in one of several "modes." The transducer is used to both generate the ultrasound beam and detect the returning echo. The number of pulses generated in a second or pulse repetition frequency is inversely related to the tissue depth. The amplitude of the signal is recorded in scales of gray, where the whitest shades reflect the strongest signal.

A-MODE DISPLAY ULTRASONOGRAPHY An ultrasonographic method that provides simple displays that are plotted as a series of peaks, the height of which represents the depth of the echoing structure from the transducer.

B-MODE ULTRASONOGRAPHY (Brightness-modulated display) B-mode ultrasonography yields two-dimensional tissue "slices" that are produced using different types of transducers, capable of scanning sequentially across a limited region or finite space. This method has a wide range of applications, including imaging of the fetus, kidneys, liver, gallbladder, uterus, heart structures, breast, prostate; screening for early ovarian cancer; evaluating liver transplant recipients both preoperatively (a narrow or thrombosed portal vein precludes transplantation) and postoperatively (to assess various complications such as rejection, infection, thrombosis, and patency of biliary tracts); and identifying gall bladder calculi. The technique is most commonly used in obstetrics, providing real-time two-dimensional images of the fetus that move in rapid succession, as in a motion picture. The "biophysical profile" has a B-mode display and measures the head (cephalometry), thorax, and abdomen, estimates fetal maturation, and identifies growth

retardation and major congenital anomalies, including anencephaly, hydrocephaly, meningocele, congenital heart disease, dextrocardia, fetal tumors,
diaphragmatic hernia, gastroschisis, omphalocele, polycystic kidneys,
hydrops fetalis, gastrointestinal obstruction and death. B-mode ultrasonography helps localize the amniocentesis needle and is of use in identifying placental anomalies including hydatidiform mole or anomalous implantation,
e.g., placenta previa. The side effects of ultrasonography are minimal
because the energy levels for diagnostic imaging are considered too low to
produce tissue destruction or major disturbances.

DUPLEX ULTRASONOGRAPHY An ultrasonographic modality that combines the standard real-time B-mode display with pulsed Doppler signals,
allowing analysis of frequency shifts in an ultrasonographic signal, which
reflect motion within a tissue, e.g., blood flow. This method is useful in evaluating atherosclerosis of the carotid arteries, arteriovenous malformations,
and circulatory disturbances in the neonatal brain

M-MODE DISPLAY ULTRASONOGRAPHY (time-motion display) A modality
in which the echo signal is recorded on a continuously moving strip of
paper, with the transducer held in a fixed position over the aortic or mitral
valves. Each dot on the display represents a moving structure; stationary
structures are represented as straight lines. M-mode was the first display to
be used in ultrasonography and continues to be useful for precise timing of
cardiac valve opening and correlating valve motion with electrocardiography, phonocardiography, and Doppler echocardiography.

Patient preparation For most applications of ultrasonography, no preparation
is required. In evaluating the fetus and pelvic structures, the patient needs to
drink as much water as possible without voiding, which can cause considerable discomfort. The purpose is to fill the urinary bladder to near capacity,
which pushes the fetus out of the bony pelvis and improves the image.

Procedure A gel is applied to the skin and the wand-like transducer is swept
across the region of interest.

Reference range Negative for anatomic abnormalities.

Abnormal values Ultrasonographic examination of different body sites is of
use in identifying cysts and other collections of fluid, structural abnormalities, tumors, and vascular lesions.

Cost The fees charged for the procedure depend on the body region, where
it is performed, and in what setting, and range from $150 to $500 or
more.

unconjugated estriol   Estriol is a major estrogen produced in pregnancy.
It is measured, in conjunction with alphafetoprotein and chorionic
gonadotropin, as an indicator of a fetus at risk for Down's syndrome, in the
abbreviated battery of tests known as the triple marker screen.

Patient preparation None required other than for drawing blood or obtaining a 24-hour urine specimen.

Procedure Estriol is measured by radioimmunoassay and high-performance
liquid chromatography.

Specimen Serum from blood collected in heparin; 24-hour urine.
Reference range

Urine

16 weeks   2 mg/24 hours.

Term   10–40 mg/24 hours.

Serum

25 weeks   3.5–10 µg/L.

Term   5–40 µg/L.

Abnormal values Less than 4 mg in 24-hour urine in later pregnancy requires immediate assessment of fetal well being. Unconjugated estriol is decreased in fetal adrenal hyperplasia, hypoplasia, and anencephaly, and increased in fetal adrenal hyperplasia

Cost $75–$125.

unidimensional echocardiography See *M-mode echocardiography*.

unstable hemoglobin See *hemoglobin*.

upper gastrointestinal endoscopy (upper GI) One of the most commonly performed endoscopic procedures, this technique allows the physician to examine and obtain diagnostic material from the mucosal surface of the upper gastrointestinal tract, from the esophagus to part of the small intestine.

Upper gastrointestinal endoscopy is useful in evaluating acute upper GI bleeding (e.g., of the esophageal veins in cirrhosis of the liver), difficulty in swallowing (dysphagia, which may be due to strictures), dyspepsia, esophageal pain, and abnormalities seen by an upper gastrointestinal radiologic study. It is also useful in identifying causes of the gastric outlet syndrome and in monitoring premalignant conditions (e.g., Barrett's esophagus, lye-induced strictures). Upper gastrointestinal endoscopy may rarely be useful in evaluating atypical chest pain or abdominal pain of unknown origin

Patient preparation Informed consent is required. Baseline coagulation studies (e.g., activated partial thromboplastin time, prothrombin time, platelet count), and certain chemistries (e.g., BUN and creatinine) should be obtained prior to the procedure. If possible, aspirin and nonsteroidal anti-inflammatory agents should be discontinued before the procedure, as should antacids which may interfere with the procedure. Dentures should be removed. Intravenous sedation (e.g., with diazepam) is routinely administered, and local anesthetic is applied to the back of the throat.

Procedure The procedure consists of the insertion of a long flexible fiberoptic endoscope (esophagogastroduodenoscope) by mouth. The mucosal surfaces of the esophagus, stomach, duodenum, and proximal jejunum are examined for the presence of changes in the form of ulceration, polyps, bleeding sites, strictures, and other changes. At the time of the procedure, "suspicious" lesions may be sampled and the specimens submitted for analysis of the cells (cytology), tissues (pathology), or fluids (e.g., microbiology to identify infections).

Specimen Fluids for cytologic examination or culture; tissue for pathological examination.

Reference range Negative for microorganisms. Negative for significant pathological or cytological changes.

Abnormal values Tissues obtained by endoscopic biopsy may demonstrate a wide range of change, including inflammation, ulcers, infection (e.g., *Helicobacter pylori*), vascular lesions (e.g., varices of the esophagus and sites of gastric bleeding), as well as benign (e.g., polyps) and malignant (e.g., cancer) tumors.

Cost $500–$700.

Comments Upper gastrointestinal (GI) endoscopy should not be performed in acute myocardial infarction, respiratory distress with decreased oxygen (hypoxia), hypotension, shock, massive upper gastrointestinal bleeding, uncontrolled hypertension, blood clotting disorders, severe coronary artery disease, recent surgery to the region, active peritonitis, perforation of organs being examined, and instability of the vertebral column. See *small intestinal biopsy, upper GI study.*

upper GI series See *upper GI study.*

upper GI study A general term for radiologic studies in which a contrast medium is administered in the upper gastrointestinal tract (esophagus, stomach, duodenum) and images are obtained. "Double contrast" studies are used to evaluate mucosal abnormalities of the esophagus, stomach, and duodenum. "Single contrast" studies are best suited for identifying gastric outlet obstruction, gastroesophageal reflux disease, hiatal hernia, and esophageal varices or cancer in the esophagus. Water soluble contrast is used to identify anastomotic leakage or gastrointestinal perforation.

Patient preparation The patient should eat nothing after midnight the night before the procedure.

Procedure The procedure consists of the administration of a barium solution ("milkshake") and the evaluation of its flow through the esophagus, stomach, and duodenum by fluoroscopy, with periodic films being taken by conventional radiologic devices.

Reference range Negative for radiologic abnormalities.

Abnormal values Changes seen include mucosal abnormalities of the esophagus, stomach, and duodenum, obstruction of the pylorus, gastroesophageal reflux disease, hiatal hernia, varices or cancer in the esophagus, anastomotic leakage, and gastrointestinal perforation.

Cost $500–$800.

Comments Barium contrast medium is a viscid radiodense material, the use of which interferes with either endoscopy or computed tomography (CT) studies. See *upper gastrointestinal endoscopy.*

urease test A colorimetric test used in microbiology to detect the presence of urease, an enzyme found in certain bacteria. In the test, bacteria in question are inoculated on a culture medium containing urea and phenolsulfonphthalein. If urease is present, as in infections by *Proteus,* a species of bacteria, a red color appears on the culture plate.

urecholine sensitivity test A clinical test in which urecholine, a cholinergic agent, is administered while the pressure in the bladder is being monitored. In the so-called "neurogenic" bladder in which there is loss or impairment of voluntary control of urination, the intravesical pressure increases by more than 15 cm above that of a control patient.

uric acid A small molecule that is a metabolite of purines, which are an integral component of DNA (deoxyribonucleic acid). Uric acid is excreted primarily by the kidneys, and to a lesser extent by the gastrointestinal tract. Increased uric acid occurs in gout, a disease of the joints, in which uric acid crystals are deposited in various tissues. Increased uric acid also occurs in situations of rapid cell turnover, such as cancer (e.g., leukemia, metastatic carcinoma, multiple myeloma), and also in alcoholism, dehydration due to diuretics, diabetes mellitus, hyperlipoproteinemia, lead poisoning, and renal failure. If no cause can be identified for the increased uric acid, it is termed idiopathic.
Patient preparation No preparation is required, other than for drawing blood or obtaining urine.
Procedure Uric acid is measured by an enzymatic digestion with uricase or by the phosphotungstate reaction.
Specimen Serum, 24-hour urine.
Reference range
Serum
   male   3.6–8.3 mg/dL.
   female   2.2–6.8 mg/dL.
Urine
   male   250–800 mg/24 hours.
   female   250–750 mg/24 hours.
Abnormal values
Increased in: gout, alcohol consumption, drugs (e.g., diazoxide, diuretics, acetazolamide, ethacrynic acid, furosemide, mercurials, epinephrine, ethambutol, nicotinic acid, corticosteroids, chemotherapeutic agents, salicylates), hyperlipidemia, hypertension, lead-induced nephropathy, Lesch-Nyhan syndrome, leukemias and other malignancies, multiple myeloma, obesity, polycystic kidney disease, psoriasis, renal failure, toxemia of pregnancy.
Cost $15–$25. See *synovial fluid analysis.*

urinalysis A low-cost test in which a urine specimen, collected at random from a patient, is examined in order to screen for various diseases. Routine urinalysis is used to detect renal disease (e.g., glomerulonephritis), urinary tract disease (e.g., bladder infection), or metabolic diseases (e.g., diabetes mellitus). Routine chemical analysis of the urine is based on the use of reagent strips (dipsticks), which are coated with material that changes color depending on the concentration of a substance of interest in the urine.

Patient preparation No preparation is required, other than for obtaining urine.

Procedure The specimen is examined by the "naked" eye or microscope, or tested with reagent strips.

Specimen Urine.

Reference range Negative for bacteria, abnormal cells, or chemical changes.

MACROSCOPIC
Color	Yellow
Odor	Urine has a unique "aromatic" odor
Appearance	Clear

ANALYTIC PARAMETERS
Specific gravity	1.002–1.040
pH	4.5–8.0
Bilirubin	None
Glucose	None
Hemoglobin	None
Ketones	None
Leukocyte	None
Nitrite	None
Protein	None
Red blood cells	None
White blood cells	None
Urobilinogen	Normal

MICROSCOPIC
Bacteria, yeasts	None
Casts	Rare hyaline casts
Crystals	Rare, usually oxalates
Epithelial cells	0–5/high-power field (40 magnifications)
Red blood cells	0–5/high-power field
White blood cells	0–5/high-power field

Abnormal values Light microscopy allows the detection of infectious agents (e.g., bacteria, fungi, parasites), crystals (which may indicate a disease of metabolism such as gout), and casts of renal tubules, which are not found (except for hyaline casts, a normal finding in the urinary sediment) in the absence of renal disease.

Cost $25–$50.

Comments Light microscopic examination of the urine of an individual who is not known to be sick rarely detects any condition that is treatable.

urinary free catecholamine test See *catecholamines.*

urine concentration test (concentrating ability test) A general term for any test in which the osmolality of the urine is measured after a certain period of fluid restriction. The ability to concentrate urine indicates adequacy of both renal and endocrine function. The responsible hormone is vasopressin (also known as antidiuretic hormone or ADH). See *specific gravity, water deprivation test*.

urine cytology The analysis of cells and debris obtained from the urine to establish a diagnosis.
Patient preparation No preparation is required, other than for obtaining urine.
Procedure Urine (containing cells from the urinary bladder) is filtered or centrifuged in order to obtain a cell concentrate. The concentrate is then examined by light microscopy by a cytopathologist.
Specimen Random "clean catch" (mid-stream) urine.
Reference range Negative for significant changes.
Abnormal values Atypical or malignant cells.
Cost $50–$75.

urobilinogens A general term for any of the breakdown products of unconjugated bilirubin which are decreased in all conditions in which liver function or biliary drainage is impaired.
Patient preparation No preparation is required, other than for obtaining urine.
Procedure Urobilinogen is determined colorimetrically.
Specimen 24-hour urine.
Reference range Less than 4 mg/24 hours.
Abnormal values
  Increased in: alcoholic cirrhosis, biliary obstruction with biliary tract infection, drugs (e.g., aminosalicylic acid, phenothiazines, sulfonamides), agents that cause hemolysis (e.g., melphalan, amphotericin B, penicillin, phenacetin, chlorpromazine, mefenamic acid), hemorrhage, intravascular hemolysis, liver damage, hepatotoxic drugs.
  Decreased in: biliary obstruction without biliary tract infection, drugs (e.g., amphotericin B, aspirin, azathioprine, chloramphenicol, chlorpromazine, colchicine, cyclophosphamide, doxorubicin, fluorouracil, indomethacin, insulin, L-dopa, mephenytoin, mercaptopurine, methotrexate, methyldopa, nitrofurantoin, penicillin, phenytoin, streptomycin, sulfonamides, tetracycline, vincristine, and others), hepatocellular damage, renal cell insufficiency.
Cost $40–$60.

urodynamic evaluation A battery of clinical tests that determine the neuromuscular responses of the urinary bladder to filling and emptying. The urodynamic evaluation consists of
  CYSTOMETRY (cystometrography) A technique used to determine bladder

capacity, pressure, presence of voluntary or involuntary contractions of the detrusor muscle (which is measured by placing warm saline solution in the bladder), integrity of the affector (sensory) limb of the detrusor reflex arc, and the bladder's compliance. Bladder compliance is the bladder's ability to stretch when filled. Cystometry may be coupled with a coordinated electromyographic evaluation of the bladder sphincter.

URETHRAL PRESSURE PROFILE (external sphincter electromyography) A procedure that measures the electrical activity of the external sphincter of the urethra. It is used to determine the functional length, resting pressure, and maximal pressure of the sphincter mechanisms.

URINARY FLOW RATE (uroflowmetry) A simple noninvasive procedure in which the volume, time required to void, and peak and average flow rates are recorded by any of a number of simple mechanical devices. The simplest of the uroflowmeters is based on gravity, which simply weighs the urine as it is passed and plots it on a graph over time.

Patient preparation For urinary flow rate evaluation, the patient should not urinate for several hours before the test. The other tests require no preparation.

Procedure For cystometry, a specialized catheter is used that is capable of both recording pressure and introducing air or carbon dioxide into the bladder to increase the pressure, thereby increasing the urge to void the urine. For external sphincter electromyography, any of a number of types (skin, anal, or urethral) of sensors are placed in the region of the external sphincter of the urethra, and the electrical activity is measured. For urinary flow measurement, the urine is measured as it accumulates in a receptacle.

Reference range Negative for any abnormalities.

Abnormal values Any changes that are suggestive of obstruction or incontinence.

Cost $800–$1000.

uroporphyrinogen I synthetase   See *porphobilinogen deaminase.*

valproic acid   An antiepileptic agent that is used to control seizure activity and massive myoclonic episodes. Because of valproic acid's narrow therapeutic range, its levels in the serum must be evaluated on a regular basis.

Patient preparation No preparation is required, other than for drawing blood; the specimen should be collected at the time of the lowest normal serum level, a time known as the "trough."

Procedure Valproic acid can be measured by enzyme immunoassay and gas-liquid chromatography.

Specimen Serum, plasma in EDTA.

Reference range 50–100 μg/ml.

Abnormal values Greater than 100 mg/ml.

Cost $75–$85. See *therapeutic drug monitoring.*

vancomycin   A "broad-spectrum" antibiotic that is effective against many gram-negative and gram-positive coccal bacteria. It is of particular use in patients whose resistant staphylococcal infections have failed to respond to penicillins or cephalosporins. Because of vancomycin's toxicity to the kidneys (nephrotoxicity) and to auditory structures (ototoxicity), it should not be administered in patients with renal failure (as it is excreted through the kidneys) and should not be used in combination with other neurotoxic or nephrotoxic antibiotics, including amikacin, cephaloridine, colistin, gentamicin, kanamycin, neomycin, polymyxin B, streptomycin, or tobramycin.

Patient preparation No preparation is required, other than for drawing blood.

Procedure Vancomycin is measured by enzyme immunoassay.

Specimen Serum. Two specimens: One obtained 30 minutes after one dose (peak) and the other just before the next dose (trough).

Reference range

| Peak | 20–40 μg/ml. |
| Trough | 5–10 μg/ml. |

Abnormal values Greater than 80 μg/ml.

Cost $160-$180 for two specimens. See *therapeutic drug monitoring.*

vanillylmandelic acid (VMA)   A breakdown product of the catecholamines epinephrine and norepinephrine, which act as neurotransmitters and hormones. Catecholamines are produced by the adrenal gland and nervous system. VMA is increased in pheochromocytomas and neuroblastomas, which are tumors of the adrenal gland and the so-called neuroendocrine system.

Patient preparation No preparation is required, other than for obtaining urine. The patient should inform the physician if he is taking any medication that would interfere with the test (see below) and, if possible, discontinue its use before providing the specimen.

Procedure VMA is excreted in the urine and quantified by a colorimetric (Pisano) method.

Specimen 24-hour urine specimen acidified with hydrochloric acid or acetic acid. The patient should rest during collection and should not take any medication.

Reference range 2.0–7.0 mg/24 hours; 1.0–6.0 µg/mg of creatinine.

Abnormal values

   Increased in: pheochromocytoma, neuroblastoma, ganglioneuroma, carcinoid tumor, drugs and hormones (e.g., epinephrine, glucagon, guanethidine [early doses], histamine, insulin, L-dopa, lithium, mephenamine, nitroglycerin, reserpine [early doses]).

   Decreased in: drugs and hormones (e.g., clonidine, disulfiram, guanethidine, hydrazine, imipramine, monoamine oxidase inhibitors, morphine, radiographic media for intravenous pyelography, reserpine).

Cost $90–$100. See *total catecholamine test.*

varicella-zoster virus (chickenpox)   A virus that belongs to the herpes family of viruses; it is classified as human herpesvirus-3. The primary or childhood form, chickenpox, presents in a characteristic fashion, commonly as a wave of itchy vesicles that spread over the entire body, healing within three to five days. In its "classic" form, chickenpox rarely represents a diagnostic dilemma. Of greater concern is the possibility that a person is exposed for the first time to the varicella-zoster virus (VZV) as an adult and does not have protective antibodies.

Patient preparation No preparation is required, other than for drawing blood.

Procedure Two specimens are drawn—one in the acute phase of the infection ("acute" serum) and the second when the patient is clearly recovering from the infection ("convalescent" serum). The levels of antibody (immunoglobulin) are evaluated by serial dilutions (titers) of serum and measured by enzyme immunoassay (ELISA), fluorescent antibody against membrane antigen (which is not widely used as it is cumbersome), complement fixation (which is not used as it is too insensitive), and others.

Specimen Serum.

Reference range Negative for antibodies by ELISA.

Abnormal values Antibodies can be detected within one to four days of acute infection. A four-fold increase in antibody titer between the acute and convalescent sera is strongly suggestive of varicella-zoster infection. *Cost* $60–$80.

varicose veins   See *Trendelenburg test* in Glossary.

vasoactive intestinal polypeptide (VIP)   A neuropeptide hormone that is present in the nerve fibers of smooth muscle and blood vessels and in the glands of the gastrointestinal and upper respiratory tract. VIP stimulates adenylate cyclase, evoking potent vasodilation, pancreatic and intestinal secretion, inhibition of gastric acid secretion, increased cardiac output, glycogenolysis, bronchodilation, and inhibition of the release of macromolecules from mucus-secreting glands. VIP deficiency may contribute to bronchial asthma, given its virtual absence in asthmatics.

Patient preparation Patient must have completely fasted (i.e., no food or water) for 10 to 12 hours prior to specimen collection. All medications should be discontinued for 24 to 48 hours.

Procedure VIP is measured by radioimmunoassay.

Specimen Plasma collected in an EDTA (lavender-top) tube. The specimen is immediately transferred to a red-top tube containing 500 mL of 10,000 KIU/mL Trasylol.

Reference range 20–53 ng/L.

Abnormal values Greater than 76 ng/L. VIP is increased in VIPoma, a pancreatic islet G-cell tumor that is morphologically identical to other G-cell tumors.

Cost $200–$220. See *watery diarrhea-hypokalemia-achlorhydria syndrome* in Glossary.

vasopressin   See *antidiuretic hormone.*

VDRL (Venereal Disease Research Laboratory test)   A reaginic screening test for syphilis. VDRL test is highly variable in tertiary syphilis and is negative in 40%–50% of cases of neurosyphilis.

Patient preparation No preparation is required, other than for drawing blood. Rarely, cerebrospinal fluid is required to detect the presence of neurosyphilis, which requires a lumbar puncture.

Procedure In the VDRL test, heat-inactivated serum is added to the VDRL antigen (a mixture of cardiolipin, lecithin, alcohol, and cholesterol), and agglutination is viewed by light microscopy at four minutes (the RPR or rapid plasma reagin test is a variant of the VDRL that is interpreted macroscopically at eight minutes). Reaginic tests are useful screens in early syphilis and are virtually always positive in secondary syphilis.

Specimen Serum, cerebrospinal fluid.

Reference range Negative.

Abnormal values Positive test results may represent biological false positivitiy, which occurs in malaria (up to 90% positive), acute infections (10%–30%), systemic lupus erythematosus (10%–20%, the classic cause of

a biological false positive VDRL test), viral hepatitis (10%), infectious mononucleosis (20%), rheumatoid arthritis (5%–10%), and others, including pneumococcal pneumonia, drug addiction, and pregnancy. Therefore, a positive VDRL test must be confirmed with FTA-ABS (fluorescent treponemal antibody absorbed).
Cost $25–$50.

venography (phlebography)   A technique used to produce fluoroscopic and/or x-ray images of the legs, which are of use in identifying blood clots in the deep veins of the legs. Blood clots in these veins may lead to occlusion of the femoral or iliac veins and may fragment, giving rise to emboli which may lodge in the pulmonary arteries, resulting in the potentially fatal pulmonary thromboembolism.
Patient preparation The patient is placed on a clear liquid diet four hours before the procedure.
Procedure The procedure consists of the intravenous injection of 50–75 ml of a radiocontrast into a vein in the foot or calf, while multiple images are obtained from various angles.
Reference range Negative for stenoses or occlusions.
Abnormal values Filling defects are seen in the presence of thromboses, compression, or occlusion.
Cost $500–$850. See *Trendelenburg test* in Glossary.

venous impedance plethysmography   See *plethysmography.*

ventilation-perfusion scan (radionuclide scan of lung)   A noninvasive radionuclide study of the ratio of pulmonary ventilation (V) to pulmonary blood flow (perfusion, Q) through the lungs. The V/QS is used to detect pulmonary embolism. Quantitative V/Q may be obtained after inhalation of the radionuclide, xenon-133 (^{133}Xe) and intravenous injection of another radionuclide, technetium-99m (^{99m}Tc). Both of these "tracers" have low levels of radioactivity.
Patient preparation All blood specimens that will be analyzed by radioimmunoassay should be obtained before the procedure.
Procedure In a commonly used protocol, the scan is performed after inhalation of ^{133}Xe and intravenous injection of ^{99m}Tc, which allows evaluation of inspiratory airflow, lung volume, presence of air trapping, and adequacy of perfusion.
Reference range A homogeneous distribution of radioactivity in the lungs.
Abnormal values A V/Q "mismatch" indicates preservation of ventilation with a defect in perfusion, a finding commonly associated with pulmonary embolism. Inconclusive studies are not uncommon and are more common in those with underlying lung disease.
Cost $800–$1000.
Comments Up to 12% of ventilation/perfusion scans are false-negatives, especially in individuals with a low risk of pulmonary embolism. A chest

X ray is also needed for proper interpretation. Synonyms include lung perfusion scan, lung perfusion scintigraphy, perfusion-ventilation scan, pulmonary scan, radionuclide perfusion scan, and V/Q scan. See *pulmonary function test*.

ventriculocardiography (spatial electrocardiography, three-dimensional electrocardiography) A refined permutation of electrocardiography that demonstrates cardiac muscle activity and myocardial damage from two points at the same time. This provides information on the direction of the heart muscle's activity as well as its force in terms of contraction and relaxation. This contrasts with standard electrocardiography, which records the force of the heart muscle activity from only one direction at a time.

Patient preparation None is required.

Procedure Electrodes are attached to four points at the same time, in contrast to two points in standard electrocardiography. It is attached to a monitor, which produces an image in a moving loop.

Reference range There is no standard or normal range.

Abnormal values Interpretation of the abnormalities seen are based on the cardiologist's experience. Vectorgram abnormalities can be used to detect myocardial infarction, an increase in the thickness of the heart muscle, and blocks in the conduction of electrical impulses known as bundle branch blocks.

Cost $300–$700.

vestibular test The vestibule is a part of the inner ear that contains tissues involved in maintaining the balance and in sending information about the state of equilibrium to the cerebellum (lower brain), where the information is processed. Abnormalities of vestibular function are manifest by dizziness, loss of balance, and nystagmus, a jittery motion of the eyes. Such cases require evaluation of both the "mechanical" (i.e., the vestibule) and the "neural processing" (nerves from the vestibule to the cerebellum and the cerebellum) parts of the vestibular system.

Patient preparation No preparation is required. Alcohol, sedatives, and tranquilizers must be withheld for two to three days before the test.

Procedure Vestibular system testing is performed by vertical and horizontal ocular recording of eye movements, nystagmus, and head position. An integral part of the testing battery is the placing of warm or cold water in the ear canal, a procedure that enhances the interpretation of alterations of the so-called vestibulo-ocular circuit. Two general forms of tests are used in practice. With falling tests, such as the Romberg test, the individual stands with the eyes closed and both feet together. This is followed by a second test in which the patient stands first on one foot, then on the other.

Reference range Negative.

Abnormal values Excess swaying implies a severe abnormality in postural sensation in the lower extremities.

Cost $800–$1000.

videodefecography   A dynamic technique for evaluating rectoanal function in which barium is injected into the rectum, and the changes that occur in response to relaxing, coughing, or straining are evaluated in "real time" by videofluoroscopy. See *defecography* in Glossary.

video electroencephalography   A method for evaluating a person with seizures in which the electroencephalographic (EEG) signal is amplified and transmitted via cable to a central station with a video image of the patient. Video EEG allows precise analysis of seizure phenomena, provides a definitive diagnosis in most (82%) patients, and can be performed in the hospital or as an ambulatory procedure at a lower cost. See *electroencephalography*.

videolaryngoscopy   A procedure in which a video camera is attached to a flexible fibroendoscope to record images; the videolaryngoscope is used to diagnose and document (medicolegally) pathologic lesions of the larynx. See *laryngoscopy*.

VIP   See *vasoactive intestinal polypeptide*.

viral culture   A laboratory test in which a specimen from a patient is placed in a culture of living cells. Unlike bacteria, viruses by definition must grow inside of a living cell and thus cannot be cultured on a nonliving growth medium. A wide range of viruses (e.g., adenovirus, enterovirus, herpes simplex, measles, mumps, myxovirus, paramyxovirus, rhinovirus, rubella, varicella-zoster, and others) can be cultured from clinical specimens, although viral cultures are not routinely performed because the therapeutic options are somewhat limited.
   Patient preparation No preparation is required, other than for obtaining the appropriate specimen from the throat, vesicle in the skin, urine, or elsewhere.
   Procedure The specimen is inoculated on a culture of living cells from various animals and tissues. After the appropriate time (one to two weeks), the cells are examined by microscopy to detect any changes in the appearance of the cell culture, known as a "cytopathologic effect." More recently, a technique known as the shell vial assay has become the method of choice for early detection of viral infection.
   Specimen Throat swab, sputum, stool, cerebrospinal fluid, or urine.
   Reference range Negative.
   Abnormal values Cytopathic effect, i.e., typical changes in the appearance of cells in culture, which are relatively specific for each virus.
   Cost $100–$250. See *shell vial assay, viral profile* in Glossary, *viral study* in Glossary.

viscosity   Viscosity is the resistance to the flow of a fluid, which in medicine refers to the thickness of the blood, or the ease with which it flows in the circulation.

Patient preparation No preparation is required, other than for drawing blood.

Procedure Viscosity is measured by a viscometer.

Reference range 1.1–1.8 relative to water.

Abnormal values If the serum viscosity is increased, the cause can then be determined by immunoelectrophoresis.

> Increased in: monoclonal gammopathies (e.g., Waldenström's macroglobulinemia, multiple myeloma), amyloidosis, cirrhosis of the liver, chronic infections, hyperfibrinogemia, rheumatoid arthritis systemic lupus erythematosus.

Cost $70–$90. See *specific gravity*.

(pattern-shift) visual evoked response (visual evoked potential) A clinical test in which the retina and optic nerve are stimulated with external visual stimuli and the effect recorded on electroencephalography.

Patient preparation No preparation is required, other than having the patient wash his/her hair before the procedure to remove the scalp oils and to facilitate the placement of the scalp electrodes.

Procedure The individual's response to a stimulus (a shifting checkerboard pattern) is recorded by electroencephalographic electrodes placed over the occipital scalp and appears 100 msec after the stimulus as a single positive peak on a graph. It is known as P-100.

Reference range No slowing of the conduction of optic nerve fibers.

Abnormal values The characteristic response, P-100 (see above), is slowed and/or its waveform altered in pathologic conditions that affect the optic nerve, including multiple sclerosis, but also glaucoma, neoplasms, ischemic, nutritional and toxic neuropathies, and pseudotumor cerebri.

Cost $50–$100.

vitamin A (retinol, carotene) A general term for fat-soluble molecules that exhibit the biological activity of trans-retinol, including retinol, carotenoids, and others. These molecules are required for the transportation of sugars in the synthesis of glycoprotein and for maintaining the mucosa covering the oral cavity and respiratory and urinary tracts, and are critical in the production of a key protein in the retina, rhodopsin. Vitamin A is stored in the liver, intestine, kidney, heart, blood vessels, and gonads, and is critical for fetal development, cell proliferation, and vision. The use of vitamin A therapy in asymptomatic children results in two-fold decrease in mortality from diarrhea, convulsions, and infection-related symptoms.

Patient preparation The specimen should be drawn from a fasting patient.

Procedure Vitamin A is measured by colorimetry, fluorometry, and high-performance liquid chromatography.

Specimen Serum. Specimen must be drawn in a chilled tube and protected from light and hemolysis.

Reference range 30–95 µg/dL.

Cost $100–$120.

vitamin B₁ See *thiamin.*

vitamin B₂ See *riboflavin.*

vitamin B₆ (pyridoxal, pyridoxine)   A water-soluble B vitamin that is present in meats, whole grains, peanuts, green vegetables, and yeast. Vitamin B₆ deficiency is a disease of malnutrition that occurs in alcoholics, in those with various inborn errors of metabolism, and in various pyridoxine-responsive syndromes. Vitamin B₆ deficiency results in pellagra, which is characterized by glossitis, weakness, seborrheic dermatitis, and irritability.
   Patient preparation No preparation is required, other than for drawing blood.
   Procedure Pyridoxine is measured by enzyme immunoassay and radioimmunoassay.
   Specimen Plasma, urine after fasting.
   Reference range Plasma 3.6–18 ng/ml; urine greater than 20 µg/g creatinine.
   Abnormal values
      Decreased in: alcoholism, drugs (e.g., isoniazid, cycloserine, penicillamine, oral contraceptives), gestational diabetes mellitus malabsorption.
   Cost $180–$200.

vitamin B₁₂ (cyanocobalamin, extrinsic factor)   A water-soluble vitamin of animal origin that is required for the synthesis of DNA. It is absorbed from the gastrointestinal tract only when it is bound to a glycoprotein known as intrinsic factor, which is produced and secreted by the gastric parietal cells. The body stores up to one year's worth of vitamin B₁₂ in the liver, kidneys, and heart. Conditions of rapid cell turnover (e.g., growth spurts in children, malignancy) require increased amounts of vitamin B₁₂.
   Patient preparation No preparation is required, other than for drawing blood.
   Procedure Vitamin B₁₂ is measured by radioimmunoassay.
   Specimen Serum, which must be separated from the cells then frozen and protected from light until analysis.
   Reference range Greater than 200 pg/ml.
   Abnormal values
      Increased in: chronic myelocytic leukemia, chronic obstructive pulmonary disease (COPD), congestive heart failure, hepatocellular disease, obesity, polycythemia vera, renal failure.
      Decreased in: atrophic gastritis, drugs (e.g., antibiotics, anticonvulsants, antimalarials, antituberculosis agents, chemotherapeutics, oral contraceptives, diuretics, oral hypoglycemics, sedatives), inflammatory bowel disease (e.g., Crohn's disease, ulcerative colitis), intrinsic factor deficiency, which causes megaloblastic anemia, malabsorption and malnutrition, parasites (e.g., *Diphyllobotrium latum*), veganism.
   Cost $70–$90.

vitamin C See *ascorbic acid.*

vitamin D A general term for steroid vitamins with the biological activity of cholecalciferol, which are present in fish liver oils, dairy products, and eggs. Vitamin D is critical for the absorption of calcium and is thus also known as antirachitic factor, as it prevents rickets, a major metabolic bone disease of children. There are several terms for the various vitamin D forms. Vitamin D_1 is a term that is no longer used, as the original vitamin D_1 was shown to consist of a mixture of vitamin D_2 and lumisterol. Vitamin D_2 is now known as ergocalciferol. Vitamin D_3 Cholecalciferol is what is usually referred to as vitamin D. It is synthesized in the skin on exposure to ultraviolet light. Vitamin D_2 is derived only from the diet. Vitamin D has a major role in the intestinal absorption of calcium, bone calcium balance, and renal excretion of calcium and therefore is measured as part of the workup for hypocalciumia, hypercalcemia, and hypophosphatemia. Specific measurement of both monohydroxy and dihydroxy forms can help pinpoint absorptive, hepatic, or renal abnormalities of vitamin D metabolism.

Patient preparation No preparation is required, other than for drawing blood.

Procedure Radioimmunoassay is used for measuring vitamin D levels.

Specimen Serum or heparin-anticoagulated plasma.

Reference range

25-Hydroxyvitamin D_3	10–40 ng/ml.
1,25-Dihydroxyvitamin D	20–76 pg/ml.

Abnormal values

Increased in: growth periods in children, hyperparathyroidism (primary), idiopathic hypercalciuria, lactation, pregnancy, tumor calcinosis, vitamin D intoxication.

Decreased in: insulin-dependent diabetes mellitus, lead intoxication, renal failure, post-menopausal osteoporosis, pseudohypoparathyroidism, uremia, vitamin D-dependent rickets.

Cost

25-Hydroxyvitamin D_3	$150–$170.
1,25-Dihydroxyvitamin D	$210–$230.

vitamin K test A test that evaluates the liver's ability to synthesize certain proteins known as vitamin K-dependent coagulation factors (prothrombin, and factors VII, IX, and X), which are enzymes involved in the formation of a blood clot. In one vitamin K testing protocol, prothrombin is measured 24 hours after injection of vitamin K, which in normal individuals increases by more than 20%. In practice, prothrombin is an adequate indicator of the status of vitamin K. See *prothrombin time.*

VMA See *vanillylmandelic acid.*

von Willebrand factor A large protein molecule, composed of multiple subunits, that is synthesized by blood vessels and platelets. The efficiency of clotting is linked to the size of the subunits (ristoctin cofactor, VIII:RCF, and von Willebrand's antigen, VIII:Ag, and the most important, factor VIII:C, the classic hemophilia A protein) of von Willebrand factor, as well as to the vascular endothelium, megakaryocytes, and platelets. Von Willebrand's disease is a relatively rare inherited bleeding disorder.

Patient preparation No preparation is required, other than for drawing blood.

Procedure Rocket electrophoresis is used to quantify von Willebrand factor levels in the blood. It is an enzyme immunoassay in which an antigen-bearing fluid is electrophoresed through agarose containing an antibody to the antigen of interest.

Specimen Plasma collected in citrated anticoagulant.

Reference range Factor VIII R:RCo and factor VIII:Ag should be 60%–150% normal.

Abnormal values Decreased in hereditary or acquired von Willebrand disease. The von Willebrand factor, like factor VIII, may be markedly increased by exercise, pregnancy, or stress.

Cost $100–$125.

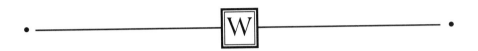

Wassermann test See *RPR test.*

water deprivation test (dehydration test) A clinical test of the ability to increase the concentration (osmolality) of urine in response to withholding water. The water deprivation test is followed by administration of vasopressin (ADH-antidiuretic hormone), also known as the water restriction-vasopressin test, which evokes a small additional (circa 9%) increase in the urine osmolality.

Patient preparation Diuretics should be discontinued. Coffee and alcohol should be avoided.

Procedure Liquids are withheld during the test. Urine is obtained at one-hour intervals for measuring specific gravity. The test is stopped when the specific gravity has stabilized.

Specimen Urine.

Reference range After 4 to 18 hours the maximum urine concentration is achieved in the normal person and the urine osmolality is two to four times greater than that of the plasma.

Abnormal values In patients with diabetes insipidus, the increase in urinary osmolality is greater than 50%.

Cost $500–$750.

Comments Because of the dangers inherent in water deprivation in certain groups of patients (those at extremes of age, or with mental disorders), water deprivation tests require close supervision. See *osmolality, specific gravity.*

Watson-Schwartz test A colorimetric test used in the differential diagnosis of porphyria. Ehrlich's benzaldehyde reagent is added to the urine, which turns pink in the presence of both porphobilionogen and urobilinogen. With the addition of chloroform or butanol, the urine remains pink in acute intermittent porphyria, which has increased porphyrinogen, which is insoluble in chloroform and remains pink from urobilinogen.

Weber test A hearing test in which a vibrating tuning fork is used to determine whether the ability to hear a vibrating tuning fork differs when the base of the tuning fork is placed on the head (bone conductance) or held freely in the air. If the sound is heard more clearly in the air, then hearing loss is conductive; if it is heard more clearly on the nondeaf side, then the hearing loss is sensorineural in nature. See *hearing (function) test, pure tone audiometry, Rinne test, Schwabach test.*

wedge biopsy   See *biopsy, wedge resection.*

wedge resection   A triangular piece of tissue that is removed in surgery, and most commonly obtained in the following two clinical situations.
   GYNECOLOGIC SURGERY The resection of a wedge of tissue from the ovary may, by an unknown mechanism, cause a woman with a condition known as polycystic ovaries or Stein-Leventhal syndrome to ovulate, and allow her to become pregnant.
   SURGICAL ONCOLOGY The resection of a wedge of tissue from the lung, containing a single mass identified by radiology. In lung cancer, if the malignancy is confined to the wedge of tissue, the surgery may result in an improved prognosis. See *biopsy, excisional biopsy.*

Weil-Felix test   A test in which agglutinins from certain strains of *Proteus vulgaris* are used to identify rickettsia, a family of small bacteria. Weil-Felix reactions vary in sensitivity and are relatively nonspecific. False-positive results are common and occur in infections by other microorganisms, e.g., leptospirosis and borreliosis, and infections of the urinary or biliary tracts.

Westergren sedimentation rate   See *erythrocyte sedimentation rate.*

Western blot (immunoblot)   An immune assay that identifies the presence of proteins of specific molecular weights. It is commonly used to confirm HIV infection after an ELISA screening assay is positive. Western blotting is also used to identify proteins in Lyme disease.
   Patient preparation No preparation is required, other than for drawing blood.
   Procedure The proteins are separated by electrophoresis, then transferred (blotted) to a nitrocellulose or nylon membrane that is then exposed to a labeled antibody, which detects the antigen (i.e., protein) of interest.
   Specimen Serum.
   Reference range Negative for protein bands.
   Abnormal values For a Western blot to be considered positive for HIV, two of the protein bands, p24, gp41, and gp160/120 must be present. False positivity in a Western blot for HIV is very rare and occurs in 0.01%–0.0007% of cases. Indeterminant or equivocal results are 100 times more common, and occur in 0.3%–0.5% of the general population. If an individual with indeterminant results is in a high-risk group, he/she usually converts within one month; low-risk individuals with a persisting inde-

terminant Western blot at three months may be regarded as negative and require no further follow-up.

Cost $100–$300.

Comments HIV-1 products, especially p24, may disappear from the serum, accompanied by a decrease in anti-HIV antibodies. See *Northern blot* in Glossary, *Southern blot* in Glossary.

wet mount A simple laboratory procedure in which a fluid (pus, exudate, vaginal discharge, sputum) or chopped tissue is mixed with a 10%–20% solution of potassium hydroxide, covered with a glass cover slip, and examined directly by the light microscope, often in a primary care setting to detect the presence of a fungi (usually dermatophytes, but also *Candida*) and less commonly tichomonads.

whole gut scintigraphy A technique in which radionuclides (indium-111 and technetium-99m) are used to evaluate the transit of foods through the stomach and small and large intestines. Patients with constipation have a slowed gastrointestinal transit time, while those with diarrhea have an increased transit time.

Wintrobe sedimentation rate See *erythrocyte sedimentation rate*.

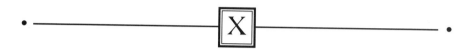

X-ray pelvimetry   See *radiologic pelvimetry*.

xylose absorption test   (D-xylose tolerance test) See D-*xylose absorption test*.

Y chromosome test   A method for detecting the male (Y) chromosome, in which dividing cells are stained with quinacrine and examined under ultraviolet light. The long arm of the Y chromosome has a typical pattern of fluorescence. The Y chromosome can also be evaluated by Southern blot hybridization, in which the DNA from the chomosome itself is analyzed. See *chromosome analysis.*

yeast culture   A test in which clinical material is obtained from a patient and grown on a nutrient-enriched medium to identify the presence of a yeast or fungus.

Yersinia enterocolitica   A bacterium that causes gastroenteritis and depression of the immune system, which can be identified by culturing the stool and by measuring titers of anti-*Yersinia* antibodies.
   Patient preparation No preparation is required, other than for drawing blood or obtaining a stool specimen.
   Procedure Stool culture and measurement of serum antibodies by immunoassay.
   Specimen Stool, serum.
   Reference range Anti-*Yersinia* antibody titers of less than 1:20 are normal.
   Abnormal values Antibody titers of greater than 1:20.
   Cost Stool culture $50–$75; antibody $50–$100.

$$\boxed{Z}$$

zetacrit (zeta sedimentation rate)   A method for determining erythrocyte sedimentation rate, which is thought to be better than the Winthrobe or Westergren methods as it is not affected by hematocrit, fibrinogen, or immunobglobulins, and there are no differences between males and females. See *erythrocyte sedimentation rate*.

zeta sedimentation rate   See *zetacrit*.

zinc   A trace metal that is essential for growth and development, and required for more than 200 enzymes (e.g., carbonic anhydrase, carboxypeptidase, DNA- and RNA-polymerases, reverse transcriptase) and proteins involved in gene expression. Zinc is present in seafood, animal proteins, unrefined grains, legumes, and nuts. Approximately 20% of dietary zinc is absorbed; its absorption is enhanced by protein-rich foods. Of the zinc in the body, 50%–60% is in muscle; 30% is in bone; approximately 90% is excreted in the feces. The recommended daily allowance is 5–15 mg. Toxic levels result from industrial exposure to zinc fumes and dusts in the manufacture of alloys, paints, synthetic rubbers, and roofing materials.

Patient preparation No preparation is required, other than for drawing blood.

Procedure Zinc is measured by atomic absorption spectrophotometry.

Specimen Serum. Blood must be collected in a special trace metal-free tube, usually with a dark blue top.

Reference range

Serum   70–120 µg/dL.
Urine   0.14–0.9 mg/24 hours.

Abnormal values

Increased in: osteosarcoma of bone, coronary artery disease, atherosclerosis.

Decreased in: acute myocardial infarction, celiac disease
drugs (e.g., estrogens, oral contraceptives, corticosteroids), hepatocellular disease, infections (e.g., acute infections), typhoid fever, tuberculosis, malignancy (e.g., lymphomas, leukemia).

Cost
  Serum $80–$90.
  Urine $80–$90.

Zung (depression) scale   An objective rating tool used by psychiatrists to evaluate depression, anxiety, hostility, phobias, paranoid ideation, obsessive-compulsiveness, and other disorders. The Zung scale consists of a multi-item questionnaire that is reported to have a 83%–97% sensitivity and 63%–82% specificity for depression. The use of this scale is declining as it is relatively insensitive to clinical improvement of a mental disorder. See *psychiatric interview* in Glossary.

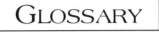

GLOSSARY

accuracy The extent to which a value obtained from a test reflects or agrees with the true value of the analyte being tested.

acid A substance that releases hydrogen ion (H+) into a solution.

acute serum Serum obtained from a person who is acutely infected with a virus, which often demonstrates an increase in immunoglobulin M antibodies against the virus. See *convalescent serum* in Glossary.

Alzheimer's disease A degenerative brain disease characterized by progressive mental deterioration, confusion, loss of memory, and progressive dementia. This extremely common condition is diagnosed based on clinical findings and confirmed by MRI and CT, which demonstrate atrophy (loss) of brain tissue.

Ames test A bacterial test that detects mutagenesis; it is used to detect and screen for compounds with carcinogenic potential.

anergy Absence of immune response to an antigen to which the host was previously sensitive. Anergy can be induced in mature CD4+ T cells by exposure to complexes of antigen and appropriate (self) major histocompatibility complex. Anergy is usually tested by loss of delayed hypersensitivity, e.g., to PPD, *Candida* antigens, or DCNB.

anticentromere antibody An antinuclear antibody found in the circulation of one-fourth of patients with certain "connective tissue" diseases, including systemic sclerosis, limited scleroderma or CREST (calcinosis cutis, Raynaud phenomenon, esophageal dysfunction, sclerodactyly, telangiectasia) complex. The antibody can be seen alone or may also

be associated with primary biliary cirrhosis. See *antinuclear antibodies.*

anticoagulant A general term for drugs used to prevent blood from clotting in the circulation. There are two different types of anticoagulants. The thrombolytic anticoagulants are used in emergencies to dissolve blood clots. Coumadin-type anticoagulants are used to prevent the formation of blood clots. Use of anticoagulants is monitored in the laboratory by measuring prothrombin time (PT) and activated partial prothrombin time (aPTT).

antigen-antibody complex The intimate association between an antigen and an antibody that bind to a specific site (epitope) on the antigen.

antipancreatic islet cell antibodies This family of antibodies may be found in the early stages of type I (also known as insulin-dependent or childhood-onset) diabetes mellitus. These antibodies attack components of the pancreatic islet cell's cytoplasm and cell surface as foreign and mount an immune response to these components. Measurement of islet cell antibodies has no clinical utility and is usually performed by scientists studying the cause of diabetes. Other antibodies identified in this disease include autoantibodies directed against insulin, proinsulin, insulin receptors, and other proteins.

antireceptor antibody A general term for an autoantibody directed against a cell receptor which is capable of altering the cell's response to the molecule that binds to the receptor, known as a ligand. Antireceptor antibodies are linked to endocrine disorders and either increase or decrease a cell's response to a particular hormone. Antibodies against the receptors for corticotropin, the H_2 histamine receptor, parathyroid hormone, beta cells of the pancreatic islets, insulin, thyrotropin (TSH), gastrin, and follicle-stimulating hormone have been identified. See *autoimmunity* in Glossary.

apparent volume of distribution (aVD)   The ratio of the total amount of drug in the body to the concentration of the drug in the plasma, or the "apparent" volume necessary to contain the entire amount of a drug if the drug in the entire body were in the same concentration as in the plasma. The aVD doesn't actually correspond to a fluid volume per se, and in the case of those drugs stored in adipose tissues, the aVD may be hundreds of times larger than the body's volume; a large aVD (e.g., amitriptyline, digoxin, imipramine, lidocaine, nortriptyline, procainamide, propranolol, thiopental) occurs when the majority of a drug is stored in tissue, while drugs with a small aVD (e.g., acetyl salicylic acid, aminoglycosides, valproic acid) are not stored in tissues. See *therapeutic drug monitoring.*

atomic absorption spectrophotometry   A highly sensitive technique used to analyze various elements, especially metals, such as aluminum, antimony, arsenic, beryllium, calcium, copper, iron, lead, lithium, nickel, selenium, thallium, tellurium, and zinc, which are present in trace amounts.

autoantibody   Any antibody that is produced by an organism against one of its own (self) antigens, including antiglomerular basement membrane antibodies, antiparietal cell antibodies, and others.

autoantigen   Any antigen (e.g., membrane, mitochondria, muscle, parietal cells, thyroglobulin) that may evoke the production of antibodies.

autoimmune disease   A condition linked to the production of antibodies against self antigens, which occurs in about 5% of the adult population. Autoimmune diseases include Goodpasture's disease, Hashimoto's disease, multiple sclerosis, myasthenia gravis, rheumatoid arthritis, systemic lupus erythematosus, and pernicious anemia.

autoimmunity   The reaction of an organism's immune system to self antigens as if they were foreign. Autoimmunity increases with age and is intimately linked to connective tissue disease and endocrinopathies. The cause is unclear.

autopsy   A postmortem examination of a body, intended to either identify any diseases that had not been detected while the patient was alive or to confirm the presence of conditions that had been diagnosed before the patient died. Types of autopsies include the following:

BIOPSY ONLY A minimalist postmortem examination. The prosecutor has permission to enter body sites and fully examine the organs but may only choose to select small fragments ("biopsies") for histologic examination.

CHEST ONLY An autopsy in which the family members have only given permission to examine the lungs and heart. This may identify an occluding thrombus in the coronary arteries or massive pulmonary thromboembolism.

COMPLETE A complete autopsy in which the chest, abdomen, and cranial cavities are examined.

HEAD ONLY A postmortem examination in which the pathology of interest is presumed to reside entirely in the cranial cavity.

NO HEAD An autopsy examining the chest and abdominal cavity without violating the cranial cavity.

autoradiography   A technique that detects the presence of radioisotopes. Autoradiography is used in molecular biology to detect radioactive probes that have bound to segments of DNA or RNA of interest. Autoradiography allows visualization of Southern and Northern blot hybridizations.

avidin biotinylated horseradish-peroxidase complex method   A commercial method for detecting antigens or antibodies in tissues. This method can be used for gene mapping, in situ hybridization, hybridoma screening, Southern blotting, radioimmunoassay, solid phase ELISA, immune electron microscopy, studies of neuronal transport, and as a means of measuring enzymatic reactions.

axial centrifugation   A method for separating serum and plasma from cells in the clinical laboratory; it is regarded as a major advance in technology because it is more rapid and reduces turnaround times for specimens.

backscatter   One of two parameters measured in flow cytometry, backscatter is detected at a 90° angle to the laser's light beam and corresponds to the fluorescence of individual cells or intracellular components stained with monoclonal antibodies. The other parameter used in flow cytometry is forward scatter, measured at 180° angle to the light, i.e., directly in front of the laser, and measures the cell's size. See *flow cytometry* in Glossary.

bacterial count A generic term for tests used to evaluate the level of contamination of drinking and recreational waters. Drinking water is assumed to be safe if no coliform organisms (bacteria normally present in the human GI tract) are found; for recreational marine or fresh waters, the EPA has suggested a geometric mean of 35 enterococcus or *Escherichia coli*/100 ml for the water to be considered safe. This is lower than the former standard of 200 organisms per 100 ml which was widely used until 1986.

basal cell carcinoma A slow-growing malignancy of the skin most common in the sun-exposed regions of the head, neck, and upper body in older individuals. See *biopsy*.

bedside testing (point-of-care testing) Evaluation of analytes in the immediate vicinity of a patient, often in a relatively critical state; devices used are often less accurate than the machines used in a hospital's laboratory but have the advantage of short turnaround time (e.g., two minutes) facilitating therapy and using minimal volumes (e.g., 250–500 ml); bedside testing may be used for pH, PO_2, PCO_2, sodium, potassium, hematocrit, glucose, calcium, and chloride. The most commonly performed bedside tests are blood glucose, blood gas, electrolytes, coagulation studies, pregnancy, and others.

beta-gamma bridge A spanning of the usually well-defined protein peaks in serum protein electrophoresis, which is seen in chronic hepatic diseases, classically in alcoholic liver disease, but also in chronic infections and connective tissue disease. See *protein electrophoresis*.

Bethesda system A system for reporting cervical and vaginal cytologic diagnoses (from pap smears) that was developed to replace the Papanicolaou system. The Bethesda system provides a uniform format for reporting results for cervical cytologic specimens and classifying noninvasive lesions. It also offers a standardized lexicon for cervical/vaginal cytopathology reports, emphasizing communication of clinically relevant information. It provides information on adequacy of specimen; presence of benign changes, including the presence of infections (e.g., *Trichomonas vaginalis, Candida, Actinomyces*, herpes simplex virus, and others); reactive changes seen in age-related atrophy, radiotherapy, IUD (intrauterine contraceptive device) use; hormonal changes; and premalignant and malignant cellular changes. The latter group includes such conditions as atypical squamous cells of undetermined significance, low grade squamous intraepithelial lesion (LGSIL) encompassing HPV and mild dysplasia/CIN 1 and high grade squamous intraepithelial lesion (HGSIL) encompassing moderate and severe dysplasia, CIN 2 and CIN 3/CIS (carcinoma in situ), and squamous cell carcinoma. Other cellular changes identified by the Bethesda system include glandular cell changes ranging from benign to malignant.

billable test A unit of productivity in the clinical and hospital (where it is known as an "ordered" test) laboratory.

binding protein (carrier protein) A general term for a protein present in the circulation that reversibly binds to molecules of various size and function (e.g., amino acids, vitamins, hormones) transporting them from the point of production to sites of use.

bioassay Any procedure that measures either the activity or amount of a substance (e.g., antibiotic, drug, hormone, vitamin) or the toxicity of a substance (e.g., a pollutant) or organism (e.g., a pathogen) of interest in an a cell or test animal.

bioavailability The presence of a substance in a form that allows it to be metabolized or to participate in biochemical reactions.

biochemical biopsy A diagnostic maneuver of uncertain clinical utility in which diagnostic chemical analyses are performed on small tissue samples (or alternatively on fluid content from cysts) to quantify analytes (e.g., hormones, metabolites) that suggest the presence of either a benign or malignant lesion.

biohazardous waste Waste products including body fluids and tissues that may carry infectious agents dangerous to humans.

biological false-positive A laboratory result that is positive in a person known to be negative for the substance being measured. The classic biologic false-positive occurs in the VDRL serological test for syphilis, which occurs in 10%–20% of patients with lupus erythematosus. See *Ulysses syndrome* in Glossary.

blank A negative control specimen required for certain assays and quality assurance in laboratory tests. Blanks assure a true negative result, allowing comparison of a possibly positive result with a known negative

blocking antibody Any immunoglobulin that

competes with another for an antigenic binding site.

block sorting test (Weigl-Goldstein-Scheerer test) A clinical test of abstract thinking that is based on the sorting of colored blocks of different sizes and shapes according to the parameter requested by the examiner. See *neurologic examination.*

borderline tumor A term used for epithelial tumors of the ovary and stromal tumors of the uterus that have a low potential for malignancy. These tumors have a survival rate that is intermediate between benign lesions and the malignant neoplasms. Other tumors of "borderline" malignant potential include adenomatous hyperplasia of the endometrium, adenomatous colonic polyps with atypia, smooth muscle tumors of uncertain malignant potential—tumors that affect the uterus, stomach, and other organs.

BRCA 1, BRCA 2 Either of the two so-called tumor suppressor genes, which if present in a woman indicate an up to 85% lifetime risk of developing breast cancer.

breast self-examination The palpation by a woman of her own breasts in order to detect tumors or cancer. Some reports suggest that breast self-examination increases the detection rate of cancer and possibly decreases mortality.

brown stains A colloquial term for immunoperoxidase stains, which are used to detect antigens in tissues. If an antigen X is present, the enzyme digests a colorless substrate into a brown pigment.

buffy coat The band of cells and cellular debris that forms between the upper layer of plasma and the lower layer of red blood cells when whole blood is spun at 5000 rpm, corresponding to leukocytes; the "buffy-crit" is usually 1%–2% and is often increased in leukemia and leukocytoses.

burr cell (echinocyte) A red blood cell with regular spines or bumps on the surface most commonly seen in uremia (a manifestation of chronic renal failure) but also in decreased potassium, gastric ulcers, cancer, venomous snake bites, and pyrokinase deficiency.

butterfly rash A photosensitive facial rash typical of lupus erythematosus that consists of reddish blush patches on the upper cheek, extending over the nasal bridge (the facial "seborrheic" region).

CAMP test A culture plate test for the presumptive identification of group B streptococci, which exhibits clearing when grown adjacent to β-lysin-producing staphylococci.

cancer screening guidelines A generic term for guidelines often promulgated by an authoritative organization (e.g., American Cancer Society) for the early detection of a malignancy that is relatively common in a particular population, the diagnosis of which in initial stages of development results in a complete cure or improved long-term survival.
  BREAST CANCER (breast cancer screening) Self-breast examination on a monthly basis, a baseline mammogram at age 40, and mammography every one to two years thereafter, depending on risk factors. See *breast self-examination* in Glossary.
  COLON CANCER The National Cancer Institute, American Cancer Society, and American College of Physicians recommend annual fecal occult blood tests for colorectal carcinoma after age 40 and flexible sigmoidoscopy every three to five years after age 50.
  PROSTATE CANCER Annual digital rectal examination after age 40 and measurement of prostate-specific antigen or acid phosphatase in the serum.
  UTERINE CERVIX CANCER (cervical cancer) Annual pap smear (Papanicolaou test) and pelvic examination after initiation of sexual activity; after three normal years the test may be reduced in frequency at the discretion of the patient's physician. See *pap smear.*

capillary electrophoresis A highly sensitive technique that allows separation of proteins, nucleic acids, and carbohydrates. It is used for analytical chemistry, biomedical research, clinical diagnosis, environmental science, food science, forensic science, and toxicology.

capillary fragility test A crude test for vitamin C (ascorbic acid) deficiency that is based on the number of petechiae (bleeding points) seen on the forearm after inflating a blood pressure cuff. The test is rarely performed because it provides little information of clinical use.

capnography The measurement and graphic display of carbon dioxide levels in the airway; capnography helps patient management by providing continuous, noninvasive monitoring of breathing in critically ill patients and early detection of important changes in respiratory status. It is used to detect a wide range of conditions including extubation of respiratory support, hypotension, massive blood loss, emphysema, chronic obstructive pulmonary disease, and pulmonary embolism.

carcinoma in situ (CIS, in situ carcinoma) A carcinoma in which all of the cytological and pathological criteria used to define malignancy have been met but which has not yet invaded beyond the epithelial or mucosal surface. CIS may regress or may be stable for a long period of time. Although the uterine cervix was one of the first locations where CIS was recognized, most other epithelia in the human body have CIS lesions. In the genital epithelia, the term intraepithelial neoplasia (IN) is used to describe the various grades of dysplasia. Grade I is the least severe and corresponds to the term mild dysplasia; grade I is followed by grade II IN (moderate dysplasia) and grade III IN (severe dysplasia), which is generally equated to carcinoma in situ. CIS is widely regarded as the lesion that immediately precedes microinvasive carcinoma. See *borderline tumors* in Glossary, *cervical intraepithelial neoplasia, intraepithelial neoplasia* in Glossary, *microinvasive carcinoma* in Glossary.

cardiac injury panel A battery of tests (lactate dehydrogenase, creatine kinase–CK, and CK-MB) used to evaluate patients who may have suffered an acute myocardial infarction.

cardiac marker A generic term for any substance that can be measured in the serum and indicates the presence of an acute cardiovascular event, usually in the form of an acute myocardial infarction; the traditional cardiac markers (the MB isoenzyme of creatine kinase–CK-MB and lactate dehydrogenase type 1-LDH1) were relatively nonspecific and are being replaced by a new generation of cardiac markers (troponin I, troponin T, and CK-MB$_2$) that more specifically reflect myocardial damage. The troponins can be measured in either an ELISA techniques or RPIA format; the subforms (CK-MB$_1$, CK-MB$_2$) are evaluated by electrophoresis followed by densitometry. See *cardiac enzymes.*

cardiac risk evaluation panel A group of tests measuring serum levels of cholesterol, triglycerides, HDL-cholesterol, and glucose to determine a subject's risk for suffering atherosclerosis-related morbidity. See *organ panel* in Glossary.

cardiac series A group of four plain chest films obtained after a barium swallow to evaluate the relative contribution of the chambers and vascular structures to the cardiac boundaries.

carryover artefact Tissue fragments from an unrelated specimen or area of the same specimen which are carried into a section of tissue being examined by the pathologist; carryovers are introduced at the time of the gross examination and are largely due to suboptimal technique by the "grosser." Once introduced, they may lead to misinterpretation of histological findings. See *"floater"* in Glossary, *sampling error* in Glossary.

cascade testing The sequential use of a group of tests to establish the diagnosis of a disease or process such as fetal lung maturity. The use of a testing cascade is required when the "gold standard" methodology is technically demanding and/or costly, and the diagnosis can under most circumstances be established by simpler or more cost-effective strategies. See *reflex diagnostic testing.*

CD4 (T4) A glycoprotein on the surface of helper (CD-4) T cells and other white blood cells. CD4 causes T cells to proliferate in response to antigens, and primitive B cells to produce immunoglobulins. CD4 also serves as the receptor for HIV.

CD4/CD8 ratio (T4/T8 ratio) The ratio of circulating T cells with "helper cell" antigens (CD4 antigen) on the cell surface to T cells with "suppressor cell" antigens (CD8 antigen). This ratio is an expression of a patient's immune competence, where a ratio of "greater than" implies an adequate immune system.

CD4 cell (CD4+ lymphocyte, T4 lymphocyte, T4 cell) A circulating T cell that helps the immune system. In AIDS patients, the number of CD4+ cells is a crude indicator of immune status and susceptibility to certain AIDS-related conditions; patients may suffer Kaposi sarcoma as the CD4+ cells fall below 300/mm³, non-Hodgkin's lymphoma below 150/mm³, *Pneumocystis carinii* below 100/mm³, and *Mycobacterium avium-intercellulare* below 50/mm³. The number of CD4+ T cells in the peripheral circulation is a critical decision point for beginning certain prophylactic therapies in patients with AIDS; antiretroviral prophylaxis less than 500/mm³, *Pneumocystis carinii* pneumonia less than 200/mm³, *Mycobacterium avium* complex, and cytomegalovirus less than 100/mm³; the gold standard method for enumerating CD4+ lymphocytes is flow cytometry. The disadvantages of measuring CD4 cell levels include low specimen throughput (±40/day) and high cost, which prevents its use in developing nations. Alternate methods for quantifying CD4+ cells are in development or implementation, including those that break apart the cells and measure the total

CD4+ (including that on monocytes) by an enzyme immunoassay.

CD8 (T8) A protein that is a marker for T cells with suppressor and cytotoxic activity; it binds to class I MHC antigens on antigen-presenting cells. See *cytotoxic T cells.*

CD8 cell (suppressor cell, cytotoxic T cell, cytotoxic T lymphocyte) A T cell with CD8 receptors on the surface that recognizes, interacts with, and destroys malignant or virally infected self cells that have certain molecules (class I major histocompatibility complex molecules) on their surface. Once the CD8 cells recognize the antigen-bearing MHC class I cells, they secrete cell products known as lymphokines, as well as enzymes, and proteins that cause target cells to burst. See the following Glossary entries: *CD4, CD4 cell, CD8.*

cell block A paraffin-embedded specimen derived from dried mucus, sputum, or debris which is present in clear fluids of pleural, pericardial, endobronchial, and other sites that cannot be processed in the usual fashion for cytological analysis.

cell-mediated immunity The arm of the immune system that acts through the "direct" cell or T-cell immunity. Cell-mediated immunity is pivotal in host defense against tuberculosis, fungi, and tumor cells and plays a key role in allograft rejection.

c-erbB-2 (HER-2/neu) An oncogene of the *erb*B oncogene family that is related to epidermal growth factor. C-*erb*B-2 expression is associated with a poor prognosis in stomach, ovarian, breast, and other cancers. The test is available in research centers.

cerebrospinal fluid A clear fluid surrounding the brain and the spinal cord; it is obtained by lumbar puncture and used to diagnose infections (e.g., meningitis) and cancers (e.g., leukemias).

chemiluminescence A reaction in which chemical energy is converted into light, allowing the detection of very low amounts of a substance of interest (e.g., DNA and RNA probes, oligonucleotides, and immune molecules).

chocolate agar (chocolatized agar) A bacterial growth medium used for *Haemophilus influenzae, Neisseria* species, and other fastidious anaerobic bacteria.

chromatography A laboratory technique in which mixtures of complex molecules are separated along a gradient of pressure or solubility between a mobile (liquid or gas) and stationary (solid or liquid) phase; the molecules are separated by absorption, gel filtration, ion exchange or partitioning, or a combination of these principles. See *gas-liquid chromatography* in Glossary, *HPLC* in Glossary, *ion exchange chromatography* in Glossary, *thin-layer chromatography.*

chromosome A component of cells that consists primarily of long, double strands of deoxyribonucleic acids (DNA) associated with RNA and histone proteins. The chromosomes contain the complete genetic information present in a living organism. The 23 pairs of human chromosomes are classified into groups that share structural similarity. The information encoded in the DNA is translated into proteins on ribosomes. See *flow cytometry* in Glossary, *ploidy analysis.*

chronic Lyme disease A neurologic condition ranging from mild (e.g., fatigue, paresthesia, arthralgia, memory loss, mood swings, and dyssomnia) to severe (e.g., spastic paraparesis, tetraparesis, ataxia, chorea, cognitive impairment, bladder dysfunction, cranial nerve deficits, myelitis, brainstem inflammation, and demyelination). See *Lyme disease.*

clinical laboratory test A general term for any test that is regarded as having value in assessing health or disease states. These tests may be divided into those that:
1. Define risk and/or disease, e.g., detection of hyperglycemia or hypercholesterolemia.
2. Classify a subject into a disease or nondisease state in which the population is bimodal with overlapping parameters, e.g., above normal without disease or high normal with disease.
3. Monitor a disease, e.g., glucose, cholesterol.

clinical pathology The field of pathology dedicated to the measurement and/or identification of substances, cells, or microorganisms in body fluids; it encompasses clinical microbiology (bacteriology, mycology, parasitology, and virology), clinical immunology, clinical chemistry, hematology, and immunohematology (blood banking).

clinical suspicion A general term for findings in a patient that suggest possible diagnoses to the physician. A clinical suspicion is a hypothesis that is then tested with appropriately targeted tests to arrive at a diagnosis.

clonal analysis Any technique used to determine whether a tissue is polyclonal and therefore reactive, or monoclonal and presumed to be malignant. Clonal analysis of lymphomas and leukemias hinges on identifying rearrangement of antigen receptor genes.

clonal expansion The proliferation of cells (arising from a single cell) that are virtually identical in structure and function to the mother cell. See *Southern blot* in Glossary, *polymerase chain reaction.*

clonality A finding that cells arise from multiple cells (i.e., polyclonal) of origin, which are reactive. Cells that arise from a single cell (i.e., monoclonal) of origin are usually malignant.

clonidine suppression test A test in which the inability of clonidine to suppress catecholamine secretion is suggestive of a pheochromocytoma.

***Clostridium difficile* colitis** A general term for colonic infections caused by *C. difficile,* which is caused by disruption of normal colonic bacteria by broad-spectrum antibiotics.

c-myc A cellular oncogene that translocates in Burkitt's lymphoma and is typically found in this condition.

coagulation factor assay Any test that measures the activity of one or more of the coagulation factors. An extrinsic factor assay is abnormal in defects of factors II, V, VII, or X. One-stage intrinsic factor assays evaluates factors VIII, IX, XI, or XII. See *coagulation panel.*

Coagulation factors

I	Fibrinogen
II	Prothrombin
III	Thromboplastin
IV	Calcium (obsolete term)
V	Proaccelerin (obsolete term)
VI	Accelerin (obsolete for Factor V)
VII	Proconvertin (obsolete term)
VIII	A composite of three separate proteins
VIII:C	Low weight component with coagulant activity, deficient in classic hemophilia
VIII:Ag	Antigenic portion of molecule
VIIIR:RCo	Supports ristocetin-initiated platelet aggregation
VIII:vWF	Von Willebrand factor, platelet adhesion
IX	Christmas factor, plasma thromboplastin
X	Stewart-Prowel factor
XI	Plasma thromboplastin antecedent
XII	Hageman factor
XIII	Laki-Lorand factor; fibrinoligane

codon A triplet of RNA nucleotides derived from DNA that translates into one of 20 amino acids.

coefficient of variation (CV) A statistical value that is used when comparing laboratory methods and instruments—the lower the CV, the greater the precision.

coin lesion A rounded, well-circumscribed, often malignant mass that measures less than four centimeters is identified by plain X rays of the lungs. The nodule may be an incidental finding in an otherwise unremarkable plain chest film. In patients with a coin lesion, details of importance include age, smoking history, geography, and previous malignancy. Causes of coin lesions include infections (e.g., abscesses, aspergilloma, histoplasmosis, and tuberculosis), benign masses (e.g., bronchial adenoma and chondroma, benign mesothelioma, neurogenic tumor, sarcoidosis, sclerosing hemangioma, rheumatoid nodules), and cancer, usually primary lung cancer.

cold nodule A focus of reduced radioisotope uptake on a ^{123}I or ^{99}mTc scintillation scan of the thyroid, which is seen in either cystic (e.g., in follicular adenomas that have outgrown their vascular supply resulting in cystic degeneration) or solid, often nonfunctional lesions; when the mass is solid by ultrasound, a biopsy is warranted because most carcinomas are cold nodules. See *hot nodule* in Glossary, *warm nodule* in Glossary.

cold scan A rounded, nonimaging region in a solid organ, e.g., the liver, when viewed by immunoscintigraphy. The significance of a "cold" vs. a "hot" scan is uncertain.

collagen vascular diseases A group of diseases characterized by arthropathies, immune complex deposition, kidney involvement, and partial or complete temporary response to corticosteroids, including dermatomyositis, mixed connective tissue disease, polyarteritis nodosa, rheumatoid arthritis, and systemic lupus erythematosus.

colonoscopic polypectomy The removal of a polyp or polypoid lesion by endoscopy. Timely removal of polyps reduces the incidence of colorectal cancer by up to 90%. In general, polyps measuring less than 1.0 cm in greatest dimension are of little clinical significance.

colorectal cancer An estimated 152,000 new cases of and 57,000 deaths due to colorectal cancer occurred in the United States in 1993. Colorectal cancer can often be detected by fecal occult blood testing. This is reported to decrease mortality by up to 30 or more percent. See *colonoscopic polypectomy* in Glossary.

colposcope A binocular microscope used in gynecology to identify lesions of the uterine cervix and to direct biopsies of the region.

column chromatography A technique for separating various molecules of different sizes. A "mobile phase" is poured through a glass or plastic column containing a stationary phase composed of solid beads, which retains molecules with certain characteristics. The molecule of interest is then washed out using a solvent.

coma panel A cost-effective group of tests used to determine the cause of a coma. The panel often measures alcohol, ammonium, calcium, creatinine, glucose, lactic acid, osmolality, phenobarbital, and drugs in the blood and urine.

commodity test Any test in a clinical laboratory that can be performed in terms of economy of scale, i.e., the higher the volume of tests of a particular type being performed, the lower the cost per unit.

competitive binding assay A method that quantifies the amount of an unknown substance in a solution, based on the variable binding of labeled and unlabeled substances to a carrier molecule with a limited and known number of binding sites.

complaint A symptom described from a patient's perspective (e.g., loss of weight, crushing chest pain, fever of unknown origin), which is often the principle reason for seeking medical attention.

complement fixation test A test that depends on the ability of serum complement to interact with antigen-antibody (Ag-Ab) complexes, which can be used to detect Ag-Ab complexes, soluble and particulate Ags, Abs, bacteria, fungi, and immunoglobulins.

computer-assisted diagnosis A generic term for any use of computer hardware and software to arrive at a diagnosis. No such system is expected to replace the diagnostic acumen of an experienced and well-trained physician. However, computer-assisted diagnosis has been used for specific clinical questions such as acute abdominal pain and may result in a 20% improvement of diagnostic accuracy and a 50% reduction in the number of perforation of the appendix and negative laparotomies.

computer-based diagnostic system Any commercially available software programs such as Dxplain, Iliad, Meditel, and QMR that attempt to simulate the clinical decision-making process and provide a diagnosis. See *computer-assisted diagnosis* in Glossary.

confidence interval A range of values for a random sample within which lies, with reasonable probability, the true value of something being studied in a given population.

confocal microscope A type of light microscope that allows results in high-resolution 2- and 3-dimensional evaluation of living cells. See *microscopy* in Glossary.

connective tissue disease (autoimmune disease, collagen vascular disease) A general term for a group of diseases that have in common various immunologic and inflammatory alterations of connective tissue. These diseases may result in the inflammation of joints, heart, muscle, kidneys, pleura, synovium, and blood vessels and include ankylosing spondylitis, dermatomyositis, inflammatory bowel disease-related arthritis, polychondritis, polymyalgia rheumatica, polymyositis, psoriatic arthritis, rheumatoid arthritis, Sjögren syndrome, systemic lupus erythematosus, systemic sclerosis, and vasculitis.

continuous-read blood culture system A device in the clinical microbiology laboratory that monitors the growth of bacteria, allowing their early detection.

control A specimen that has known or standardized values for an analyte, which is processed at the same time as an unknown specimen. The "control" specimen is either known to have the substance being analyzed (i.e., "positive" control) or known to lack a substance of interest (i.e., "negative" control).

convalescent serum Serum from a person who has been previously infected with a virus, which often demonstrates an increase in immunoglobulin G antibodies against the virus. See *acute serum* in Glossary.

copayment A shared payment by the patient and the insurance provider for a health care service; copayments range from $10 to 20% of the service's cost.

core window The timespan during which a hepatitis B-infected patient has detectable hepatitis core antigen (HBc) in the serum but has yet to produce detectable levels of hepatitis B surface antibody. See *window period* in Glossary.

Corvac™ tube (barrier tube) A proprietary blood collection tube that contains a silicone-based material. After collection, the specimen is spun, the cells and sludge in the blood are "driven" through the silicone, and the serum is easily removed for analysis of a wide range of chemical components.

Coulter™ A proprietary cell counter that functions on the principle of the electrical impedance of particles. The Coulter counter allows automated loading of specimens and electronic classification of broad categories of conditions, including the increase or decrease of red blood cells, white blood cells, and platelets in the circulation. A newer device, the Cell-Dyn, has entered the marketplace as a direct competitor.

counterimmunoelectrophoresis A rapid immunoassay that detects minute quantities of an antigen by forming a precipitin line in a gel between an antibody and antigen of different electrophoretic mobilities.

counterstain A stain of a different color (e.g., red) after a primary stain (e.g., blue); counterstains are used to differentiate among various cellular elements.

C-peptide suppression test A test used to identify the causes of hypoglycemia, based on the finding that beta cell secretion in the pancreas (as measured by levels of C peptide) is suppressed during hypoglycemia to a lesser degree in those with insulinomas than in normal persons. The test requires that the serum glucose be greater than or equal to 60 mg/dL and that the data be adjusted for weight and age.

crossmatch (serologic) An agglutination test that determines donor-recipient blood compatibility. Cross matches are of two types: major crossmatch, in which patient serum (which may contain antibodies) is cross-reacted against the donor's red blood cells, and minor crossmatch, in which patient red blood cells are incubated with donor serum.

The latter is of less clinical significance and reveals donor antibodies against low-incidence antigens.

crush preparation (squash prep) A rapid cytologic smear that is prepared by crushing (i.e., squashing) small tissue fragments between two glass slides, which are then either fixed in 95% ethanol and stained with H&E (hematoxylin and eosin) or air-dried and stained with Diff-Quik®.

curbside consultation (sidewalk consultation) An informal and unofficial consultation obtained in one of two different contexts, either by a layperson who may "corner" a physician for an opinion about a medical condition, diagnostic modality, or therapeutic option, or a physician asking a colleague in another specialty for the best method for managing a particular clinical problem

cut-off A term that most commonly refers to a critical value for an analyte above or below which the value is considered abnormal.

cystic fibrosis The most common inherited (autosomal recessive) condition in whites. It affects 1 in 1600 whites and 1 in 17,000 blacks and is characterized by abnormalities of the secretions of the exocrine (pancreas, bronchial, intestinal, salivary, lacrimal, and sweat) glands. Involvement of the intestinal glands before birth result in an increased thickness of stools during the perinatal period, a finding once termed mucoviscidosis, another name for cystic fibrosis. Patients who survive childhood suffer from chronic lung disease and malabsorption due to pancreatic involvement and rarely survive beyond age 50.

cytomorphometry (histomorphometry) The quantitative measurement of cellular features.

cytopathologic effect The typical changes that occur in virally infected cells in culture, which is a means of identifying a virus in a clinical specimen.

darkfield microscopy A type of light microscopy in which an object is illuminated at an oblique angle and appears bright against a dark background (all light reaching the eye is reflected). Darkfield microscopy is the preferred method for identifying spirochetes such as *Treponema pallidum,* which causes syphilis.

dawn phenomenon Early morning hyperglycemia that is not preceded by hypoglycemia; it is related to increased insulin requirements in insulin-dependent diabetes mellitus, possibly the result of nocturnal pulses of growth hormone.

deceleration A periodic slowing the the fetus' heart rate in response to uterine contractions.

decision level(s) An alternative to reference values, representing values for laboratory test results which, when exceeded, require a response by the clinician. See *panic values* in Glossary.

"decorate" A verb referring to positive staining by the immunoperoxidase method; when a cell or tissue has an antigen of interest, such as cytokeratin, it is said to be "decorated" when stained with (usually) monoclonal antibodies to cytokeratin. See *immunoperoxidase method* in Glossary.

deductible The amount of out-of-pocket expenses an insured individual must pay before the benefits of an insurance policy or health care plan begin. After the deductible has been paid, the insurer assumes any further costs.

deep vein thrombosis A postoperative condition in which there is clotting of blood within veins, most often of the legs. These clots may break free, a process known as embolism, and lodge in various arteries, reducing the blood flow to the organs supplied by these arteries and causing regional necrosis (death). Deep vein thrombosis occurs in nearly one-half of total hip replacements without anticoagulation, and 2%–3% of these evolve to fatal pulmonary thromboembolism. The diagnosis of deep vein thrombosis can be made by Doppler velocimetry, impedence plethysmography, compression ultrasonography (real time B mode), magnetic resonance venography, radionuclide venography, thermography, and venography.

defecography A technique for evaluating rectoanal function; a small amount of barium is injected into the rectum, and lateral radiographs are made as the patient relaxes or strains while seated on a special commode. See *videodefecography*.

defensive medicine A style of patient management defined as measures taken to document clinical judgement in case there is a lawsuit; such measures include informed consent (a document indicating that a patient understands the intended outcome and potential risks of a procedure), documentation (the formal paperwork by a physician that justifies his reasoning for managing a patient in a particular way), and aggressive medical workups, including over-ordering of diagnostic tests to exclude unusual diseases.

delta agent A virus causing a form of hepatitis first described in southern Italy. HDV is dependent on hepatitis B virus (HBV) for packaging its genome into viral particles; HDV requires that the patient be previously infected by HBV. Patients with delta viremia are positive for HBsAg, anti-HBc, and usually HBe. HDV is found in IV drug abusers, hemophiliacs, and AIDS patients, is often associated with fulminant hepatitis, and is endemic in many parts of the world. See *hepatitis D virus*.

delta bilirubin (biliprotein) A bilirubin fraction that is tightly bound to albumin with a serum half-life of 17 days; it is detected only in patients with conjugated hyperbilirubinemia in whom it represents a substantial fraction of the direct-reacting bilirubin; the existence of the delta bilirubin fraction explains the slow resolution of hyperbilirubinemia after hepatitis or after surgical correction of biliary obstruction.

delta osmolality The value representing the difference between the calculated and the measured (by freezing point depression) osmolality. A delta omolality of greater than 40 mosmol/kg often presages a poor clinical course, as it indicates the accumulation of osmotically active metabolites or toxins. See *osmolality*.

developmental milestone Any of a series of activities, e.g., raising the head, rolling over, walking or other significant points in a child's physical and/or mental development that may be used to assess maturation and detect developmental delay.

developmental "red flag" Any number of objective findings that indicate a delay in achieving developmental milestones. Developmental red flags in the assessment of infants, toddlers, and preschoolers fall into five major areas:
1. Gross motor skills, e.g., does not roll over (five months), can't hop (four years).
2. Fine motor skills, e.g., doesn't hold rattle (five months), can't copy a circle (four years).
3. Language skills, e.g., not babbling (six months), doesn't understand prepositions (four years).
4. Cognitive skills, e.g., doesn't search for dropped object (seven months), doesn't know colors or any letters (five years).
5. Psychosocial development, e.g., does not smile socially (five months), in constant motion, resists discipline, does not play with other children (three to five years).

developmental screening test Any of a number of tests or questionnaires for evaluating a child's achievement of developmental milestones.

diabetes panel A battery of cost-efficient laboratory tests used to evaluate patients with a "working diagnosis" of diabetes mellitus and to determine the level of long-term glucose control and related conditions. The panel includes carbon dioxide, cholesterol, chloride, creatinine, fasting glucose, hemoglobin A_1c, potassium, sodium, and triglycerides.

diagnosis of exclusion A disease that is extremely rare and often unresponsive to therapy. Diagnosis should only be seriously considered when all other possible conditions have been completely excluded.

diagnosis-related groups See *DRGs* in Glossary.

diagnostic accuracy The closeness of the results of a diagnostic test to the actual clinical state, which is reflected in high sensitivity, high specificity, high positive and negative predictive values.

diagnostic "overkill" The use of excessive or overlapping tests that merely confirm a diagnosis (e.g., ordering a magnetic imaging study of the brain when a previous computed tomography has already identified an intracranial mass).

diagnostic test A generic term for any test intended to establish the presence of a particular disease or pathologic entity that is not known to be present in a patient. See *management test* in Glossary, *screening test*.

diagnostic yield A general term for the likelihood that a test or particular procedure will provide information needed to establish a diagnosis.

diaphanography (transillumination of the breast) An obsolete technique in which light is directed through the breast and the transmitted light photographed. The denser the tissues, the darker they appear on the film. Diaphanography is less reliable than mammography and does not accurately distinguish cancer from benign mastitis.

diazo reaction A method for measuring bilirubin, which consists of mixing bilirubin with diazotized sulfanilic acid (the diazo reagent) to produce reddish-purple azodipyrroles.

"diff" (white blood cell differential, differential count) A colloquial term for the differential count of circulating leukocytes (white blood cells), which is usually generated by an automated cell multichannel instrument.

differential brushing A technique for localizing radiographically occult lung cancer by obtaining specimens individually from each branch of the tracheobronchial tree.

differential diagnosis A list of conditions that is known to cause a particular clinical sign or symptom.

differential growth medium A medium that has various integrated organic compounds and salts that favors the growth of certain bacteria.

digitalis A cardiac glycoside found in the foxglove plant. Synthetic derivatives—digoxin and digitoxin—are the most popular of the cardiac glycosides.

digital mammography The production of mammographic images without film, which results in greater resolution and clarity than that obtained by conventional film mammography. Digital mammography is used as a screening technique, allowing faster, earlier, and more accurate detection of early breast abnormalities.

dipyridamole-thallium scintigraphy A diagnostic procedure that permits the assessment of myocardial blood flow in patients who are unable to undergo exercise testing. See *dipyridamole-thallium SPECT* in Glossary.

dipyridamole-thallium SPECT A diagnostic test (dipyridamole-thallium single photon-emission computed tomography) that is a refinement of dipyridamole-thallium scintigraphy. DT SPECT allows assessment of myocardial perfusion without requiring exercise testing. Cardiac risks may be more accurately determined, however, by studying previous clinical evidence of coronary artery disease, and by studying other factors, such as advanced age, obesity, presence of diabetes, and hypertension.

direct diagnosis The diagnosis of a disease based on well-established and constant mutations that are directly detectable on DNA, such as sickle cell anemia and a_1-antitrypsin, both of which have point mutations that are identical in all patients.

DNA (deoxyribonucleic acid) A large molecule consisting of a backbone of sugars (deoxyribose) esterified to phosphate groups linked to nucleotides in the form of purines (adenine and guanine) and pyrimidines (cytosine and thymine). Chromosomes are composed of two strands of DNA wrapped in a double helix. Analysis of DNA is the definitive means of identifying a person's blood and body fluids for legal purposes.

DNA amplification Any method used to increase the copy number of a sequence of DNA. See *polymerase chain reaction.*

DNA analysis A general term for any technique used to analyze genes and DNA. These methods include chromosome analysis, DNA hybridization, in situ hybridization, polymerase chain reaction (PCR), restriction fragment length polymorphism (RFLP) analysis, and Southern blot hybridization.

DNA fingerprinting A technique based on the analysis of short, genomic sequences (minisatellites) that are highly specific. The likelihood that two individuals have the same DNA fingerprint is estimated to be approximately one in 30 billion and thus is more specific than restriction fragment length polymorphism analysis. (See *RFLP.*) DNA fingerprinting is useful in paternity testing, human genome mapping, and forensic medicine where it is increasingly used to identify criminals. See *chromosome analysis, DNA* in Glossary.

DNA ploidy analysis The determination of the number of single copies of a complete haploid (n) set of chromosomes present in a particular cell population. For most organisms a diploid set (2n) is normal and is a "soft" criterion that supports a cell population's relative normalcy; in some malignancies it is regarded as a positive prognostic feature in cancer of the bladder, colon, kidney, and ovary, but not small cell carcinoma of the lung. DNA ploidy analysis is most efficiently performed using a flow cytometer. See *flow cytometry* in Glossary, *ploidy analysis, proliferation index* in Glossary.

DNA probe A small, single-stranded fragment of cloned, biotin-labeled, or radio-labeled DNA that is complementary to a DNA molecule of interest; it can be detected by dot-blotting a sample of properly prepared blood, by in situ hybridization of tissues, or by Southern blot hybridization when the complementary strand of DNA is immobilized on a membrane.

documentation A generic term for any formal record of patient-physician contact with dates (and often times) that "documents" various aspects of patient management. In certain types of patient care, such as cosmetic surgery, photographs are used as documentation.

Doppler effect A physical principle based on the decrease in oscillation frequency of an object emitting sound or energy waves as it passes a point of measurement.

Doppler sonographic imaging (Doppler ultrasonography) Any of a group of imaging methods that takes advantage of the Doppler shift principle, a change in pitch resulting from the relative motion between an ultrasound source and an observer.

Doppler velocimetry A technique used to assess preterm fetuses with growth retardation, reducing the need for repeated fetal-blood monitoring, which is invasive and carries a risk of hemorrhage.

DORA (Directory of Rare Analyses) A book published by the American Chemical Society that catalogs uncommonly ordered clinical tests and the laboratories performing them. DORA tests include forensic ABO grouping, acetylcholinesterase, quantitative hepatitis C, lead in paint, latex-specific IgE platelet typing, meconium, drug screening, selenium, silicone, *Giardia lamblia* antibodies, and 1900 others.

dosimetry The science that measures and calculates the dose and type of radiation administered to a patient with a disease requiring radiotherapy; it is used for particular malignancies.

dot blotting A rapid hybridization technique for semiquantifying a specific RNA and DNA fragment. See *DNA hybridization, Southern blot* in Glossary.

dot-DAT (dot blot-direct antiglobulin test) A type of Coombs test in which IgG is immobilized on a solid phase, and the patient's red cells are coincubated on the solid phase. Subjective interpretation is eliminated because the test is not placed on a scale (1+ to 4+) as for the usual Coombs test.

dot-ELISA (dot-enzyme linked immunosorbent assay) A semiquantitative test used to detect the presence of a particular antigen by "dotting" it on support medium and probing it with an antibody raised against the antigen, followed by the use of a detection system.

double-blinded study A clinical study in which both the patients and researchers are unaware of whether a patient is in the treatment or experimental drug arm or in the placebo arm of the study.

double immunodiffusion assay A semiquantitative method for detecting an antibody (or antigen) in a system. A known antigen is placed in a well cut in a block of agar, and a test serum is placed in a second well. The two molecules migrate in a centrifugal fashion. If an antibody and its antigen are present in the system, a precipitation line that is detectable by Coomassie blue staining appears.

DRGs (diagnosis-related groups) A system of classifying patients according to diagnosis, length of hospital stay, and therapy received. DRGs are used to contain costs.

drug of abuse A general, nonspecific term for virtually any agent that can be used (usually self-administered) outside of the context for which it was originally intended. This definition is usually synonymous with illegal "recreational" drugs (e.g., marijuana, cocaine, heroin) but may also encompass controlled prescription drugs that are abused, as well as alcohol and nicotine.

dry chemistry The use of dry chemical technology (e.g., Ektachem™) to laboratory parameters. Because it does not require a water source or drainage, dry chemical methods are best suited for point-of-care testing.

dry tap A needle biopsy of bone marrow in which either blood without clot or no material at all is obtained. Dry taps are due to fibrosis, necrosis, or an extremely packed marrow and occur in 5%–10% of marrow biopsies. At least 60% of dry taps prove to be malignant; most are leukemias, but dry taps may be seen in lymphoma, myeloma, and metastatic carcinomas. Benign disease (e.g., iron deficiency, marrow hypoplasia, hemosiderosis, granulomas, and pernicious anemia) account for the remaining dry taps.

DSM-IV (Diagnostic and Statistic Manual of Mental Disorders) A document produced by the American Psychiatric Association in Washington, D.C. that standardizes the criteria used to diagnose psychiatric disorders.

dysplasia A term that signifies defective growth. It is used by pediatricians for the altered growth of tissues of an extremity and by pathologists for a histologic lesion that has premalignant potential. As used in diagnostic medicine, dysplasia refers to a histological lesion with premalignant potential that affects epithelial linings, particularly squamous epithelium of the uterine cervix, oral cavity, upper respiratory tract, penis, anus, and elsewhere; epithelial dysplasia may be induced by HPV, especially types 16, 18, 31, and 33 and is identical to the term intraepithelial neoplasia.

dysplastic nevus A premalignant skin lesion that is characterized by irregular macules—numbering from a few to the hundreds—with a central papule, dark color, and nodular elevations. See *skin biopsy*.

EA rosettes (erythrocyte-antibody rosettes) Clusters of sheep red blood cells around monocytes sensitized with sheep erythrocyte hemolysin, which occurs when a portion of the hemolysin molecule attaches to the Fc receptor on cell surfaces.

EAC rosettes (erythrocyte-antibody-complement rosettes) Cell clusters formed by B cells and monocytes when sheep erythrocytes have been sensitized with a heterophile antibody in the presence of complement proteins.

EDTA (ethylenediaminetetraacetic acid, edetic acid) A chelating agent that binds divalent (e.g., arsenic, calcium, lead, and magnesium) and trivalent cations and is used to treat lead and other heavy metal intoxication. EDTA is added to specimen tubes to transport specimens in laboratory medicine for analysis in chemistry (e.g., CEA, lead, and renin); in hematology, where it is the preferred anticoagulant for blood cell counts, coagulation studies, hemoglobin electrophoresis, and erythrocyte sedimentation rates; and in transfusion medicine where it prevents hemolysis by inhibiting complement binding.

electrocochleography A test for measuring sound-evoked cochlear potentials. It is part of the battery of auditory-evoked potential tests used to diagnose inner ear disease. There are three types of electrocochleography—transtympanic, tympanic, and extratympanic. This method is used to diagnose Meniere's disease, sudden hearing loss, and perilymphatic fluid leaks.

electron microscopy A technique used to examine thin sections of tissues and cells at magnifications far greater than that which can be obtained by simple light microscopy.

electronystagmography A battery of neurologic and neuro-otologic examinations that record eye movements. These tests are used to separate vestibular and oculomotor deficits of the central nervous system from peripheral vestibular system disease.

electrophoresis The separation of proteins according to the amount that they migrate when subjected to an electrical current.

ELISA (enzyme-linked immunoassay) ELISA is a type of immunoassay used to detect the presence and/or quantity of a wide range of antigens or antibodies. ELISA has replaced most radioactive methods (particularly RIA or radioimmunoassay) for detecting the presence of antigens or antibodies of interest because disposal of radioactive waste is a major problem. In ELISA, the binding of an antigen to a specific portion of its antibody is seen by linking the antibody to an enzyme. A noncolored compound is placed in solution with the antigen-antibody-enzyme complex. If the immune reaction occurs, the enzyme acts on the compound, producing a color change, the intensity of which can be measured by a spectrophotometer.

embryoscope A narrow-bore device, which is a modification of an arterioscope, used to perform embryoscopy.

EMIT (enzyme-multiplied [or mediated] immunoassay technique) A proprietary immunoassay (Syva Corp, Palo Alto) used for therapeutic drug monitoring (e.g., antiepileptic, antiasthmatic, antineoplastic, and cardioactive agents), detection of "abuse" drugs (e.g., cannabinoids and cocaine metabolites), and hormones (e.g., thyroxine). See *ELISA* in Glossary.

endoscopic ultrasonography A technique in which an echoendoscope is used to identify masses smaller than can be seen by conventional imaging modalities.

enteroclysis study A radiologic study in which a contrast medium is instilled by a nasogastric tube in the small intestine, and images are obtained. Enteroclysis studies were once used to identify early tumors of and metastases to the small intestine, mucosal defects (as occur in Crohn's disease), and the source of occult small intestinal bleeding. The procedure has fallen into disuse. See *upper GI study.*

epithelial Pertaining or referring to an epithelium.

epithelium A highly cellular nonvascularized layer of tissue that covers the free surfaces of organs and body sites; most epithelia derives from the ectoderm, a layer of primitive tissue present in the early embryo; epithelia include squamous epithelium of the skin, mouth, esophagus, anus, and lower female genital tract, the gland-rich mucosa of the gastrointestinal tract, nasopharynx, trachea, and upper respiratory tract, and the transitional epithelium of the urinary tract.

esoteric testing The analysis of "rare" substances or molecules that are not within the realm of the routine clinical laboratory. See *DORA* in Glossary.

executive profile A battery of laboratory parameters that may be measured annually in executives in order to detect any disease.

false negative A laboratory result from a patient known to have a particular disease, which is negative or does not detect the presence of an analyte that is usually abnormal in the disease of interest. See *false positive.*

false positive A laboratory result from a patient known *not* to have a particular disease, which is positive or detects an analyte that is usually normal. See *false negative.*

fast CT imaging A type of computed tomography that provides information about cardiac anatomy, pulmonary and coronary arteries, myocardial perfusion, and microcirculation. See *spiral computed tomography.*

feedback loop A system of checks and balances that exists in the endocrine system, where elevation of releasing hormones by the hypothalamus and stimulating hormones by the pituitary gland result in decreased secretion of hormones by the endocrine glands (e.g., the thyroid, adrenal gland, ovaries, and other so-called "end organs").

fibrin clot A semisolid mass of molecules formed after fibrinogen is acted upon by thrombin. See *partial thromboplastin time.*

finger-to-nose test A test of voluntary motor function in which the person being tested is asked to slowly touch his nose with an extended index finger. The test evaluates coordination and is altered in the face of cerebellar defects. See *heel-knee test* in Glossary.

FISH (fluorescent in situ hybridization) A hybrid of three technologies—cytogenetics, fluorescence microscopy, and DNA hybridization—used to determine cell ploidy and to detect the presence or absence of chromosome segments. FISH is used in cytogenetic studies, where probes for particular chromosomes (e.g., chromosomes 21) or chromosomal regions are used for the prenatal diagnosis of common syndromes (e.g., trisomy 21) or to detect early stages of lymphomas. FISH is simpler, less labor intensive, and faster (48 hours vs. 2–3 weeks) than classic cytogenetics.

flame photometry   A laboratory technique used to identify elements (e.g., sodium, potassium, lithium, barium, and calcium).

flipped pattern   An inversion of the ratio of lactate dehydrogenase (LD) isoenzymes LD$_1$ and LD$_2$ Normally the LD$_1$ peak is less than that of the LD$_2$, a ratio that is inverted (flipped) in 80% of myocardial infarctions within the first 48 hours. The flipped pattern also occurs in renal infarcts, hemolysis, hypothyroidism, and gastric cancer.

"floater"   Extraneous tissue fragments accidently introduced onto a histological glass slide of material from person B, which come from paraffin-embedded material floating on a water bath from patient A. Floaters are a serious and not uncommon problem in surgical pathology.

flotation method   A simple method for isolating parasite eggs; when shaken with water, feces sink, while hookworm and other parasite eggs float.

flow cytometry   A laboratory procedure based on laser-induced excitation and fluorescence of cells that have been labeled with monoclonal antibodies raised against cell surface and intracellular antigens, then tagged with fluorochrome markers; the cells can be sorted by size, intensity, and type of fluorescence, and DNA ploidy can be analyzed. The flow cytometer is used to diagnose clonal expansion (seen in lymphomas or leukemias), monitor immune status (the helper-suppressor ratio, a commonly used parameter in AIDS patients for adjusting the dose of zidovudine and other drugs), analyze DNA ploidy (generally, anaplastic tumors are more aggressive and have greater aneuploidy), and measure the growth rate of a cell population (which reflects the percentage of cells in the S growth phase). See *helper:suppressor ratio, ploidy analysis.*

fluorescence microscopy   A type of light microscopy in which a tissue or cell of interest is stained with a fluorochrome and illuminated by ultraviolet or short-wave visible light. The light is projected onto the specimen by halogen-quartz, mercury, or xenon lamps and re-emitted at another wavelength. Fluorescence microscopy thus contrasts with conventional microscopy because the tissue emits fluorescent light upon returning from an excited to a ground state. The technique is used to detect the presence of antigens or antibodies (including circulating autoantibodies), immune deposits in glomerulonephritis, and for chro-

mosome analysis. See *microscopy* in Glossary.

fluorescence polarization immunoassay (FPIA)   A highly sensitive assay in which a drug of interest is linked to a fluorescent probe molecule. When a solution containing immune reactants is excited with polarized light, the fluorescent molecule emits polarized light; if it is "stationary" (i.e., not tumbling in solution) and locked in a complex with the drug and antidrug antibody, it does not fluoresce.

footprinting   A method for detecting interaction between regulatory (promoter) proteins and DNA (DNA footprinting), as well as DNA and RNA (RNA footprinting).

formaldehyde   A highly toxic gas that is irritating to the respiratory and conjunctival mucosa. See *formalin* in Glossary.

formalin   A solution of formaldehyde gas in water that acts as a disinfectant and, when buffered, "fixes" tissues for examination by a pathologist.

forward angle light scatter   The amount of light scattered by a particle in flow cytometry, which reflects its size. See *backscatter* in Glossary, *flow cytometry* in Glossary.

four cell diagnostic matrix   A simple decision-making model for evaluating the relative merits of a diagnostic test; the matrix compares the ability of various methodologies to diagnose the presence of a disease, defining such terms as false negativity and positivity, sensitivity, and specificity.

functional residual capacity   The volume of air that remains in the lungs after a normal (i.e., not forced) expiration.

fungal serology   Infections with fungi cause the formation of antibodies just as viral infections do. There are serologic tests to detect the specific antibodies directed toward the fungi. The most common fungi (and the diseases they cause) are *Aspergillus* (aspergillosis), *Coccidioidomyces* (coccidioidomycosis), *Cryptoccocus neoformans* (cryptococcosis), *Histoplasma capsulatum* (histoplasmosis), *Blastomyces dermatitidis* (blastomycosis), *Candida albicans* (candidiasis), and ringworm. In addition to serologic tests, fungal cultures can be obtained. Specimens for cultures include skin scrapings, biopsies, and blood.

galactose-1-phosphate uridyl transferase   An enzyme that converts galactose to glucose during lactose metabolism, the deficiency of which causes the most common and severe form of galactosemia.

gammopathy An abnormal increase in the production of immunoglobulins. Monoclonal gammopathies are usually malignant and include multiple myelomas, Waldenström's disease, chronic heavy-chain disease; they may also be benign, appearing in amyloidosis and monoclonal gammopathy of undetermined significance. Polyclonal gammopathies are usually benign and appear in inflammatory conditions, such as angioimmunoblastic lymphadenopathy, cirrhosis, leishmaniasis, rheumatoid arthritis, systemic lupus erythematosus, and tuberculosis; they may also be seen in lymphomas, Hodgkin's disease, and metastatic adenocarcinoma.

gas chromatography-mass spectrometry (GC-MS) A technique combining gas chromatography with mass spectrometry that is used to analyze complex biological specimens. Both techniques require that the compounds being analyzed are in a gaseous state.

gas-liquid chromatography A type of chromatography that is a highly sensitive and specific analytic method for quantifying substances in toxicology and in research.

gas washout technique A method that uses inert gases (nitrogen, helium, neon, and xenon) to measure the airways and lung volumes.

gated blood pool scanning A radionuclide technique used in cardiology to calculate cardiac output, right and left ventricular ejection fractions, stroke volume ratio (which identifies valve regurgitation at rest and during exercise), and abnormalities of regional wall movement.

gating A process in which the observer selects a level of electronic signal above which a certain action is allowed, as in flow cytometry where only those lymphocytes that fall within a "gated" region are counted, while those outside this region are not.

gel (agar gel) A semisolid medium made from seaweed agar that is used as a support in various areas of the clinical and research laboratory. Gels are used in clinical chemistry for serum protein electrophoresis, in hematology for separating hemoglobins, in immunology for antigen-antibody reactions, in microbiology (where various nutrients are added to the agar to enhance or select for the growth of certain bacteria and fungi), and in molecular biology for separating DNA, RNA, and proteins by electrophoresis.

gel filtration chromatography (Molecular sieve chromatography) A column chromatographic technique in which gel particles of a certain size and porosity comprise the stationary phase, allowing the fractionation of a solution of molecules according to size, shape and rate of diffusion into the gel; larger molecules pass through the column and are eluted before smaller molecules.

gene The classic definition of a gene as a unit of heredity carrying a single trait and recognized by its ability to mutate and undergo recombination is primitive. As currently defined, a gene is a segment of DNA nucleotides that encodes a sequence of messenger RNA capable of giving rise to a functional (enzyme, hormone, receptor) polypeptide.

gene rearrangement The shuffling of genetic material, where introns (intervening sequences) of DNA are removed and exons are spliced together to form mRNA from which new proteins are formed. Gene rearrangement is a process typical of antigen receptor genes in which gene segments are juxtaposed or rearranged.

giant cell A general term for any of a number of markedly enlarged cells which may occur in benign or malignant lesions; although they are highly nonspecific, their presence in the proper setting supports the diagnosis of certain diseases.

Gleason grading system The most widely used system for stratifying the histologic features of prostate cancer. This system divides lesions into five groups of decreasing glandular differentiation, from well-differentiated carcinoma (grade 1) which has a relatively good prognosis, to poorly differentiated carcinoma (grade 5) which is usually an aggressive malignancy. See *Gleason score* in Glossary, *prostate biopsy, prostate cancer* in Glossary, *prostate-specific antigen.*

Gleason score A value derived from the Gleason grading system that is the sum of the two most predominant histologic patterns seen in prostate cancer. It is relatively predictive of the clinical outcome; as a general rule prostate cancers with lower Gleason scores are less aggressive and are associated with longer survival. See *Gleason grading system* in Glossary, *prostate biopsy, prostate cancer* in Glossary, *prostate-specific antigen.*

globulin Globulin is a protein measured as part of total protein on automated chemistry analyzers. It is calculated from the total protein and albumin levels.

GMS stain (Gomori-Grocott methenamine silver stain) A stain used in histology and cytopathology for identifying fungi and *Pneumocystis carinii*.

GNR (gram-negative rods) Bacilli that do not absorb the gram stain are popularly known as GNRs. The most common GNRs of clinical importance are of the coliform family *Enterobacteriaceae* (e.g., *Escherichia, Proteus, Pseudomonas, Salmonella, Shigella*). Growth of GNRs usually implies fecal contamination as in peritonitis induced by appendicitis, a ruptured diverticulum, or a gunshot wound.

gold-sol curve (Lange's colloidal gold test) An obsolete and nonspecific method for measuring protein in cerebrospinal fluid.

gold standard The best diagnostic or therapeutic modality for a condition, against which any new tests or therapies are compared. A gold standard is loosely equivalent to a "standard of practice" and may be described in textbooks, having withstood the test of time.

gout A painful condition affecting the joints that is caused by the deposit of uric acid crystals in joints and other tissues.

gram stain A stain used in the laboratory to evaluate specimens submitted for culture. A portion of the specimen is smeared on a glass slide and stained with the two coloring agents that constitute the gram stain. The gram stain is examined under the light microscope to determine the specimen's adequacy and the presence of bacteria. A positive gram stain can reveal information as to the type of bacteria; a stain is termed as gram-positive if it stains blue-purple or gram-negative if it has pink-magenta color.

great vessels A general term for the major blood vessels that enter and leave the heart, including the superior and inferior vena cava, pulmonary arteries and veins, and the aorta.

gross dictation A formal "script" generated by a pathologist to describe surgically excised tissues; it provides details on size, shape, morphology, color, and consistency. The pathologist may choose not to submit tissue in certain cases (e.g., uncomplicated hernias or a fractured femoral head in an older person).

half-life ($T_{1/2}$) The amount of time required for a substance to be reduced to one-half its previous level by degradation, decay (radioactive half-life), by metabolism (biological half-life), or by elimination in a system (e.g., half-life in serum).

HAT medium (hypoxanthine, aminopterin, and thymidine) A culture medium used in the production of monoclonal antibodies.

head and neck cancer A general term for a malignancy of the head and neck, which usually refers to squamous cell carcinoma of the oral cavity, pharynx, and larynx. Most are related to tobacco consumption.

heel-knee test A test of voluntary motor function in which the person being tested is asked to slowly touch the knee with the heel of the opposite leg. The test is part of a complete neurological examination and is used to evaluate coordination; it is altered in the face of cerebellar defects. See *finger-to-nose test* in Glossary.

Heinz bodies Inclusion bodies seen in red blood cells that correspond to denatured proteins, especially hemoglobin. Heinz bodies are seen in glucose-6-phosphate dehydrogenase deficiency, thalassemias, unstable hemoglobin syndromes, and irreversibly sickled cells.

hemagglutination A serological reaction used to screen for the presence of various antigens. A latex bead is coated with an antigen "X" and incubated with an antibody having a weak affinity for antigen "X" but a stronger affinity for the antigen X of interest. If X antigen is also present in the test serum, the linking antibody will bind to X rather than "X," thereby causing a nonagglutinating reaction (i.e., a positive reaction). A negative result appears as "clumping" of the latex particles. Hemagglutination is used in transfusion medicine to detect antigens on the red blood cell surface and in microbiology to identify hepatitis B virus, leptospirosis, rubella, and other microbes.

hemagglutination inhibition reaction An immune reaction in which an agglutination is prevented or inhibited. In this test a positive result is generated when an antigen-antibody reaction does not occur because an antigen or antibody is present in the reaction systems that prevents the red blood cells from agglutinating. The reaction is used to identify viruses, including rubella, rubeola, variola, herpesviruses, cytomegalovirus, Epstein-Barr virus, adenovirus, influenza, mumps, and parainfluenza. The technique is also used to identify bacteria (e.g., *Neisseria gonorrhea, Streptococcus pneumoniae, Vibrio cholera, Rickettsieae*), and parasites.

hematoxylin   A natural-dye stain used to examine tissues by light microscopy; it is the major "workhorse" stain in histopathology, staining nuclei and calcium-bearing material a blue-purple color. Hematoxylin is usually used with eosin, the so-called counterstain, which stains other tissues and cell components pink.

hemoglobinopathy   A defect in production of either α or β hemoglobin, which may be quantitative or qualitative, congenital, or (rarely) acquired. While the more common hemoglobin defects (e.g., HbS, HbC, and thalassemias) cause a characteristic clinical picture, some rare hemoglobin variants are not accompanied by clinical disease.

hemolytic disease of the newborn   A condition in which red blood cells undergo hemolysis due to an incompatibility of fetal antigens with the maternal immune system. The condition is caused by the production of maternal IgG antibodies in response to the fetal erythrocytes that enter the maternal circulation. If the IgG response and the sharing of circulations (as occurs in low-grade feto-maternal hemorrhage) is intense, erythroblastosis fetalis occurs. A dangerous feature of this condition is hemolysis, which if intense, results in excess unconjugated (indirect) bilirubin that overloads the infant's liver. Because of the immaturity of the blood-brain barrier, the bilirubin deposits in the basal ganglia of the infant's brain, causing cell death, and kernicterus.

heparin   An anticoagulant that inhibits activated factors IXa, Xa, XIa, XIIa, and thrombin and decreases local anti-thrombin-III, promoting its inactivation by neutrophil elastase. The interaction of heparin with endothelial cells results in the displacement of platelet factor 4, which in turn inactivates heparin.

heparin neutralization assay   A rarely performed test that may be used to monitor heparin therapy or to differentiate effective heparin therapy from the presence of circulating anticoagulants (e.g., fibrin degradation products) as the cause of increased thrombin time.

hepatic function panel   A standard battery of laboratory tests used to evaluate the baseline status of the liver. It often includes serum albumin, total or direct bilirubin, alkaline phosphatase, alanine aminotransferase, and aspartate aminotransferase.

hepatitis   A general term for any inflammatory process involving the liver which is classically caused by hepatitis A (HAV) and hepatitis B (HBV) viruses. HAV is usually acquired through the oral-fecal route, has a shorter incubation period, and is rarely associated with long-term morbidity; HBV is usually acquired through parenteral (intravenous) contact, has a longer incubation period, and is linked to hepatocellular carcinoma. Other viral hepatitides include hepatitis non-A, non-B (many of which are due to hepatitis C), hepatitis D (delta agent), hepatitis E, CMV (cytomegalovirus), Coxsackie-virus, herpesvirus, infectious mononucleosis (caused by Epstein-Barr virus), measles, mumps, rubella, rubeola, bacteria, parasites, and fungi. Noninfectious forms of hepatitis may be induced by chronic or acute alcohol use, drug reactions, various chemical agents and toxins, hyperthermia, and radiation.

hepatitis E virus   (HEV, enteric non-A, non-B hepatitis)   Hepatitis E is an RNA virus transmitted by the oral-fecal route and implicated in major epidemics where sanitation is poor, the drinking water contaminated, and the population malnourished. There are currently no FDA-approved laboratory tests available for HEV.

hepatitis non-A, non-B   All hepatitides that cannot be accounted for by known viruses are called non-A, non-B hepatitis. Until testing was available for hepatitis C, non-A, non-B virus was the most common cause of transfusion-transmitted hepatitis. The diagnosis of non-A, non-B virus infection is one of exclusion (i.e., one that is made when laboratory tests for all the other types of hepatitis viruses are negative). Those hepatitides that are attributed to nonviral causes (e.g., toxins, drugs, and others) are known as nonviral hepatitis.

hepatitis panel   A standard battery of laboratory tests that is cost effective in evaluating the clinical and immune status of a person with possible hepatitis. The hepatitis panel includes HBsAg, HBsAb, HBc-IgM, HBc-IgG, HAV-IgM, HAV-IgG, and HCV Ab. The acute hepatitis panel includes hepatitis B surface antigen (HBsAg), antihepatitis B surface antigen (anti-HBs), antibody to hepatitis B core antigen (anti-HBc), anti-HBe, antihepatitis A (IgM), and antihepatitis C. The chronic hepatitis (carrier) panel includes the above but not antihepatitis A assay.

hepatobiliary scan   A test used to identify biliary cystic duct obstruction, which appears as a filling defect in the region of the gallbladder. The test has a high rate of false-positivity because many of the patients with acute acalculous cholecystitis have fasted for prolonged periods of time. While the test is highly sensitive, its lack of specificity in fasting, critically ill patients at greatest risk for acute acalculous cholecystitis limits its use to excluding this condition rather than confirming it.

(human) herpesvirus-1 (HHV-1, herpes simplex-1) A herpesvirus that typically affects the body above the waist and is responsible for most cases of oral herpes and fever blisters. It is often accompanied by stomatitis, conjunctivitis, necrotizing meningoencephalitis, and encephalitis.

(human) herpesvirus-2 (HHV-2, herpes simplex-2, HS-2) A herpesvirus that is most commonly transmitted sexually and primarily affects the body below the waist, causing venereal, vulvovaginal, and penile herpetic ulcers.

herpesvirus-3 (HHV-3) Herpes varicella-zoster has two clinical forms: acute HHV-3 infection (chickenpox) and chronic HHV-3 infection (shingles).

herpesvirus-4 (HHV-4) See *Epstein-Barr virus.*

herpesvirus-5 (HHV-5) See *cytomegalovirus.*

herpesvirus-6 (HHV-6 Human B cell lymphotropic virus, HBLV) A recently discovered virus that infects 90% of the U.S. population early in life, causing a fever and rash. Although it is usually nonaggressive, it may cause severe hepatitis and roseola (exanthem subitum) with acute infectious mononucleosis-like symptoms; it is a major cause of febrile seizures, emergency department visits, and hospitalization. Perinatal transmission may result in asymptomatic, persistent, or transient neonatal infection. It is a major cause of acute febrile illness in young children and may be associated with varied clinical manifestations and viremia. Increased concentration of HHV-6 DNA occurs in pneumonitis in immunocompromised patients (e.g., bone marrow recipients with graft-versus-host disease) which may be due to reactivation. Testing for HHV-6 is regarded as an esoteric test and must be sent to a reference laboratory.

herpesvirus-7 A poorly characterized herpesvirus associated with roseola infantum (exanthem subitum), and like HHV-6

(HHV-6A and HHV-6B) it replicates within CD4+ T cells.

herpesvirus-8 See *Kaposi sarcoma-related herpesvirus* in Glossary.

heterophile antibody An antibody, usually an IgM agglutinin produced in one species of animal, that is capable of reacting against the antigens (usually red blood cells) of another, unrelated species. These antibodies are classically seen in humans with infectious mononucleosis where the antibodies react with sheep erythrocytes. High titers of heterophile antibodies also occur in serum sickness.

heterophile agglutination test This test is used primarily for the diagnosis of infectious mononucleosis, but has been largely replaced by rapid screening tests.

"high dry" field A colloquial term used by pathologists for 400x magnification, the combined result of a 10x ocular and 40x objective. "High dry" fields are generally used to study nuclear details and to count mitotic figures in the evaluation of certain malignancies.

high-grade squamous intraepithelial lesion (HGSIL, HSIL) A lesion defined by certain cytopathologic findings (e.g., cells occur singly or in syncytia-like sheets, increased nuclear:cytoplasmic ratio, nuclear hyperchromasia) that translate into moderate-to-severe dysplasia (CIN 2 to 3/carcinoma in situ) of the uterine cervix, a precancerous lesion. In contrast to low-grade squamous intraepithelial lesions, the diagnosis of HSIL requires that the clinician take further action, usually to excise a portion of the cervix by cone biopsy.

high-power field A unit of measurement, usually understood to be a "high dry" field, used by pathologists to assess a tumor's growth rate, which by extension, indicates its aggressiveness. The number of mitotic figures per HPF serves to determine the prognosis of certain tumors, particularly in Hodgkin's disease and smooth muscle tumors of the stomach and uterus.

histamine A small molecule that causes contraction of the smooth muscle of the bronchioles and small vessels, increased vascular permeability, and secretion by nasal and bronchial mucous glands. Histamine is responsible for the symptoms of hay fever, urticaria, angioedema, and the bronchospasm of anaphylactic reactions.

histopathologist (anatomic pathologist) A physician who has undergone a formal training period (in the United States, three or more years) in histopathology who is eligible or certified by the American Board of Pathology to interpret histologic slides prepared from diseased tissue.

Holter monitor A portable device that records electrocardiograms; it is worn for a given period of time, usually 24 hours, by an individual with suspected cardiovascular disease. During this period the patient records any unusual stresses as well as all normal activities. The Holter is used to identify unrecognized heart disease and can help identify individual stresses (e.g., personal problems) that may affect the heart.

"home brew" product A product that a laboratory develops in-house from existing products or from components already on the market; it is not intended for commercial manufacture, sale, or distribution.

home testing (do-it-yourself testing) Any form of diagnostic evaluation using a simple kit or test that is available over-the-counter in a pharmacy and intended to be self-administered. Home tests are designed to allow an unskilled individual to detect the presence of a substance of interest in the urine or, less commonly, in the blood.

hook effect An artefact occasionally seen in the immunoradiometric assay (IRMA) that appears when the hormone being measured is present in very high concentrations. The hook effect requires that two different concentrations be measured.

hospital autopsy A postmortem examination performed in a hospital or medical facility that is motivated by interest in a person's cause of death and initiated by a family member. Unlike an autopsy performed in the context of forensic science, which is driven by concern about whether the death occurred by unnatural causes, permission to perform a hospital autopsy must be given by the closest living relative.

hot nodule A focal increase in radioisotope uptake on a ^{123}I scintillation scan in a solid organ (e.g., the liver or thyroid) when viewed by immunoscintigraphy. In the thyroid, hot nodule(s) often correspond to a toxic nodular or multinodular goiter in which functional thyroid lesions suppress TSH (thyroid-stimulating hormone) synthesis. Hot nodules therefore rarely correspond to malignant lesions; the significance of a "hot" vs. "cold" scan is uncertain. See *cold*

nodule in Glossary, *warm nodule* in Glossary.

"hot seat" A location in some academic departments of pathology that provides tentative diagnoses for all tissues received from the previous day's surgery and endoscopic procedures.

hot spot A region of DNA where mutation and recombination occur at a much higher-than-normal rate.

HPLC (high-performance liquid chromatography) A highly sensitive analytic method in which analytes are placed at high pressure in a chromatography column to separate them, allowing highly specific identification. HPLC is used in industrial and clinical laboratories for pharmacology, toxicology, therapeutic drug monitoring, and analysis of hormones, including catecholamines, small peptides, and steroids. It is commonly used in sports medicine to detect abuse of anabolic steroids. HPLC may be used in tandem with various forms of liquid chromatography (e.g., gel filtration, adsorption, partition, and ion exchange).

HTLV (human T-cell leukemia/lymphoma virus) A family of retroviruses that produces a DNA copy from viral RNA by using reverse transcriptase. The HTLVs are capable of immortalizing and transforming T cells and causing T-cell leukemias. The HTLV family is transmitted by blood and mucosal contacts.

HTLV-III (human T-cell leukemia/lymphoma virus, type III) HTLV-III is an obsolete name for what is now known as HIV-1 (human immunodeficiency virus, type I), which has been intimately linked to AIDS.

hybridization The formation of a complex of complementary nucleotides; hybridization methods are a group of techniques for determining the relatedness or sequence "homology" between two strands of nucleic acids (e.g., DNA, RNA), allowing precise identification of relatively short (up to 20 kilobases) segments or sequences of DNA (Southern blot) or RNA (Northern blot). See *dot blotting* in Glossary.

hydroxybutyric dehydrogenase An enzyme once used in the diagnosis of myocardial infarction that has fallen into disuse because more sensitive tests are available.

hyperemia test (Moschcowitz test) A rarely used clinical test for artherosclerosis of the leg, in which a tourniquet is used to render the leg bloodless, after which the compression is released, and the speed at which a normal, healthy-pink color returns to the leg is compared to that of a normal person.

hyperlipidemia A general term for any condition with an increase in circulating fatty acids, triglycerides, and cholesterol which is linked to an increase in carrier lipoproteins (hyperlipoproteinemia) and the presence of degradative enzymes, including lipoprotein lipase. An increase in the lipids in the circulation causes cardiovascular disease, the major cause of death in older adults. 30%–40% of the population is sensitive to dietary cholesterol, and increased dietary cholesterol may increase the cholesterol in the circulation. Increased lipids occur in secondary hypercholesterolemia, which is seen in acute intermittent porphyria, cholestasis, hypothyroidism, and pregnancy. Secondary hypertriglyceridemia is seen in diabetes, acute alcohol intoxication, acute pancreatitis, gout, bacterial sepsis, glycogen storage disease I, and contraceptive use.

hyperlipoproteinemia A general term for an increase of lipid-carrying proteins in the circulation. Hyperlipoproteinemias have been traditionally divided into five clinical forms which have variable hereditary components and different responses to dietary and pharmacologic intervention.

hypertension An abnormal increase in systemic arterial blood pressure which affects approximately one-fourth of Americans. Hypertension is defined as a systolic blood pressure of greater than 160 mm Hg and/or diastolic blood pressure of 95 mm Hg; it is classified according to the intensity of increased diastolic blood pressure:

CLASS I (MILD)
Diastolic pressure 90–104 mm Hg.
CLASS II (MODERATE)
Diastolic pressure 105–119 mm Hg.
CLASS III (SEVERE)
Diastolic pressure more than 120 mm Hg.

Evaluation of hypertension requires clinical history for patient and family history, two blood pressure determinations, fundoscopic examination, identification of bruits in the neck and abdominal aorta, evaluation of peripheral edema, peripheral pulses, residual neurologic defects in stroke victims, chest films to determine cardiac size, and laboratory parameters to rule out causes of secondary hypertension.

hypertension panel A battery of serum tests used to evaluate a person with hypertension.

The panel measures BUN/creatinine, chloride, CO_2 content, free urinary cortisol, potassium, sodium, thyroxine, vanillylmandelic acid, urinalysis, and bacterial colony count. Causes of secondary hypertension include:

AGING
CARDIOVASCULAR Open heart surgery, coarctation of aorta, increased cardiac output (anemia, thyrotoxicosis, aortic valve insufficiency).
CEREBRAL Increased intracranial pressure.
ENDOCRINE Mineralocorticoid excess, congenital adrenal hyperplasia, glucocorticoid excess (e.g., Cushing's syndrome, hyperparathyroidism, acromegaly).
GYNECOLOGIC Pregnancy, oral contraceptives.
NEOPLASIA Renin-secreting tumors, pheochromocytoma.
DECREASED PERIPHERAL VASCULAR RESISTANCE Arteriovenous shunts, Paget's disease of bone, beri-beri.
RENAL DISEASE Vascular, parenchymal.

hypogammaglobulinemia A state characterized by a decreased production of proteins that migrate in the gamma region of a protein electrophoretic gel. Hypogammaglobulinemia may be congenital, as in Bruton's disease or other B-cell defects, or acquired, as occurs in chronic lymphocytic leukemia, which may be accompanied by monoclonal gammopathies.

hypoglycemia A decrease in circulating glucose, which is often a symptom of endocrine disease such as hypopituitarism, Addison's disease, adrenogenital syndrome, islet cell tumors, factitious insulin ingestion, nonpancreatic neoplasms, hepatic disease, and glycogen storage disease. Hypoglycemia may be associated with preclinical diabetes mellitus, follow gastrectomy, or be related to alcohol ingestion or therapeutic drugs, including sulfonylureas, oral hypoglycemic agents (e.g., chlorpropamide, tolbutamide), aspirin, phenformin, and insulin.

hypophysis The gland that regulates the endocrine system. It is divided into the anterior lobe (adenohypophysis), which contains the cells producing ACTH, FSH, growth hormone (GH or somatotropin), LH, and TSH; the intermediate lobe, which produces MSH; and the posterior lobe (neurohypophysis), which is controlled by the hypothalamus and produces antidiuretic hormone (vasopressin) and oxytocin.

hypothalamic-pituitary-adrenal axis A tightly linked interdependent endocrine unit that, in concert with the systemic sympathetic and adrenomedullary systems, comprises a major peripheral limb of the stress system, the main function of which is to maintain basal and stress-related homeostasis. The hypothalamus and pituitary gland (adenohypophysis) form the central part of the axis and are active even at rest, responding to various blood-borne or neurosensory signals, including small molecules known as cytokines. At the highest level, corticotropin-releasing hormone (CRH) and noradrenergic neurons innervate and stimulate each other.

hypothalamic-pituitary "axis" A group of feedback systems that coordinate the activity of the major peptide hormones. The hypothalamus synthesizes releasing hormones that act on the pituitary, which in turn evokes end-organ responses. The five axes include the hypothalamic-pituitary (HP) adrenocortical-ACTH-adrenal gland axis, HP-FSH/LH-gonadal axis, HP-TSH-thyroid gland axis, HP-growth hormone-somatotroph axis, and the hypothalamic-lactotroph-breast axis.

icterus index A term for the relative yellowness of the serum, an indicator of jaundice due to elevated bilirubin secondary to diseases of the gallbladder or liver.

IDL (intermediate-density lipoprotein) A plasma lipoprotein composed of protein, phospholipid, cholesterol, and triglycerides, which transports cholesterol from the intestine to the liver. Once IDL arrives in the liver, the lipid is removed by hepatic lipoprotein lipase to form low-density protein.

image analysis The evaluation and interpretation of objective features of cells or tissues (e.g., optical density of the nucleus, smoothness of the cell or nuclear membrane). Image analysis encompasses a constellation of manual (e.g., imaging cytometry, DNA ploidy analysis), computer-assisted (e.g., morphometry), and automated microscopic techniques linked to expert systems (e.g., PapNet, used to screen pap smears of the cervix). These techniques are used to analyze tumors, immune dysfunctions, and physiological phenomena.

imaging center A facility that has the equipment necessary to produce various types of radiologic and electromagnetic images, as well as the professional staff to interpret the images obtained. Imaging centers are often free-standing and financially independent, but they may be affiliated with a health care facility or hospital, operated on a fee-for-service basis, and owned by a group of investors, some or all of whom may be radiologists. See *imaging.*

immune complex assay Any of a number of nonspecific assays that were once used to monitor autoimmune diseases. Because these tests are expensive and contribute little to the treatment of disease, they are no longer routinely used.

immune complex disease A condition caused by circulating antigen-antibody (immune) complexes (ICs) which, in the presence of mild antigen excess, lodge in small vessels and filtering organs of the circulation. In immune complex disease, the size of the complexes is critical: large ICs are insoluble and are rapidly degraded in the body, small ICs circulate without eliciting a reaction, and medium-sized ICs activate the complement cascade. Immune complexes appear in lupus, periarteritis nodosa, scleroderma, rheumatoid arthritis, temporal arteritis, Behçet's disease, Reiter's disease, Wegener's granulomatosis, Sjögren syndrome, ankylosing spondylitis, bacterial infections (*Neisseria meningococcus, N. gonorrhoeae,* streptococcus, leprosy, syphilis, salmonellosis), viral infections (HBV, infectious mononucleosis, CMV, subacute sclerosing panencephalitis, dengue), malignancy (carcinoma, melanoma, leukemia, lymphoma), inflammation (inflammatory bowel disease, optic neuritis, idiopathic glomerulonephritis, interstitial pneumonitis), neurological conditions (multiple sclerosis, myasthenia gravis, Guillain-Barré disease), bullous pemphigoid, diabetes mellitus, intestinal bypass, pemphigus, primary biliary cirrhosis, Henoch-Schönlein syndrome, sickle cell anemia, and thrombotic thrombocytopenic purpura.

immune electron microscopy A technique that uses ferritin-labeled antibodies to study the structure of various intracellular organelles by an electron microscope.

immunoassay Any assay that measures an antigen-antibody response, the sensitivity of which varies according to the method. The least sensitive immunoassay is immunoelectrophoresis, followed by agglutination, single-agar diffusion double-agar diffusion, nephelometry, enzyme immunoassay, complement fixation, immunofluorescence, ELISA, and RIA, in order of increasing sensitivity. ELISA and RIA are sensitive to less than 0.001 ng/ml. See *ELISA* in Glossary, *radioimmunoassay* in Glossary.

immunocytochemistry The application of immune reactions in analyzing the presence of antigens or antibodies in cells (immunocyto-chemistry) or tissues (immunohistochem-istry). Immunocytochemistry reactions are based on a "sandwich" method which relies on the binding of biotin to biologically active molecules and the affinity that avidin has for biotin. The antigens of interest are detected by either a fluorescent molecule or an enzyme, bathing the tissues in the final step with an enzyme-linked chromogen.

immunodiffusion assay A technique that detects an antigen or antibody in serum or other flu-ids of interest. If there is an affinity between the antigen and antibody, precipitation occurs as the two diffuse toward each other. See *radial immunodiffusion* in Glossary, *rocket electrophoresis* in Glossary.

immunofluorescence A method in which a fluo-rochrome dye is linked to a participant (i.e., an antigen or antibody) in an immune reac-tion. If the component of interest is present, the fluorochrome dye will remain in the reac-tion milieu, "tagging" the immune partici-pant for qualitative (e.g., immunofluores-cence microscopy) or quantitative (e.g., by flow cytometry) evaluation.

immunogen A synonym for antigen.

immunofluorescence microscopy A technique in which tissues and cells are examined by a flu-orescent light microscope to detect the pres-ence of immunoglobulins, complement, and other immune molecules. In direct immuno-fluorescence, an antihuman antibody with a fluorescent tag such as fluoresceinated isoth-iocyanate (FITC) is incubated directly with an antigen of interest. In the more sensitive indi-rect method, unlabeled antihuman antibody is first incubated with the antigen, then with an antibody that has a fluorescent tag allowing "amplification" of the signal. Immunofluor-escence microscopy is used to study immune deposits in Berger's and Goodpasture's dis-eases and hemolytic uremic syndrome and to study the epidermal-dermal junction in bul-lous pemphigoid, pemphigus vulgaris, and dermatitis herpetiformis. See *antinuclear antibodies, microscopy* in Glossary.

immunonephelometry A diagnostic technique that detects relatively small antigen-antibody aggregates in a solution. Nephelometry con-trasts with turbidimetry, which detects large clumps and particles in a system based on a drop in light from a direct beam of light.

immunopathology 1) The discipline that stud-ies the relationship of immune reactions to the pathogenesis, diagnosis, and treatment of disease. 2) A generic term for any defect or lesion induced by the immune system.

immunoperoxidase method A technique that detects antigens in tissue sections through a series of incubations.

immunotyping (immunophenotyping) A me-thod for identifying cell surface or cytoplas-mic antigens which allows detection of clonal-ity and classification of B- or T-cell tumors.

inaccuracy The difference between the mean of a set of repeated measurements and the true value of the analyte. In general, inaccuracy is evaluated by comparing a reference method of known accuracy with a new method, usually using a specified number of patient samples.

incidental finding ("incidentaloma") An inciden-tally discovered mass or other lesion that is detected by computed tomography, MRI, or other modality performed for an unrelated rea-son. The "classic" incidentaloma is a mass of the base of the brain located in the sella turca, which may be accompanied by visual disturbances and altered pituitary hormone secretion. Most sub-jects with incidentalomas remain asymptomatic; some may have a pituitary adenoma or chemod-ectoma. See *Ulysses syndrome* in Glossary.

incisional biopsy A surgical procedure to remove part of a lesion that is submitted for pathologi-cal evaluation. See *biopsy, excisional biopsy.*

index of suspicion A term used in various med-ical fields to indicate how seriously a particu-lar disease process is being considered as a diagnosis. For example, there would be a high index of suspicion that rapid weight loss in an elderly patient would be due to pancreatic cancer and a low index of suspicion that it would be due to AIDS.

indicator enzyme Any enzyme (e.g., alkaline phosphatase, peroxidase) used to detect the presence of a particular substance. An indica-tor enzyme acts by catalyzing a reaction in which a colorless substrate is digested, yield-ing a colored material that can be quantified or semiquantified by a spectrophotometer.

indirect immunofluorescence A two-step tech-nique that is a modification of the indirect antiglobulin (Coombs) test in which the anti-gen reacts with a primary antibody. The pri-mary complex then reacts with an antibody that has been labeled with a fluorescent tag. Because the indirect method eliminates the need to purify and conjugate antibodies to a particular antigen, it is widely preferred to direct methods.

indium-111 labeled leukocyte scan A rarely performed technique used to identify local aggregates of white blood cells (WBCs) which accumulate in an infection or inflammation (as occurs in the cardiac muscle after a heart attack). The technique consists of labeling WBCs with indium-111, a radioactive tracer, and taking pictures of the body with a gamma camera.

infertility The involuntary inability to conceive, which contrasts to sterility, the complete inability to reproduce. One-half of infertility is due to female factors, e.g., fallopian tube defects, uterine and cervical pathology, vaginal disease, amenorrhea, anovulation, nutritional and metabolic defects, immunologic defects, and ovulatory defects; half of infertility stems from male factors including decreased sperm production, abnormal sperm, ductal obstruction, ejaculatory defects (psychogenic or anatomic), or immunologic defects. See *hemizona assay, sperm penetration assay.*

inflammatory bowel disease A general term for several conditions including Crohn's disease, ulcerative colitis, and idiopathic inflammatory bowel disease. Patients with inflammatory bowel disease often have two or more of the following: visible abdominal distension, relief of pain upon defecation, and looser and more frequent bowel movements when the pain occurs. See *irritable bowel disease* in Glossary.

informed consent A general term for a voluntary agreement by the patient to allow performance of specific diagnostic or therapeutic procedure. A procedure performed without valid informed consent makes the physician liable for a lawsuit with a formal charge of assault and battery. The following should be discussed with the patient: the risks and benefits of a proposed treatment or procedure, alternative treatments or procedures and their risks and benefits, and the risks and benefits of doing nothing.

infrared spectrometry The analysis of points on the infrared spectrum which can be used for analyzing solids, liquids, or gases.

in situ hybridization A method for detecting the presence of a sequence of DNA, mRNA, or proteins in their native (natural) location within a cell or tissue. In situ hybridization is a three-step process in which DNA from the target and the probe are denatured, the probe hybridizes to the target DNA, and the

amount of hybridization is measured. Cells or tissues are heat- or acid-fixed on a glass slide, denatured with 70% formamide, and bathed in a solution containing a label that is complementary to the mRNA in the tissue. If complementary strands are present, they will hybridize in the cells or tissue, linking to each other, which can be detected by autoradiography (or other techniques), then counterstained with a standard histological stain to delineate cellular, histological (tissue), or other architectural landmark. The amount of DNA probe hybridized is directly proportional to the amount of DNA complementary to the probe present in the specimen. See *hybridization* in Glossary, *Southern blot* in Glossary.

in situ PCR A form of polymerase chain reaction (PCR) in which the reaction occurs directly on/in a cell or tissue mounted on a glass slide.

intelligence quotient (IQ) A ratio that compares a person's cognitive skills with that of the general population. IQ is usually calculated as the mental age divided by the chronological age, multiplied by 100. These tests are thought to measure the complex interplay between attention, processing, and retrieval of information and the execution of the processes that are regarded as the domain of intelligence. Various tests are used to measure IQ; those that measure performance (i.e., nonverbal skills) rather than purely verbal ability are regarded as providing more objective information about a person's intelligence. There are nearly 20 IQ tests in current use, making it difficult to compare IQs and to standardize the criteria used to define intelligence. IQ tests are loosely divided according to the age being tested and whether the test must be given by a person skilled in the administration of the test or by a nonprofessional. See *psychological testing.*

ADULT
20–35   Severe mental retardation
36–51   Moderate mental retardation
52–67   Mild mental retardation
68–83   Borderline mental retardation
90–110   Average
140+   Gifted (genius)

"interesting" disease A general term for any clinical or pathologic nosology that is rare, difficult to diagnose, challenging to treat, poorly understood pathogenically, or any combination of the above.

interference microscopy A type of light microscopy that is used to examine unstained, transparent, or reflecting specimens (e.g., living cells and tissues). The image produced is similar but superior to that produced in a phase-contrast microscope. See *microscopy* in Glossary.

interferon Any of a family of immune regulatory proteins (immunomodulators) produced by T cells, fibroblasts, and other cells in response to DNA, viruses, mitogens, antigens, or lectins. Interferons increase the bactericidal, viricidal, and tumoricidal activities of macrophages. See *interleukin(s)* in Glossary.

interleukin(s) A family of factors produced by lymphocytes, monocytes, and other cells that induce growth and differentiation of lymphoid cells and hematopoietic stem cells. See *interferon* in Glossary.

internal standard A standardized, stable, and constant substance added to a chromatographic sample that neither interferes with nor has a molecule signature overlapping that of the molecular species being analyzed. Internal standards serve as a positive control. See the following entries in the Glossary: *blanks, control, quality control*.

interventional radiology A subspecialty of general radiology that provides either diagnostic information (e.g., CT-guided "skinny" needle biopsies and dye injection for analysis of various lumina and tracts such as arteriography, cholangiography, antegrade pyelography) or therapeutic options (e.g., percutaneous nephrostomy or biliary drainage).

intracardiac electrophysiological studies A study of the state of the cardiac conduction system which is performed by introducing multipolar catheter electrodes into the vascular system and positioning them in various parts of the heart, allowing simultaneous recording of multiple leads. The catheters record local electrical activity.

intraepithelial neoplasia An in situ carcinoma that is confined to an epithelial surface, e.g., those that line the female genital tract. Intraepithelial neoplasia may superficially penetrate adnexal glands, and measure less than 3 to 5 mm in thickness. The term intraepithelial neoplasia is adjectively modified according to the site of origin, e.g., anal intraepithelial neoplasia, vulvar intraepithelial neoplasia. See *CIN*.

invasion The penetration of a basement membrane by a neoplastic process, which usually implies a malignancy with metastatic potential.

ion exchange chromatography A form of chromatography in which anions or cations in a mobile phase are separated by interactions with a stationary phase composed of beads of different porosities.

ionizing radiation All particles capable of producing ions, including alpha particles, beta particles, gamma rays, X rays, neutrons, high-speed electrons or protons, and other high-energy particles. See *electromagnetic spectrum, nonionizing radiation*.

iron stores The amount of bone marrow iron. Iron stores are a crude indicator of a disease state and are graded on a scale of 0 (no discernable iron) to 4+ (heavy clumps of hemosiderin). A marked decrease or absence of marrow iron occurs in chronic disease, hemorrhage, decreased iron intake, hypochromic anemia, and polycythemia vera. A marked increase in bone marrow iron may be due to conditions affecting red blood cell production (e.g., β-thalassemia, hemolytic anemia and sideroblastic anemia), the liver (e.g., hemochromatosis, alcoholic cirrhosis, viral hepatitis), and other diseases (e.g., porphyria cutanea tarda, Gaucher's disease) and increase the risk of acute myocardial infarction.

irritable bowel syndrome (spastic colon) A heterogeneous group of chronic functional disorders that affect the large intestine and are characterized by colicky pain, general malaise, and increased frequency of bowel movements. Six symptoms have been identified that are more common in IBS than in other gastrointestinal disorders: abdominal distension, relief of pain with bowel activity, more frequent stools with the onset of pain, looser stools with the onset of pain, passage of mucus, and a sensation of incomplete evacuation. Irritable bowel syndrome is thought to be related to psychophysiologic stress. It is most often seen in anxious 20–40-year-old females. All diagnostic tests—including barium enemas, biopsies, and levels of gastrointestinal hormones are negative—and thus it is a disease of exclusion. See *inflammatory bowel disease* in Glossary.

isoelectric focusing A technique that separates proteins by charge along a pH gradient, allowing them to migrate to a point where their overall electric charge is zero or neutral. Isoelectric focusing is used to detect abnormal hemoglobins, myoglobin, and glycohemoglobin and to separate amylase and alkaline phosphatase isoenzymes. Although not widely used in the clinical laboratory, this technique is beginning to take the place of routine electrophoresis.

isotope A radionuclide of an element having the same atomic number (i.e., number of protons) as another but differing in atomic mass (i.e., number of neutrons).

isotype A subtype of an immunoglobulin that is present in all normal individuals, regardless of race.

jitter The electrical variability in the interval between two action potentials of successive discharges of the same single muscle fiber. Jitter is due to variation in the synaptic delay at the branch points in the distal axon and the neuromuscular junction.

Jones' criteria A set of criteria for the diagnosis of acute rheumatic fever. Acute rheumatic fever is diagnosed with two (or more) major criteria or one major and two minor criteria, assuming there is previous evidence of group A streptococcal infection.
MAJOR CRITERIA: Carditis, erythema marginatum, polyarthritis, Sydenham's chorea, subcutaneous nodules.
MINOR CRITERIA: Clinical findings include previous rheumatic fever or known rheumatic heart disease, arthralgia, or fever. Laboratory findings: Increased acute phase reactants, erythrocyte sedimentation rate, antistreptolysin O, C-reactive protein, increased P-R interval on EKG.

Kaposi sarcoma-related herpesvirus (herpes virus 8) An as yet-uncharacterized infectious agent, presumed to be a herpesvirus, which is believed to be the cause of both "classic" and AIDS-associated Kaposi sarcoma and body cavity-based lymphomas.

kD (kilodalton) A unit of protein size; a 100 kD protein has approximately 850 amino acids.

kernicterus The staining of certain portions of the infant brain by bilirubin that has penetrated the blood-brain barrier. Kernicterus is classically linked to Rh hemolytic disease of the newborn, in which the immune system of a mother who does not have the RhD antigen on her red blood cells comes in contact with the infant's red blood cells and forms antibodies against them. This causes a brisk hemolysis and increased bilirubin. Serum levels of 20 mg/dL or greater pose a high risk for kernicterus and are a medical emergency. Severe kernicterus has a high mortality rate, and affected infants are characterized by lethargy, poor feeding, hypertonicity, seizures, and apnea. Survivors often have dental dysplasia, cerebral palsy, and hearing loss.

kidney panel A battery of tests that is most cost-effective in evaluating the kidney's functional status, including albumin, BUN/creatinine, chloride, CO_2 content, creatinine clearance, glucose, potassium, total protein, sodium, 24-hour urinary creatinine, and protein. See *organ panel*.

koilocytosis An abnormality of the superficial cells of the uterine cervix and less commonly of the mouth and elsewhere. Koilocytosis is induced by human papillomavirus (HPV) infection, and while not a pre-malignant lesion per se, it is typically seen in HPV infection and some serotypes of HPV (types 16 and 18) that are premalignant. Its presence should alert the clinician about possible future malignancy. Koilocytotic changes may also occur in atrophy-related vascular degeneration of the cervix (as seen in menopause) or in non-HPV infections such as trichomoniasis, *Gardnerella vaginalis*, and candidiasis.

label An enzyme or a radioactive isotope of a normal molecule that replaces a nonradioactive molecule, which is used to mark or indicate the presence of a protein or molecule of interest, using an identification system such as immunoperoxidase staining or RIA.

labeling index A measurement of the mitotic activity of a cell population, which is defined as the number of cells in the S phase of the growth cycle divided by the total cells in the population.

laboratory error A nonspecific term for any error in results or result reporting attributed to a clinical laboratory or its workers. Currently, instrument technology has advanced to the point of full automation, and results are transferred and reported by computer; in this setting, it is appropriate to divide the steps at which laboratory error occurs into preanalytical, analytical, and postanalytical components.

laboratory test A general term for the analysis of one or more specimens from a subject in a site (laboratory) dedicated to assuring accurate and timely results. Laboratory tests are performed to detect (screen for or diagnose) a disease or exclude its presence, determine the severity of a disease, monitor its progress and response to therapy, and determine prognosis.

β-lactamase An enzyme present in some bacteria that results in resistance to antibiotics containing the beta-lactam ring, which includes penicillins and cephalosporins. The most commonly performed β-lactamase test is the chromogenic substrate test.

Lancefield precipitation test An immunoprecipitation test used to determine the subtype of streptococci, based on the presence of specific carbohydrates.

laser An instrument that is widely used in medicine, as both a diagnostic and therapeutic tool. Lasers are being increasingly used in dermatology for coagulation-bleaching of tattoos and port-wine nevi, endoscopy for coagulating vascular malformations, and gynecology. In the laboratory, lasers serve as the light source in flow cytometry and spectrophotometry.

late phase reaction A secondary immune response in asthmatics after an antigenic challenge or to irritants such as cold air, ozone, and viruses. Neutrophils release histamine, stimulating secondary mast cell and basophil degranulation and evoking bronchial hyperreactivity. The late phase reaction differs from the primary immune response in that prostaglandin PGD2 is not produced.

latex agglutination test Any assay that uses visible agglutination as an end-point to detect a reaction between particles and an analyte. In the usual latex agglutination test, an antibody is bound to latex beads in a solution that is placed in contact with the material of interest. Latex agglutination tests have been a mainstay in the clinical laboratory (e.g., for detecting rheumatoid factors) and have become increasingly popular because they can be formatted in a one-step process, making them ideal for home testing (e.g., pregnancy testing).

lawn plate A bacterial culture plate in which the organisms are inoculated, then grown to confluence (a "lawn") on a nutrient medium (e.g., blood agar). Lawn plates are used to detect minimum bactericidal concentration of antibiotics (MIC). See *minimum inhibitory concentration* in Glossary.

LE cell A neutrophil characteristically seen in the synovium or peripheral blood in patients with lupus erythematosus; the cytoplasm is distended by a red-purple homogeneous or "glassy" inclusion ("hematoxylin" body) with an eccentric nucleus, corresponding to phagocytosed deoxyribonucleoprotein (DNA-histone complex). LE cells are also seen in scleroderma, drug-induced lupus erythematosus, and lupoid hepatitis.

Lee-White clotting time A test formerly used to evaluate the whole blood clotting system and monitor heparin therapy. Because of the intra- and interlaboratory variability in end points, this test is being phased out.

"left shift" An increase in the peripheral blood smear of immature granulocytes with decreased nuclear segmentation (i.e., "band" forms) due to increased production of the myeloid series in the marrow, caused by acute infection.

leishmanin (skin) test (Montenegro test) A largely abandoned test that consists of the intradermal injection of leishmanin, a sterile, non-species-specific preparation. The reaction is interpreted at 48–72 hours and indicates the presence of hypersensitivity (but not immunity) to leishmania antigens.

lepromin skin test A clinical test of delayed hypersensitivity that consists of the intradermal injection of lepromin, a crude preparation from the nodules of lepromatous patients. The first phase of the reaction (formally known as the Fernandez reaction) is manifest as erythema and induration which peaks at 24–48 hours; the second phase (formally known as the Mitsuda reaction) is manifest as nodule formation, which peaks at 3–4 weeks. The lepromin reaction is nonspecific, because most normal individuals have a positive reaction.

leukocyte bactericidal test An assay of the ability of neutrophils to cause lysis of bacteria, which is decreased in chronic granulomatous disease, glucose-6-phosphate dehydrogenase, and myeloperoxidase deficiency. In individuals with normal granulocytes, 90% of the bacteria are killed in 30 minutes.

leukocyte common antigen (CD45) A single-chain glycoprotein used as an immunoperoxidase marker for differentiating between poorly differentiated carcinoma.

Liebermann-Burchard test A labor-intensive, quantitative chemical reaction for measuring cholesterol. Enzymatic methods have virtually replaced chemical methods in clinical laboratories for determining cholesterol.

ligase chain reaction (LCR) A DNA amplification technique for detecting minimal amounts of a known DNA sequence. This is similar in principle to the polymerase chain reaction (PCR).

likelihood ratio The frequency that a test result

is positive in individuals with a particular disease.

Limulus (amebocyte) lysate test (*Limulus* lysate assay detection system) A highly sensitive laboratory test based on the ability of bacterial lipopolysaccharide or endotoxin, a component of gram-negative bacterial wall, to activate horseshoe crab (*Limulus polyphemus*) amebocyte lysate (LAL) in the presence of calcium to form an active serine protease. The protease converts a soluble protein into an insoluble complex. The assay is used to detect the presence of small numbers of gram-negative bacteria in clinical specimens (e.g., in cerebrospinal fluid) and pharmaceuticals.

linear staining A pattern of immune deposition described as continuous, smooth, thin, delicate, and ribbon-like; linear deposits of IgG and C3 are seen in patients with either antiglomerular basement membrane disease or Goodpasture's syndrome when viewed by immunofluorescent microscopy. Linear staining in the skin corresponds to IgA deposition at the dermal-epidermal junction in bullous dermatosis, which is seen by indirect immunofluorescence.

linkage analysis The study of the association between the inheritance of a condition in a family and a particular chromosomal locus. For traits affected by only one gene, linkage will precisely locate the gene of interest on a chromosome.

lipid panel A standard panel of laboratory tests used to evaluate the baseline lipid status, which often includes total serum cholesterol, directly measured lipoprotein, HDL-cholesterol, and triglycerides.

lipid profile An abbreviated battery of tests performed on an automated chemical analyzer that includes total cholesterol, LDL-cholesterol, HDL-cholesterol, and triglycerides. The profile helps stratify patients according to their risk of atherosclerosis-related disease.

lipoprotein A family of lipid-carrying, water-soluble proteins which includes chylomicrons; high-, intermediate-, low-, and very low-density lipoproteins that are responsible for the transportation of cholesterol; phospholipids; and triglycerides throughout the circulation. The lipoprotein fractions determine the risk for coronary artery disease; elevated LDL increases its risk, and increased HDL decreases that risk. Direct measurement of HDL, LDL, cholesterol, and triglycerides has in large part supplanted electrophoresis.

HDL high-density lipoprotein is synthesized in the liver and intestine and is responsible for cholesterol metabolism. The higher the HDL-cholesterol level, the lower the risk of myocardial infarct; HDL is used to screen for atherosclerosis.

IDL intermediate-density lipoprotein is a metabolic intermediate formed by the action of lipoprotein lipase on chylomicrons and VLDL.

LDL low-density lipoprotein, when increased, indicates a greater risk for atherosclerosis and coronary artery disease.

VLDL very low-density lipoprotein has triglycerides as its main lipid component.

lipoprotein(a) [Lp(a)] A lipoprotein with a wide range (20–760 mg/L) of serum levels that has a lipid content similar to LDL. Lp(a) is a so-called acute phase reactant and is elevated in certain acute conditions (e.g., acute myocardial infarction and thromboembolism).

liver function tests (LFTs) A battery of biochemical determinants measured in the serum that reflect the liver's metabolic reserve capacity. LFTs include those that:
1. Measure the liver's ability to excrete endogenous (bilirubin, bile acids, ammonia) or exogenous (drugs, dyes, galactose) substances and perform metabolic functions, including conjugation and synthesis of proteins.
2. Measure substances elevated in liver disease, inflammation or necrosis (elevation of transferases and other enzymes, vitamin B_{12}, iron, and ferritin) or biliary tract obstruction (bilirubin, cholesterol, enzymes, and lipoprotein-X).

liver panel A battery of cost-effective tests used to evaluate the liver's functional status, including its ability to produce proteins, metabolize toxic substances, and detect inflammation. A liver panel measures transferases (ALA, AST, γ-glutamyl transferase), alkaline phosphatase, total bilirubin, conjugated bilirubin, total protein, albumin, and prothrombin time. See *liver function tests* in Glossary.

liver-spleen scan A scintigraphic imaging technique in which a radiopharmaceutical is injected intravenously in order to visualize metabolically active, radioisotope-labeled, potentially malignant masses of 2 cm or larger present in the liver and spleen. This scan helps determine the size of the liver and spleen, the presence of dysfunction, and the presence of focal lesions.

load A group of specimens, the testing on which is usually performed in a batch analyzer.

loading test Any test in which excess quantities of a particular substance (e.g., drug, protein) are administered to a patient to determine the ability to metabolize that substance.

locomotion index (leukotactic index) A measurement of the ability of leukocytes to migrate in response to chemotactic stimuli. Chemotaxis is decreased in the congenital lazy leukocyte syndrome or in the presence of circulating chemotactic factor inactivator, which is increased in cirrhosis, lepromatous leprosy, sarcoidosis, lupus erythematosus, Hodgkin's disease, and hairy cell leukemia.

Lombard (voice-reflex) test A clinical maneuver used to determine whether a person is feigning unilateral deafness, in which one side is exposed to masking noise. A person with claimed hearing loss will increase the intensity of his voice above the masking noise, whereas a person with true hearing loss will not increase his voice intensity.

long-acting thyroid stimulator (LATS) An antithyroglobulin autoantibody that mimics thyrotropin, which is produced by most patients with Grave's hyperthyroidism.

lot A batch of a manufactured product (e.g., chemicals, drugs, reagents, or specimen tubes) that were produced or packaged from one production run and simultaneously subjected to quality control testing.

low-grade squamous intraepithelial lesion (LSIL) A lesion defined by an array of cytopathologic findings that translate into either HPV infection or mild dysplasia (cervical intraepithelial neoplasia grade 1 or CIN 1) of the uterine cervix (a diagnosis made on histologic examination of biopsied tissue). In contrast to high-grade squamous intraepithelial lesion, the diagnosis of LSIL does not force the clinician to take further action, and he/she can either excise a portion of the cervix by cone biopsy or by LEEP or follow the patient to exclude progression of disease. See *high-grade squamous intraepithelial lesion.*

lupus band test (lupus test) The lupus band test is relatively nonspecific as similar bands also appear in acne rosacea, anaphylactoid purpura, atopic and contact dermatitides, autoimmune thyroiditis, early bullous pemphigoid, cold agglutinin syndrome, dermatomyositis, facial telangiectasia, hypocomplementemic vasculitis, lepromatous leprosy,

polymorphous light eruption, primary biliary cirrhosis, drug-induced lupus erythematosus, pyoderma gangrenosum, rheumatoid arthritis, and scleroderma. See *antinuclear antibodies.*

Lyme embryopathy A complex of congenital malformations (syndactyly, cortical blindness, intrauterine fetal death, prematurity, and neonatal rash) described in infants born to women with Lyme disease while pregnant.

lymphadenopathy Enlargement of the lymph nodes by virtually any cause. See *benign lymphadenopathy.*

lymphocyte A white blood cell formed in lymphoid tissues (e.g., thymus, spleen, lymph nodes, tonsils, and elsewhere). Lymphocytes comprises an average of 34% of the normal WBCs in the peripheral circulation, with counts ranging from 1500 to 4000/mm^3. Lymphocytes are divided into B cells and T cells, corresponding to the humoral and cell-mediated arms of the immune system, and these arms must interact before lymphocytes can participate in the immune response. Activation of lymphocytes in immune defense requires a complex series of specific interactions in which an antigen is reduced to a minimum, presented to the T cells in the appropriate context, and recognized as foreign. Once the immune system develops a "memory" for the antigen, re-exposure to that antigen will result in a cascade of responses and the production by mature B lymphocytes (plasma cells) of an antibody directed against the antigen. See *T cell* in Glossary, *lymphokines* in Glossary.

lymphokines A group of nonspecific, hormone-like polypeptides secreted by various cells of the immune system during an antigen response, which either enhance or suppress the immune system. Lymphokines are produced by activated T cells and natural killer cells; they promote cell proliferation, growth, and/or differentiation and regulate cell function by acting on gene transcription and in inflammation. Lymphokines include γ-interferon, interleukins IL-2 to IL-6, granulocyte-macrophage colony-stimulating factor, and lymphotoxin. See *interferons* in Glossary, *interleukins* in Glossary.

macroglobulin A general term for any large serum protein detected by sharp points in a protein electrophoresis.

macrophage A type of white blood cell that interacts with protein and polysaccharide antigens and "presents" these antigens to T cells. There are three types of macrophages: those that circulate in the blood (monocytes); those that remain in certain tissues (tissue macrophages, which are abundant in the lungs, liver, brain, and skin); those that arise in the presence of local inflammation (histiocytes). Macrophages secrete various substances that enhance the immune response to infectious agents and malignant cells. These substances include enzymes, interleukins, complement proteins, and regulatory proteins.

make-a-picture story A psychological test in which a person creates a story with fictional characters using cut-out figures, animals, and objects to illustrate the story.

malabsorption A condition in which nutrients from the gastrointestinal tract are not absorbed in the appropriate manner or quantity. See *D-xylose tolerance test*.

malignant An adjective pertaining or referring to either a neoplasm (e.g., malignant lymphoma) or a pernicious process (e.g., malignant hypertension). The one absolute criteria for malignancy is the presence of metastasis, i.e., the seeding of tumors to other sites in the body.

malignant cell A cell that is in a state of permanent proliferation and is capable of metastasis. Malignant cells are defined by various changes in structure and function. These changes enable malignant cells to invade normal tissues and grow independently from the immune system's control; normally, the immune system prevents cells from dividing rapidly and from developing in other parts of the body.

malnutrition A general term for a number of nutritional deficiencies which may be related to poverty, alcohol, mental disorders, infection (e.g., tuberculosis), or cancer, or may occur in a hospital setting when a patient is receiving all his/her nutrients intravenously. Once diagnosed, the severity of the malnutrition and type of nutritional deficiency must be determined through a battery of laboratory tests, including measurement of serum levels of folic acid, iron, magnesium, protein, and vitamin B_{12}.

management test A general term for any test specifically intended to guide the therapy of a disease (e.g., diabetes mellitus, hypertension) known to be present in a patient. See *diagnostic test* in Glossary, *screening test*.

mandatory reporting The obligatory reporting of a particular disease to a health authority. Mandatory reporting is a responsibility of health professionals for communicable diseases and for abuse (e.g., child abuse, spousal abuse). In infectious diseases, the state boards of health maintain records and collect data on diseases that represent a hazard to the public.

mass spectroscopy (mass spectrometry) An analytical method for measuring molecular mass and structure, in which a specimen is ionized and passed through either an electron beam (for liquid samples) or spark (for solids). Mass spectroscopy may be coupled with gas chromatography to increase the method's sensitivity.

McMurray's test A clinical test used to identify the presence of a torn meniscus. The patient lies on his/her back with the knee completely flexed. The examiner rotates the foot fully outward while slowly extending the knee. A painful click in outward rotation indicates a torn medial meniscus; a painful click in inward rotation indicates a torn lateral meniscus.

Meckel's diverticulum scan (ectopic gastric mucosa scintigraphy) A rarely performed clinical test in which the radionuclide technetium-99m is administered orally, and abdominal images are obtained using a gamma camera. This technique can be used to identify acid-secreting cells outside of the stomach, a finding typical of Meckel's diverticulum, a developmental defect of the small intestine.

medical laboratory technician A person who is trained to perform most laboratory tests but is not authorized to report on or perform the most technically demanding tests. See *medical technologist* in Glossary.

medical technologist A laboratory worker with at least four years of formal college or university education (a bachelor of science degree in medical technology), who is trained in the performance of various techniques in clinical pathology, including hematology, microbiology, chemistry, blood banking, immunology. See *medical laboratory technician* in Glossary.

medium (microbiology, growth media) Liquid or solid matrix (e.g., agar) with nutrients that support the growth of microorganisms. Differential media are often solid and contain various chemical and other substances, e.g., colorants, that may be produced by certain microorganisms, aiding in their identification. Enrichment media are often liquid and contain specific nutrients giving one or more of the microorganisms a growth advantage. Selective media are those in which nutrients are added to either promote or slow the growth of one or more group of bacteria, giving the desired organisms a "selective" growth advantage.

melanoma (malignant melanoma) A highly malignant tumor of melanocytic cells that most often arises in the skin and is diagnosed by biopsy. Any dark area or spot on the skin that undergoes a change in color or increase in size should be seen by a physician experienced in examining pigmented lesions. The vast majority of pigmented lesions are benign, e.g., birthmarks. See *biopsy.*

metabolic acidosis A condition in which there is decreased pH in the circulation due to either an increase in acids or the loss of bicarbonate.

metabolic alkalosis A condition in which there is increased pH due to either a decrease in acids or an excess of bicarbonate.

metastasis The spread of a malignant neoplasm and eventual development into a secondary focus of malignancy.

metastatic tumor cell A cell that has undergone multiple changes allowing it to invade, disseminate, implant, survive, and grow at sites distant from the site of origin. See *malignant cell* in Glossary.

method of choice A general term for any diagnostic or therapeutic maneuver that is preferred in practice, based on its ease of performance or diagnostic efficiency.

methyl red test A test used in clinical microbiology to differentiate among *Enterobacteriaceae*, a family of bacteria. *Enterobacter aerogenes* and *Klebsiella* species are negative.

microinvasive carcinoma A superficially invasive epithelial (squamous) cell malignancy, which has a specific significance in gynecologic pathology. In the uterine cervix, microinvasive carcinoma penetrates less than 5 mm from the base of the epithelium or less than 7 mm in horizontal spread. See *carcinoma in situ* in Glossary.

microscopic hematuria (microhematuria) Hematuria that is so minimal that it can only be confirmed by light microscopic examination of the urine. See *urinalysis.*

microscopy The examination of a tissue or cell

of interest using a light microscope with an incandescent light bulb. The light microscope can be modified by changing the light source (e.g., with a fluoresent lamp to detect immune reactions) or by modifying the path of the light itself (e.g., with polarization filters to detect various crystals seen in synovial fluid in gout). The "workhorse" light microscope in today's laboratory is binocular and compound, having 10x to 15x (x meaning magnifications) ocular lenses and multiple objectives on a rotating "nose-piece" ring. Histopathologists often use the terms "scanning" power for 25x to 40x, "low" power for 100x, "high" power for 400x, "high dry" power for 600x, and "oil" for 1000x.

Millon clinical multiaxial inventory (test) A psychological test which consists of questions that provide information for classifying a person's personality type into one of 20 categories; the test has been used in diagnosing personality disorders in the Diagnosis and Statistical Manual of the American Psychiatric Association. See *DSM-IV* in Glossary.

Mills' test A test for lateral epicondylitis (tennis elbow) which is positive if pain is evoked in the lateral epicondyle of the humerus by extension of the forearm, when the wrist is flexed and the forearm is fully pronated.

minimum bactericidal concentration (antibiotic susceptibility testing) The lowest concentration of an antibiotic that kills at least 99.9% of the bacteria in specimen. Minimum bactericidal concentration reflects a bacterium's susceptibility to an antibiotic.

minimum inhibitory concentration (MIC) The minimal amount of antibiotic necessary to inhibit bacterial growth from a clinical isolate, which serves as a form of antimicrobial susceptibility testing. In a laboratory test, the lowest concentration of an antibiotic to be administered to a patient is extrapolated from the amount of inhibition of bacterial growth in culture. This is most commonly determined by the diameter of nongrowth surrounding a paper disk impregnated with antibiotics, the so-called "disk diffusion test." Note: in vitro sensitivity to an antibiotic does not guarantee response to that antibiotic in a patient.

mirror test A crude clinical test used to obtain material from the trachea; the patient coughs on a mirror held in place in the upper larynx.

miscall A diagnostic error, as in a pathologist miscalling a benign tumor as malignant. See *laboratory error* in Glossary, *misdiagnosis* in Glossary.

misdiagnosis The incorrect diagnosis of a morbid condition. By itself, misdiagnosis is insufficient to result in a successful lawsuit for malpractice if the physician can support the contention that he exercised reasonable and prudent medical judgement in arriving at a diagnosis in accordance with accepted medical standards.

mixed agglutination reaction A method used in the blood bank to detect cross-reacting antigens on different types of cells. "Indicator" cells that were previously coated with antibodies are added to test cells; the reaction is positive if aggregates containing both cell types are formed or if the indicator cells bind to the test cells bound to a glass slide.

molecular biology Molecular biology seeks to understand the mechanisms controlling gene expression in physiological and "disease" states; ultimately, it may provide the tools necessary for diagnosing and treating genetic diseases. See *DNA* in Glossary.

molecular genetic analysis A nonspecific term for the detection or diagnosis of a disease by analysis of segments of DNA or RNA, rather than by indirect methods. See *molecular biology* in Glossary.

molecular medicine A general term for the application of the techniques of molecular biology to clinical medicine. Molecular medicine encompasses "diagnostic" methods (e.g., Southern blot hybridization, DNA amplification by PCR), the use of agents produced by recombinant DNA techniques (e.g., biological response modifiers and vaccines), and more recently the insertion and manipulation of the genome itself.

molecular prognostication A general term for the use of the techniques of molecular biology to determine the prognosis of a malignant, premalignant, or other disease process.

monoclonal antibody (MAb) A highly specific antibody that is formed either naturally (e.g., in cold hemagglutinin disease, plasma cell dyscrasia) or can be produced synthetically in a laboratory by fusing an immortal cell (mouse myeloma) to a cell producing an antibody against a desired antigen.

monoclonal immunoglobulin A protein produced by clonally expanded immunoglobulin-producing cells, as seen in various malignancies, such as multiple myeloma, Waldenström's macroglobulinemia, and leukemia. Monoclonal immunoglobulin production may occur in other malignancies (e.g., adenocarcinoma and carcinomas of the bladder, cervix and liver), as well as angiosarcoma and Kaposi sarcoma.

monocyte A type of white blood cell that is present in the circulation and comprises 2%–5% of the circulating white blood cells. Monocytes contain enzymes and certain surface proteins that enhance the immune system.

Morton's test A clinical maneuver used to identify metatarsal pain, which is positive when lateral pressure across the forefoot elicits pain.

motility test A test used in the clinical laboratory to detect the movement of bacteria on soft agar, which is indirect evidence of the presence of flagella, (found in many *Enterobacteriaceae)*, other gram-negative organisms, *Bacillus* species, *Corynebacterium* species, and *Listeria* species.

mRNA (messenger ribonucleic acid) The reverse template "message" from DNA that is required for protein synthesis. Under most circumstances, the "message" flows from the DNA to the RNA, which is then translated into protein.

mucicarmine stain A stain used in surgical pathology that is strongly positive in biopsies of the gastrointestinal tract and certain fungi, particularly *Cryptococcus neoformans.*

multiple myeloma A malignancy composed of tumor cell aggregates in the bone marrow and in extramedullary sites. The most characteristic feature of multiple myeloma is the presence of a prominent increase in monoclonal immunoglobulins, often light chains, which are identified in serum and urine.

multiple puncture test A general term for any of a number of now-abandoned tests for sensitivity to tuberculin, which is due to past exposure to tuberculosis.

multiple sclerosis A demyelinating disease in which infiltrating white blood cells cause a breakdown of the myelin (the insulating layer of lipid that covers nerves). Multiple sclerosis is most common in young female adults, affecting 1 in 2500 in the United States, and is more common in cold-to-temperate climates. It is characterized by waxing and waning or slowly progressive neurologic changes, with tingling of nerves, gait and visual defects, muscular weakness, absent abdominal reflexes, hyperactive tendon reflexes, cerebellar ataxia, retrobulbar neuritis, loss of proprioceptive sense, spastic weakness of legs, and vertigo. The cause of MS is uncertain, although it is thought to be autoimmune in nature. Diagnosis is based on the clinical suspicion, the finding of multiple defects by CT and MRI, oligoclonal elevation of IgG in the cerebrospinal fluid (present in 90% of patients), and "evoked potentials" by electroencephalography in the visual cortex and brainstem. All of these tests are nonspecific and must be correlated with the clinical findings. The definitive diagnosis of multiple sclerosis requires a brain biopsy, although this is rarely performed.

mumps skin test An obsolete and nonspecific clinical test for immunity to mumps antigens, which has been replaced by serologic tests of specific mumps immunoglobulins.

Murphy's kidney punch (Murphy's test) A clinical test in which the examiner makes jabbing thrusts under the patient's 12th rib(s), evoking pain and/or tenderness in the presence of renal inflammation or infection.

myasthenia gravis An autoimmune disease characterized by weakness and muscle fatigue. The neuromuscular junctions in myasthenia gravis have fewer acetylcholine receptors, simplified synaptic folds, and widened synaptic spaces. The condition is characterized by ptosis, diplopia, weakness, and fatigability of skeletal muscles; it may be associated with thymoma, thymic hyperplasia, other autoimmune diseases or phenomena (e.g., thyroiditis, Graves disease, rheumatoid arthritis, and lupus erythematosus). The diagnosis is established by the anticholinesterase test (Tensilon test), repetitive nerve stimulation, assay for anti-acetylcholine receptors, and single fiber electromyography

mycobacteria (*Mycobacterium*) A genus of bacteria of the family *Mycobacteriaceae* that contains the tuberculosis bacteria, *Mycobacterium tuberculosis*. See *acid-fast stain, tuberculosis test.*

mycosis A general term for a fungal infection. The most common fungal infections are the various clinical forms of candidiasis, caused by *Candida* albicans. *Candidiasis* occurs in the vagina in adult women, in the mouth in children, and the esophagus in patients with AIDS and other immunocompromised states.

Naffziger's test A clinical test used to identify compression of nerve roots in the cervical spine, which is based on an intensification of the pain and paresthesias ("tingling") of the hand and fingers; the examiner exerts pressure on the scalenus anterior muscles.

natural antibody (normal antibody) An antibody present in the circulation, without there being known previous exposure to the antigen; anti-A and anti-B of the ABO blood group are the only naturally occurring antibodies that are virtually always present in subjects who lack the relevant antigen.

natural killer cell (NK cell) A type of white blood cell (null cell or large granular lymphocyte) comprising 3%–5% of peripheral leukocytes, that has an intrinsic ability to kill various cells (e.g., virus-transformed fibroblasts, solid or hematopoietic tumor cells, microorganisms, embryologic, marrow and thymic cells).

negative predictive value The proportion of subjects with a negative test result who do not have a disease. See *positive predictive value* in Glossary.

neonatal panel/profile A battery of low-cost laboratory tests performed on the serum and urine of newborn infants to identify potentially treatable diseases or abnormalities. The typical neonatal panel/profile measures albumin, (total) bilirubin, blood group (ABO and Rh), BUN (blood urea nitrogen), calcium, electrolytes (sodium, potassium, chloride), carbon dioxide, and glucose. See *neonatal screen.*

neoplasm Any autonomous proliferation of cells, classified according to:

BEHAVIOR Benign, borderline, or malignant.

DEGREE OF DIFFERENTIATION Well-differentiated (i.e., the neoplastic cell simulates its parent or progenitor cell) or poorly-differentiated (i.e., the neoplastic cell is bizarre and grows aggressively).

EMBRYOLOGIC ORIGIN Epithelial, lymphoproliferative, mesenchymal, neural crest, etc.

GROSS APPEARANCE Well-circumscribed or infiltrative; benign neoplasms are generally slow-growing, well-circumscribed, often invested with a fibrous capsule, and often only symptomatic if they compromise a confined space (e.g., massive meningioma of the cranial cavity) or encirclement of vital blood vessels; malignant neoplasms are often aggressive with increased mitotic activity, necrosis and invasion of adjacent structures and metastatic potential. See *metastasis* in Glossary.

nephelometry A technique that measures the

concentration of substances by means of light scattering by the suspended particles. It is most commonly used to detect immune complexes when the participating antigen or antibody is unknown. See *turbidimetry*.

neuraminidase (exo-α-sialidase, acylneuraminyl hydrolase) An enzyme located on the extracellular portion of membrane-bound glycoproteins, glycolipids, and proteoglycans. Neuraminidase and hemagglutinin are located on the "spikes" of influenza virus.

neuraminidase inhibition test A laboratory method used to identify strains of influenza virus based on the ability of specific antibodies to inhibit the enzymatic activity of types of neuraminidase present on the outer coat of influenza viruses.

neuroendocrine system A system derived from the primitive neural crest which is composed of neuroendocrine cells and neuroepithelial bodies. Each organ has a neuroendocrine component, and neuroendocrine components are scattered throughout the body.

neuron-specific enolase (NSE) An enzyme that is present in neurons, neuroendocrine cells and tumors, astrocytomas, medullary carcinoma of the thyroid, pituitary adenomas, and endocrine neoplasms of the pancreas and gastrointestinal tract. NSE is also present in benign and/or non-neuronal tissues and tumors (meningioma, fibroadenoma, breast, kidney, and ovarian cancer, and rarely in lymphomas).

neurotransmitter Any of a number of small molecules present at synapses or neuromuscular junctions that are capable of transmitting an electrical impulse by binding to a receptor. Virtually any molecule capable of modifying neural signals may act as a neurotransmitter.

neutralizing antibody (neutralization assay) An immunoglobulin produced by the host as a defense against bacteria, reducing its infectivity. Neutralization assays are used in the laboratory as serologic tests to detect an individual's previous exposure to a specific microorganism. Alternatively, the patient's serum or body fluid can be tested for the presence of an antigen (e.g., a virus) by performing a neutralization assay with a standardized antibody or antitoxin.

neutron activation analysis A highly sensitive method for quantifying elements in nanogram amounts.

ninhydrin test A rarely used term for the use of the ninhydrin reagent to stain amino acids in paper chromatography, thin-layer chromatography, and column chromatography.

NMR spectroscopy A technique that analyzes the magnetic structure of molecules, which is used in research to analyze the three-dimensional structure of proteins.

noninvasive (non-interventional) An adjective referring or pertaining to any form of therapy in which the integrity of mucocutaneous barriers is not violated.

normoblast An immature nucleated red blood cell (erythrocyte).

Northern blot A technique used in research to detect the presence of specific messenger RNA (mRNA) molecules, which "translate" the information encoded by DNA into proteins. See *polymerase chain reaction, Southern blot* in Glossary, *Western blot*.

nuclear medicine A field of medicine that uses radioisotopes to diagnose (diagnostic nuclear medicine) and treat disease.

nuclease A general term for any enzyme that cleaves the phosphodiester bond of polynucleotide chains (i.e., nucleic acids DNA and RNA) which are produced by most biological systems; nucleases can be either exonucleases or endonucleases.

nucleic acid A molecule that is either a double-stranded chain of DNA nucleotides (carrying genetic information) or a single-stranded chain of RNA (critical in protein synthesis). The individual units of nucleic acids are pyrimidine nucleotides (cytosine, thymine, and uracil) and purine nucleotides (adenine and guanine).

5′-nucleotidase A membrane enzyme that hydrolyzes 5′-phosphate groups of nucleotides; it is produced primarily in the liver and present in both the liver and bile ducts.

nucleus The cell "organelle" that contains the genetic material (DNA) and the replicative and transcriptional machinery (RNA and binding proteins) necessary to copy genomic information and encode the structural and functional proteins required for cell function.

oat cell carcinoma A subtype of small cell carcinoma of the lung that is characterized by a dense hyperchromatic oval nucleus, often with a vague central groove and minimal cytoplasm. Oat cell carcinomas have neurosecretory granules containing hormones. They are highly aggressive, with a three-month survival without therapy, often accompanied by cerebellar degeneration; 80% have metastases to the brain.

obturator test (obturator sign) A clinical test evaluated on a person who is lying on his/her back with the right hip and knee flexed and rotated internally and externally. Pain in the right lower quadrant is due to irritation of the medial internal obturator muscle and is "classically" associated with appendicitis but may also occur in right pelvic abscesses.

occult blood Blood that is inapparent to the naked eye. When used by health professionals, the term is understood to mean blood in the stool, which may be an early indicator of colorectal cancer, but it also may be seen in amebiasis, heavy metal poisoning, and acute ischemia. See *occult blood testing.*

occult infection An infection that is first recognized by secondary manifestations. Occult infections are most often caused by a bacterial infection in an obscure site, such as an abscess of the subphrenic or other intraabdominal region.

occult primary malignancy (occult cancer, unknown primary) A malignancy of unknown origin that is asymptomatic and first manifests itself as metastases or secondary (paraneoplastic) phenomena. The finding of an occult primary cancer is often associated with a poor prognosis. Occult primary cancers are problematic for the physician treating the patient, because appropriate therapy requires that the primary cancer be eliminated, and many remain obscure despite an aggressive diagnostic workup. Certain malignancies metastasize with greater than expected frequency. For example, of occult primary malignancies occurring in the brain, up to 85% of the primary cancers arises in the lungs

oncogenic virus Any DNA virus (e.g., human papillomavirus) or RNA virus (e.g., retrovirus) that is capable of causing malignant transformation of cells.

one-stage factor assay Any of a number of coagulation studies intended to detect deficiencies of a specific coagulation factor.

ONPG test (O-nitrophenyl β-D-galactopyranoside test) A test used in microbiology to detect b-galactosidase, which is present in *Escherichia coli* and *Pseudomonas cepacia.*

opiate A family of drugs of abuse, some of which are used therapeutically. This group includes codeine, morphine, and heroin.

opportunistic Pertaining to or referring to a microorganism that may be part of the normal nonpathogenic flora, which causes disease should the opportunity arise, e.g., through a compromise of the host's immune status.

opportunistic infection An infection caused by a microorganism, usually bacterial, that is part of the normal "flora" and becomes pathogenic when the host's immune system is compromised by an unrelated disease, e.g., AIDS, chemotherapy, or diabetes mellitus.

organ panel A battery of tests intended to evaluate one specific organ system, such as the thyroid gland.

osmotic fragility The susceptibility of red blood cells to water-induced rupture. Since the red blood cell membrane has limited distensibility, cells with weaker membranes are more susceptible to rupture, as occurs in hereditary spherocytosis. Osmotic fragility is also increased in hereditary elliptocytosis and in aging red blood cells. Osmotic fragility is decreased in jaundice, iron therapy, thalassemia, sickle cell anemia, and after splenectomy.

osteoporosis A condition characterized by the loss of bone. Osteoporosis is the most common disease of elderly females and causes more than 100,000 fractures per year in the United States (vertebrae 54%, hip 23%, distal forearm 17%). The typical patient at high risk for osteoporosis is female, white, elderly, thin, and immobilized. Primary involutional osteoporosis is divided into type I ("postmenopausal") osteoporosis, which is relatively common and primarily affects older women, and type II ("age-related") osteoporosis, which is less common. Secondary osteoporosis is "driven" by nonosseous factors, which may be related to therapy, surgery (early oophorectomy, orchiectomy, subtotal gastrectomy), drugs (corticosteroids, anticonvulsants, heparin, L-thyroxine), endocrine (hypogonadism, increased adrenocortical, parathyroid, or thyroid activity), gastrointestinal (alactasia, malabsorption), bone marrow (mastocytosis, metastatic malignancy, multiple myeloma), osseous disease (osteogenesis imperfecta, Marfan syndrome, rheumatoid arthritis), and other diseases, e.g., immobilization, chronic obstructive pulmonary disease.

oxidase test A color test used in microbiology to detect the presence of intracellular enzymes and cytochrome oxidase in bacteria.

The test is based on the production of p-phenylenediamine and is used to identify anaerobes and facultative anaerobes, in which it is present.

p53 A tumor-suppressing protein encoded by the proto-oncogene p53. In its native form, p53 inhibits cell growth and transformation by activating the transcription of genes that suppress cell proliferation.

pan-B-cell marker Any of a number of antigens present on the surface of all normal B cells (lymphocytes). CD19 is considered the best pan-B cell marker and, like surface immunoglobulins, indicates that the cells are of B lineage and therefore involved in the production of antibodies. Other pan-B cell markers are CD20 and CD24. Testing for pan-B cell markers is generally a tool for evaluating patients with unusual immune defects. See *pan-T-cell marker* in Glossary.

panic values Laboratory results from patient specimens that must be reported immediately to the clinician; they are often of a nature requiring urgent therapeutic action.

PANIC VALUES

ANALYTE	SI UNITS	US UNITS
Calcium	<1.65 mmol/L	<6.6 mg/dl
	2.22 mmol/L	12.9 mg/dl
Glucose	<2.60 mmol/L	<46 mg/dl
	26.9 mmol/L	484 mg/dl
K⁺	<2.8 mmol/L	<2.8 mEq/L
	6.2 mmol/L	6.2 mEq/L
	8.0 mmol/L	
	if hemolyzed	
Na⁺	<120 mmol/L	<120 mEq/L
	158 mmol/L	158 mEq/L
CO₂ in	<11 mmol/L	<11 mMol
plasma	40 mmol/L	40 mMol

pan-T-cell marker Any of a group of antigens present on the surface of all normal T cells (lymphocytes). The presence and ratios of T-cell markers indicate a person's immune status. In AIDS patients, the ratio of helper T cells (designated as CD4 or T4 cells) to suppressor T cells (CD8 or CD8 cells) is closely monitored because a decrease in this ratio is commonly associated with clinical deterioration and worsening of disease. See *flow cytometry* in Glossary, *helper:suppressor cell ratio*, *pan-B-cell marker* in Glossary.

pap "mill" A general term for a laboratory that encourages cytotechnologists to screen an unlimited number of pap smears by paying them on a per-case basis. Pap mills became a focus of national attention when evidence mounted that the high volume

(200 or more cases a day per screener) resulted in an increased number of missed malignant and premalignant lesions. Most states have enacted legislation limiting the number of pap smears that one technologist can screen a day.

PapNet See *image analysis* in Glossary.

paraffin section (permanent section) A thin (4–7 millimeter in thickness) section of tissue obtained by a biopsy or other surgical procedure, surrounded by paraffin, which is processed by various steps, sliced with a microtome, stained, then mounted on a glass slide and examined by light microscopy. In contrast to the "frozen section" (or quick section), in which a tissue is examined within minutes of its removal from a patient, "paraffin section" tissues are available for interpretation by the pathologist in no less than six to eight hours. The tissues are fixed in formalin and bathed in a series of solutions (in order, after formalin, 70% alcohol, 95% alcohol, 100% alcohol, and xylene) that dry the tissue and allow its infiltration with paraffin, the optimal embedding material for histologic evaluation of tissue. See *biopsy, frozen section, hematoxylin* in Glossary.

parakeratosis The finding of parakeratotic cells on an epithelial surface, which is usually benign and is a protective reaction to inflammation or chronic trauma. It occurs in uterine prolapse or pessary-induced irritation and may also occur in human papilloma virus (HPV) infections of the cervix, squamous intraepithelial lesions, or squamous cell cancer.

paraneoplastic syndrome A family of conditions caused by the indirect effects of malignancy, which may be the first sign of a neoplasm or its recurrence. Paraneoplastic syndromes occur in more than 15% of all malignancies, are due to the production of hormones and other factors, and often regress with adequate treatment of the primary tumor. The range of expression is broad and includes tumor-related weight loss, hormonal effects, peripheral neuropathy, myopathy, central nervous system and spinal cord degeneration and inflammation, leukemoid reaction, reactive eosinophilia, peripheral cytoses or cytopenias, hemolysis, disseminated intravascular coagulation, thromboembolism, renal dysfunction, nephrotic syndrome, uric acid nephropathy, gastrointestinal symptoms (anorexia, vomiting, protein-losing enteropathy, malignant hepatopathy), bullous mucocutaneous lesions, ichthyosis, acanthosis nigricans, dermatomyositis, lactic acidosis, hypertrophic pulmonary osteoarthropathy, hypertension, and amyloidosis.

paraprotein A general term for any immunoglobulin produced in excess quantity, usually in a malignant neoplasm.

passive immunity A transient immune resistance to various organisms due to the presence of antibodies produced by another organism. Passive immunity is either congenital (e.g., as seen in neonates as a result of the transplacental transfer of IgG of maternal origin) or active (e.g., antibodies are administered to a person with an infection known to respond to a particular immune globulin).

PAS stain (periodic acid-Schiff stain) A stain commonly used in pathology, which is based on the periodic acid-Schiff reaction. Many substances and cells are PAS-positive, including mucosubstances (positive in the gastrointestinal tract), fungi, parasites, lipofuscin, polysaccharides, glycogen, glycolipids, and glycoproteins. The PAS stain is of use to the pathologist attempting to identify the origin of certain tumors, such as those that have metastasized to the liver.

Paul-Bunnell-Davidsohn test An immune test for infectious mononucleosis, which is based on the presence of sheep red blood cell agglutinins (known as heterophil antibodies) in patients with infectious mononucleosis. The Paul-Bunnell-Davidsohn test is more complex than the one-step monospot test for infectious mononucleosis and has waned in popularity. See *Epstein-Barr virus, monospot test.*

peak (peak level) The maximum serum level of a free or unbound drug, a value used to monitor drug therapy, where success depends on maintaining as high a level of the drug in the blood as possible while maintaining the drug below toxic levels. The "peak" is usually measured ±1/2 hour after an oral dose of a drug. See *trough* in Glossary.

performance test A general term for any nonverbal, activity-based test used to evaluate intelligence. Performance tests have the advantage of being relatively independent of "cultural bias" and a person's language skills. Five subtests of the Wechsler Adult Intelligence Scale are performance tests. See *psychological test.*

perfusion scan A radionuclide study used to determine the adequacy of the blood flow through the lung, usually as part of a ventilation-perfusion scan. The early part of the test is known as the wash-in, which is followed by equilibrium and wash-out. See *ventilation-perfusion scan.*

peroxidase reaction The formation of a blue precipitate from a dye complex, which occurs when cells or tissues containing certain proteins (e.g., hemoglobin and peroxidase) are incubated with hydrogen peroxide. The peroxidase reaction is a critical part of the benzidine, guaiac, and orthotoluidine tests. The reaction is used in the hematology laboratory to differentiate acute myelocytic leukemia from acute lymphocytic leukemia in patients undergoing a "blast crisis," a phase of acute deterioration. The reaction is important because the treatment hinges on determining which is the cell of origin in the leukemia.

pH All living and nonliving systems operate in acid, basic, or neutral environments, which requires an appropriate balance between the acids (expressed as hydrogen ions) and bases in the bicarbonate ions in the body. A number of components in the circulation (hemoglobin, protein, phosphate, and bicarbonate) serve as buffers to prevent swings in the pH. In addition, the kidneys and lungs either excrete or exhale the excess component that is preventing the pH from being maintained as optimal (near neutral). See the following Glossary entries: *metabolic acidosis, metabolic alkalosis, respiratory acidosis, respiratory alkalosis.*

pharyngitis A general term for inflammation of the mucosal surfaces of the oropharynx, regardless of the cause. See *throat culture.*

phase contrast microscopy A type of light microscope that converts differences in the refractive index as light passes through an object into variations of light intensity, allowing structural details to be seen in unstained living cells. See *microscopy* in Glossary.

phenolphthalein test A rarely performed test for laxative abuse that quantifies the amount of phenolphthalein (present in over-the-counter laxatives) excreted in the urine by thin-layer chromatography.

phospholipid A general term for a lipid containing phosphorus, e.g., lecithins and sphingomyelin.

photodocumentation The use of photography to record and document various aspects of patient management.

photon absorptiometry A technique in which the

density of a bone is determined by measuring the absorption of a beam of X rays or gamma rays passed through it. See *bone densitometry.*

phycocyanin A photosynthetic protein obtained from algae that is used as a tracer in immunofluorescence assays.

phycoerythrin A photosynthetic protein that is a bright fluorescent tracer allowing discrimination between the yellow-orange signal of a positive immune reaction and the greenish autofluorescent background.

phytohemagglutinin (PHA) A protein that is a lymphocyte mitogen (i.e., it stimulates cells to divide). PHA is used in vitro to measure lymphocyte-mediated cytotoxicity, as a nonspecific immune stimulant for in vitro studies of mononuclear cells, and for evaluating cytokine production. It is mitogenic for T cells (lymphocytes) and stimulates CD4 ("helper") T cells more than CD8 ("suppressor") T cells. It is a weaker mitogen for B cells. The degree of response to PHA in respective cells can be measured by the cell's production of interleukin 2.

Pirquet test An obsolete scarification test for tuberculosis.

plasma A clear yellow fluid that comprises 50%–55% of the blood volume; plasma is 92% liquid, 7% protein, and less than 1% inorganic salts, gases, hormones, sugars, and lipids. Fibrinogen- and coagulation factor-depleted plasma is termed "serum."

plasminogen activation A critical reaction in biological systems in which plasminogen is converted into plasmin by tissue- or urokinase-type plasminogen activators. Plasminogen activators are linked to the regulation of blood vessel formation, embryogenesis, inflammation, ovulation, and metastasis.

pneumothorax The presence of air in the pleural cavity, which is a complication of various endoscopic and surgical procedures in the thoracic cavity.

polarization A laboratory technique in which fluids and tissues are analyzed for the presence of crystals that have an intrinsic ability to change the direction of light passing through them. Polarization is used to identify monosodium urate crystals in synovial fluid in gout, or other crystals in the urine. See *microscopy.*

Politzer's test A seldom-used test that detects

the presence of Eustachian tube obstruction, in which a vibrating tuning fork is placed in front of the nostrils. In the absence of obstruction, the sound is perceived as being louder upon swallowing.

polyacrylamide gel electrophoresis A type of high-resolution electrophoresis that is performed on a polyacrylamide gel and used to determine the size of proteins.

polyclonal antibody Any of a number of immunoglobulins produced by multiple, usually nonmalignant clones of cells that have been stimulated by an antigen which may evoke multiple clonal expansions, each responding to a different site on the antigen. See *monoclonal antibody* in Glossary.

polyp A general term for any raised tumor mass, commonly understood to be derived from the overlying surface covering (epithelium) of a particular tissue. Polyps are often neoplastic, either benign or malignant, and are of greatest interest in the colon, female genital tract, nasopharynx, and stomach.

Porter-Silber chromagen A general term for any glucocorticoid detected by the Porter-Silber reaction, which includes 11-deoxycortisol, cortisol, cortisone, and some 17-hydroxicorticosteroids.

positive predictive value The number of true positives divided by the sum of true positives (TP) and false positives (FP), a value that represents the proportion of subjects with a positive test result who actually have the disease; this is also known as the "efficiency" of an assay. See *negative predictive value* in Glossary.

potato-dextrose agar A nonselective growth medium for the growth of yeasts and molds, including *Aspergillus niger, Candida albicans, Saccharomyces cerevisiae,* and *Trichophyton mentagophytes.* It is less popular than Sabouraud's medium.

PPD (protein purified derivative) The antigenic material used to detect previous exposure to tuberculosis. See *Mantoux test, tuberculin tests.*

precautions A general term for those activities intended to minimize exposure to an infectious agent. In practice, when a patient is designated as requiring precautions, both he and his specimens (body fluids and waste products) are handled with increased circumspection by his caregivers, as the term carries the implication that he is infected with a contagious or dangerous organism, such as hepatitis B or HIV-1.

precipitation test (precipitin reaction) A general term for any test in which the endpoint is the formation of an insoluble antigen-antibody complex that precipitates out of solution.

precision A measurement of the reproducibility of a test or assay, i.e., its capability of producing the same results when performed on the same specimen under the same conditions.

predictive value (P value) A value that predicts the likelihood that a particular result from a clinical test correlates with the presence or absence of a disease process. See *negative predictive value* in Glossary, *positive predictive value* in Glossary.

pre-existing condition Any injury, illness, or medical condition that a person had before obtaining a health insurance policy, which might preclude that person from being approved for insurance.

preferred provider organization A form of managed health care in which a limited number of health providers (physicians, hospitals, and others) provide services to a defined group of clients for a negotiated fee-for-service rate that is below the "market value" for the service(s).

probe A segment of DNA or RNA that measures up to several hundred base pairs in length and spans the region of a gene's point mutation or gene rearrangement. Probes are used in molecular biology to identify the presence of a segment of DNA or RNA of interest in cells and tissues. See *in situ hybridization* in Glossary.

procedures manual A book that delineates the diagnostic procedures performed by a clinical laboratory, explained with sufficient detail so that a procedure may be performed by a person unfamiliar with it.

products of conception The aggregate of tissues of fetal origin present in pregnancy, including chorionic villi and/or fetal tissue, required to make the definitive diagnosis of intrauterine pregnancy.

profile A panel of screening tests used to establish a baseline of normalcy for either a certain population (e.g., executive profile) or for a limited group of analytes (e.g., lipid profile). See *organ panel* in Glossary.

progesterone receptor A progesterone-binding protein complex found in the cytoplasm of certain cells. The presence of progesterone receptors is of interest to oncologists because up to 80% of patients with breast and endometrial cancers with these receptors respond favorably to hormone therapy. See *estrogen receptor.*

proliferation index The sum of events occurring in the S and G_2M phases of the cell cycle, which is expressed as a fraction of the total cell population. See *flow cytometry* in Glossary.

prostate cancer A common malignancy; 106,000 new cases are diagnosed in the United States per year, causing 30,000 deaths. 35%–50% of men over 70 years of age have prostate cancer. Its behavior is difficult to predict—many individuals with prostate cancer die of natural deaths and/or old age. Screening for PSA, digital rectal examination, and transrectal ultrasonography increases the rate of detection but may not decrease mortality due to prostate cancer in asymptomatic individuals. See *digital rectal examination, Gleason's grading system* in Glossary, *prostate biopsy, prostate-specific antigen.*

proton NMR spectroscopy (water-suppressed proton, NMR spectroscopy) A laboratory technique that averages the methyl and methylene line widths in the NMR spectra of plasma lipoproteins. This technique was reported to be a useful cancer screen in asymptomatic subjects, a finding that was not confirmed in subsequent studies.

proverbs test A clinical test used to evaluate abstract thinking based on the ability to explain the meaning of a proverb (e.g., "haste makes waste," "a stitch in time saves nine"), which is an expression of intelligence that deteriorates in dementia.

prozone phenomenon A reduced reaction that occurs when antibodies are present in excess and inhibit antigen-antibody reactions. The prozone phenomenon occurs when an antigen-antibody reaction is measured by immunoprecipitation and immunodiffusion.

pseudoallergy An adverse, nonimmune, anaphylaxis-like reaction of sudden onset, often associated with food ingestion, which may be due to an anaphylactoid reaction, intolerence (e.g., psychogenic response), metabolic defect (e.g., enzymatic deficiency, tyramine), and toxicity (e.g., tetrodotoxin). True allergies to foods are hypersensitivity reactions caused by release of histamines evoked by IgE; most true allergies are linked to eggs, milk, peanuts, nuts, fish, soy beans, and shrimp. See *RAST.*

pseudohypertension Blood pressure that is measured as higher than the actual blood pressure, due to markedly calcified ("pipestem") brachial arteries. It is most common in the elderly who have extensive atherosclerosis. If not identified, pseudohypertension may be misinterpreted as requiring therapy.

pseudomembranous colitis An acute illness, often accompanied by severe diarrhea, that may follow antibiotic therapy with ampicillin, clindamycin, metronidazole, and others. These antibiotics eliminate the patient's native bacterial flora, resulting in a "superinfection" by *Clostridium difficile*, which is responsible for virtually all cases of pseudomembranous colitis. The condition may occur in "compromised" hosts, the elderly, or those with a background of colonic obstruction, leukemia, major surgery, uremia, spinal injury, colon cancer, burns, infections, shock, heavy metal poisoning, hemolytic-uremic syndrome, cardiovascular ischemia, Crohn's disease, shigellosis, necrotizing enterocolitis, and Hirschsprung's disease. The diagnosis of *C. difficile* colitis can be made with a stool-cytotoxin assay, which is both highly sensitive and specific, but relatively costly. ELISAs are less expensive, but less sensitive.

pseudovitamin An organic substance that does not meet the accepted definition of a required human vitamin. Pseudovitamins include substances that are true vitamins, but not in humans; substances first described as vitamins, but no longer regarded as such; and "factors" in blood, vegetables, fruits, or minerals that have been termed "vitamins" by various persons. See *vitamins* in Glossary.

psychiatric evaluation A general term for the assessment of a person's mental, social, and psychological functionality. See *psychiatric interview* in Glossary.

psychiatric history A person's mental profile, which includes information about the patient's chief complaint, his or her present illness, psychological adjustments made prior to the onset of disease, individual and family history of psychiatric or mental disorders, and his/her early developmental history. See *psychiatric interview* in Glossary.

psychiatric interview The psychiatric interview is the psychiatrist's main tool for assessing a patient who may be suffering from a mental disorder. In the interview, there is a free flow of information from the patient that forms the basis for therapy. The psychiatric interview is used to understand how the individual relates with his environment and determines social, religious, and cultural influences in the person's life, conscious and unconscious motivations for behaviors, ego strengths and weaknesses, coping strategies, mental support systems and social networks, points of vulnerability, aptitudes, and achievements.

pulmonary thromboembolism (pulmonary embolism, PTE) Blockage of the pulmonary arteries by blood clots, most of which arise in the deep leg veins, causing an estimated 4% of all hospital deaths in the United States each year. Pulmonary thromboembolism is underdiagnosed because the classic clinical signs of dyspnea, chest pain, and hemoptysis are absent, or the patient may be comatose or sedated and unable to communicate. PTE is found at autopsy in 30%–65% of patients who die from severe burns, trauma, or fractures.

pulsed field gel electrophoresis A technique of molecular biology that is used to separate segments of DNA into several hundred to several thousand kilobase pairs in length.

purine One of the "building block" molecules (adenine and guanine) for ribonucleic acids; purines are attached to pyrimidine bases, which are linked to each other either with a single strand of ribose (forming ribonucleic acid) or with a double strand of deoxyribose (forming deoxyribonucleic acid). See *pyrimidine* in Glossary.

pyrimidine One of the "building block" molecules for ribonucleic acids; pyrimidines form either ribonucleic acid (which integrates uracil and cytosine pyrimidine bases) or deoxyribonucleic acid (which integrates thymidine and cytosine bases). Normally, pyrimidines only pair with purines, and not with pyrimidines. See *purine* in Glossary.

pyruvate kinase deficiency An inherited condition affecting Northern Europeans in which the lack of pyruvate kinase in the red blood cells results in chronic hemolytic anemia. One-third of cases present in the neonatal period with jaundice, requiring phototherapy; in older children, pyruvate kinase deficiency may range in severity from asymptomatic, to requiring occasional blood transfusions, to resulting in jaundice and splenomegaly.

quality control (QC) A series of mechanisms intended to ensure the accuracy, reliability, and consistency of data, assays, or tests used in laboratory medicine. QC methods differ in each laboratory, are delineated in the laboratory's procedures manual, and require standardized solutions containing glucose, cholesterol, electrolytes, and other substances that are obtained by pooling specimens from individuals known to be normal for the parameter being measured.

quantify Determine the quantity of; to measure.

quinidine Quinidine is an antiarrhythmic drug that reduces myocardial excitability, conduction velocity, and contractility. See *therapeutic drug monitoring.*

radial immunodiffusion A simple method for quantifying serum proteins (e.g., apolipoproteins, complement proteins, immunoglobulins, and others).

radiation The combined processes of emission, transmission, and absorption of highly energetic waves and particles on the electromagnetic spectrum. Types of radiation include alpha radiation, beta radiation, and gamma radiation. Well-known effects of radiation include changes in the cells, especially those with rapid turnover, e.g., the colon and hematopoietic tissues.

radioimmunoassay (RIA) A test that measures various hormones, such as human chorionic gonadotropin (β-HCG), insulin, and thyroid-stimulating hormone (TSH). RIAs are being increasingly replaced by ELISA (enzyme-linked immunoassays), which are easier to perform because the reagents are more easily stored and do not involve radioactive waste.

radionuclide (radioactive isotope, radioisotope) An artificial or natural nuclide with an unstable nuclear composition that decomposes spontaneously by emission of electrons (β-particles) or helium nucleus (α-particle and γ-radiation), ultimately achieving nuclear stability. Radionuclides are used as labels, for radiation therapy, or as sources of energy.

radon (radon-222) A naturally occurring radioactive gas linked to an increased incidence of malignancy, including leukemia, childhood cancer, myeloid leukemia, renal cell carcinoma, melanoma, and prostatic carcinoma in adults. In the United States, 13,000 cases of lung cancer per year are attributed to radon gas exposure.

random error The scattering of values in a test system around a point known to be a correct value. Random errors in the laboratory can be due to variations in line voltage, lamp output,

or amount of fluid drawn in pipettors or dispensors.

rape kit A collection of receptacles (cups, envelopes, plastic bags, tubes), disposable items (cotton swabs, napkins, pipettes), and tools (sterile comb for pubic hairs, sheets) used to obtain specimens from a rape victim, in order to establish details in a forensically acceptable fashion about the perpetrator and the manner of the rape. See *semen analysis.*

reagin An obsolete general term for IgE, referring to IgE as both an initiator of the immediate hypersensitivity reaction and as a nonspecific antibody produced in syphilis.

receptor An integral membrane-bound protein with a highly specific recognition or target site. When a ligand (e.g., an antigen, drug, hormone, or virus) binds to its respective receptor, the cell responds by activating a membrane-bound enzyme, producing "second messengers."

recombinant DNA technology The constellation of techniques that comprise "genetic engineering," in which a gene producing a protein of interest from one organism is spliced into the genome of another organism. See *polymerase chain reaction.*

recreational drug A general term for any agent (most of which have significant psychotropic effects) used without medical indications or prescription in the context of social interactions. Recreational drugs overlap with the "classic" drugs of abuse (e.g., heroin, cocaine) in that their use is illegal and described as "recreational" only if there is no component of addiction. See *drugs of abuse* in Glossary.

"red flag" An indicator (e.g., an asterisk that is usually printed in red and generated in the laboratory) when an analyte's value falls "out of range," i.e., above or below a laboratory's predetermined values for normal. See *decision level* in Glossary, *panic values* in Glossary.

reducing substance A general term for any substance that "reduces" copper ions. The normal level of reducing substances in the urine is 0.5–1.5 mg/dL. An increase of reducing substances usually indicates an increase in glucose and galactose. Copper is also reduced by other sugars (e.g., arabinose, fructose, lactose, maltose, ribose, and xylose), endogenous metabolites (e.g., ascorbic acid, creatinine, cysteine, glucuronic acid, hippuric acid, homogentisic acid, ketone bodies, oxalaic acid, and uric acid), or exogenous substances (e.g., cinchophen, formaldehyde, isoniazid, nalidixic acid, probenecid, salicylates, and sulfanilamide). Assays for reducing sugars may be false positive by the copper reduction test, in the presence of endogenous or exogenous substances.

red urine "disease" A general term for any clinical condition associated with red urine; it includes hematuria due to glomerulonephritis, bladder tumors, foreign bodies or calculi, infection, inflammation, thrombosis, and other conditions. Less common causes of red urine include trauma-related myoglobinuria or hemoglobinuria, porphyria, pyrrolinuria, ingestion of beets, phenolsulfonphthalein, fuchsin, aniline dyes in candy and food, anthraquinolone laxatives, deferoxamine, rifampin, isoniazid, and aspirin.

Reed-Sternberg cell A large binucleated cell with large, dark, "owl-eyed" nucleoli surrounded by a clear halo; these cells are diagnostic for Hodgkin's disease and are most abundant in the lymphocyte-depleted type.

reference laboratory A general term for any (usually for-profit) laboratory dedicated to performing a broad menu of tests at a distance from the patient, usually outside of the hospital. The referring of clinical specimens is an increasingly common practice for various reasons, including space, cost, volume, staffing, and technology.

reference man A hypothetical male whose anatomic, biochemical, laboratory (chemistry, hematology), and physiologic values represent the norm. A reference man is an idealized entity that serves to standardize experimental results and relate biological insults to a common base. See *reference range*.

reference manual A test menu produced by a laboratory that includes information on patient and specimen preparation, causes for specimen rejection, interpretation of results, information on test panels (batteries of tests for a particular disease or organ system), billing information, and name(s) of specialized laboratories where the laboratory sends specimens requiring tests not being performed in-house.

reference method Any extremely accurate analytical technique used as a "gold standard" against which other tests measuring the same analyte are compared. As a general rule, reference methods have one or more feature that prevents them from being used on a routine basis.

reference range A set of values for an analyte being measured in a patient, which is regarded as encompassing the usual maximum or minimum for the given analyte. In order for a laboratory to produce accurate results, it must be certain that the normal results are consistent and fall within a range of "normalcy," and that the results that fall outside of this reference range are abnormal. In establishing the reference range, most laboratories pool sera from patients who have "normal" values for the analyte being measured. The table below indicates the criteria that are examined when a laboratory establishes its reference range.

ESTABLISHING A REFERENCE RANGE
1. The reference subjects should be normal, healthy, and if indicated, subdivided according to age, sex, or other parameters.
2. The laboratory should use a consistent protocol in which the precision, reliability, and accuracy are delineated, preferably on the same instrument. The sample should be obtained under "standard" conditions, i.e., pre- or postprandial, drawing a similar volume of blood into the collection tube, where each test tube has a standard amount of anticoagulant and thus differences in volume would yield differences in coagulation studies.
3. The range for the reference value should be broad enough to encompass most normal subjects.
4. The statistical methodology and decisions for "tail cutoffs" must be clearly and logically delineated.
5. The range must allow for updating of patient pool, new clinical data, and new methodologies.
See *decision levels* in Glossary, *panic values* in Glossary.

referral center A large university-based tertiary-care hospital that performs tests and therapeutic procedures beyond the expertise of community hospitals.

relapse The worsening or reappearance of cancer, often leukemia. The most common sites of relapse are in the bone marow, testes, and central nervous system. See *remission* in Glossary.

remission The regression of symptoms or lesions in a malignancy—most commonly referring to the disappearance of a tumor by radio- or chemotherapy—and amelioration of clinical symptoms, which may be temporary, partial, or complete. A complete remission of long enough duration (e.g., two years in childhood lymphocytic leukemia) is termed "permanent remission" or cure. See *relapse* in Glossary.

residue The functional "unit" in a polymer (e.g., an amino acid in a protein or a nucleotide in a sequence of DNA).

respiratory acidosis A condition in which there is a decrease in pH due to excess carbon dioxide (CO_2) retention. Causes of respiratory acidosis include hypoventilation due to drugs, central nervous system depression, cardiac or pulmonary disease, or neuromuscular defects. Respiratory acidosis is characterized by slow deep breathing, somnolence, confusion, myoclonus with asterixis, coma, and increased intracranial pressure. See the following Glossary entries: *metabolic acidosis, metabolic alkalosis, respiratory alkalosis.*

respiratory alkalosis A condition in which there is a increase in pH due to excess CO_2 excretion. Causes of respiratory alkalosis include hyperventilation (e.g., due to anxiety, hypoxia, drugs, fever, increased air temperature) and incorrect ventilator settings. Respiratory alkalosis is characterized by rapid, deep breathing, paresthesia, twitching, nausea, vomiting, and coma. See the following Glossary entries: *metabolic acidosis, metabolic alkalosis, respiratory acidosis.*

reticulocyte An immature red blood cell (RBC) found in the peripheral circulation for 24–48 hours after its release from the bone marrow until it develops into a mature RBC. Reticuloctes contain organelle remnants that are not present in mature RBCs and usually indicate an increased production of red blood cells, which may occur after therapy for iron-deficiency anemia. See *reticulocyte count.*

retrovirus An RNA virus that is capable of inserting and expressing its own genetic information in a host genome by transcribing its own RNA into DNA integrated into the host genome. Retroviruses include human T-cell lymphotrophic viruses and HIV-1 (human immunodeficiency virus-1).

reverse transcriptase An enzyme of retroviral origin that is capable of copying genomic RNA into DNA, catalyzing the synthesis of DNA using retroviral RNA as a template.

RFLP (restriction fragment length polymorphisms, restriction site polymorphism) RFLPs correspond to any of a number of local normal variations in the DNA sequence of a person that may be detected by enzymes known as restriction endonucleases, which cut DNA at very specific sites. These individual variations or polymorphisms (i.e., RFLPs) in DNA occur approximately 1 per 200–500 base pairs and cause the genome to be cut at different sites, yielding fragments of different lengths that are unique to each individual; the likelihood of two people having the same RFLPs is estimated to be one in one billion. RFLPs may then be identified by electrophoresis. See *polymerase chain reaction, Southern blot* in Glossary.

RIA See *radioimmunoassay* in Glossary.

rim pattern (peripheral rim pattern, shaggy pattern) An immunofluorescent pattern that is arranged peripherally along the nuclear membrane, due to the deposition of antibodies directed against double-stranded DNA. High antibody titers (greater than 1:200) are often present in the sera of patients with lupus erythematosus and other connective tissue diseases. See *antinuclear antibodies.*

Robertsonian translocation (centromeric fusion) A chromosomal rearrangement seen in 4% of cases of Down syndrome (trisomy 21). It occurs between chromosomes 13, 14, 15, 21, and 22, where a segment from the long arm of one chromosome is translocated to another chromosome, most commonly to chromosome 14. The risk of having a second child with a Robertsonian-type Down syndrome is 10%–15% for a maternal carrier and 5% for a paternal carrier of the translocation.

robust Pertaining or referring to any method (or procedure) that is relatively insensitive to violations in the method's required rules.

rocket electrophoresis A one-dimensional enzyme immune assay in which an antigen-bearing fluid is electrophoresed through agarose containing an antibody to the antigen of interest. Rocket electrophoresis is used to quantify von Willebrand factor levels in the blood and derives its name from the sharp projectile-like spikes of the immunoprecipitin.

Rorschach test A type of personality test in which ten ink blots are presented to an individual for interpretation of what he/she sees. The "ink blot test" generates an enormous amount of data, much of which requires subjective interpretation. First used in 1921, the Rorschach reached its peak of popularity in the 1950s but continues to have currency among psychologists. See *psychological test.*

rosette A term for a garland-like arrangement of structures, cells, or bodies around a central point or blood vessel, usually seen by light microscopy.

round cell   A general term for a relatively small white blood cell with a single, round-to-oval nucleus, which includes lymphocytes, monocytes, plasma cells, and occasionally histiocytes.

sampling error   An "error" that occurs in a diagnostic work-up when insufficient, inadequate, or nonrepresentative material is ob-tained for analysis, usually from a biopsy or, less commonly, a cytology specimen. Sampling errors are well-known causes of false negative results.

sandwich method   A general term for any technique used to identify an antigen or antibody by "sandwiching" a molecule of interest (X) between two other standardized molecules (Y and Y′) that recognize molecule X immunologically or serve as immune recognition sites. See *immunoperoxidase method* in Glossary.

sarcoidosis   A systemic granulomatous disease of unknown cause, which involves the lungs, lymph nodes, skin, liver, spleen, and parotid glands. By light microscopy, the lesions are similar to tuberculosis, but lack cell death (necrosis).

scanning power   The lowest magnification (20x to 25x) power used in diagnostic tissue pathology, which allows the surveying of tissues and pattern recognition. See *high-power field* in Glossary, *microscopy* in Glossary.

Schick test   A clinical maneuver, now of historic interest, that was once used to detect immune responsiveness to diphtheria toxin. Evaluation of previous exposure to *Corynebacteria diphtheriae* (the bacterium that causes diphtheria) is now performed with an assay for diphtheria antitoxin.

scintillation   The sporadic emission of quanta (flashes) of visible or ultraviolet light by fluorescent substances after they have been excited by a photon or ionizing (radioactive) particle. Scintillation is integral to radioimmuoassays because there is one scintillation (flash of light) for each ionizing event, allowing for precise quantification of the incident radiation. See *radioimmunoassay* in Glossary.

SCRIMP technique   (SCRape/IMPrint method) A proposed method by which a working summary of the findings of an autopsy can be rendered in rapid time; it consists of scraping pathological tissues and imprinting them on a glass slide.

secondary antibody   A general term for the second antibody used in a "sandwich" method (e.g., ELISA) or immunoperoxidase method.

The secondary antibody is "raised" against the species of animal (e.g., rabbit, goat) used to make the primary antibody. See *sandwich method* in Glossary.

second opinion   A formal or informal advice sought from a second health professional as to the correctness of a diagnosis and/or appropriateness of a recommended therapy.

Seleny test   (keratoconjunctivitis test)   A laboratory procedure used to determine the ability of various bacteria to invade tissues.

sequencing   The process of determining the primary order of nucleotides in a segment of DNA or RNA, or of the amino acids in a protein.

seroconversion   The development of antibodies detectable in the serum following exposure to a particular organism or antigen, by a person who had not been previously exposed to a particular antigen. Seroconversion often indicates current infection (and transmissibility) of an infectious agent.

seronegative   The lack of antibodies or other immune markers in the serum that would indicate exposure to a particular organism or antigen. In an immunocompetent person, exposure to an immunogenic antigen results in a seroconversion and the person is said to be seropositive; seronegativity therefore implies the capacity for immune responsiveness or seroreactivity. See *anergy* in Glossary.

seropositive   The presence of antibodies or other immune markers in the serum that would indicate prior exposure to a particular organism or antigen.

serum half-life   The amount of time a drug or hormone remains in the circulation until its level is reduced to half the initial amount as a result of metabolic breakdown.

"sharps"   Any sharp object (e.g., syringe needles, scalpel blades, broken test tubes, glass) that may contain human blood, fluids, and tissues with pathogenic organism. See *biohazardous waste, universal precautions.*

short draw   A general term for a tube of blood drawn for analysis that has less than the recommended volume.

SI   (Systeme International d'unites, International System)   The international system for standardization of units of measurement, which is a refinement and extension of the metric system.

sigmoidoscope A rigid or flexible device for examining the sigmoid colonic mucosa. Because of its simplicity, the rigid sigmoidoscope is of use in examining the anorectum and distal sigmoid colon. For higher lesions, the flexible sigmoidoscope reduces patient discomfort, has a two- to four-fold greater diagnostic yield than the rigid sigmoidoscope, and allows evaluation, photography, and biopsies of the large intestine to the cecum. See *endoscopy*.

significance A measure of the deviation of data from a statistical mean or middle value. Significance is defined by a probability (p) value; a p of 0.05 indicates a 5% possibility (or 1 chance in 20) that a data set will differ from a mean and 19 chances in 20 that the data set will not.

skin cancer A general term for any malignancy of the skin, which is often divided into: NON-PIGMENTED SKIN CANCER, e.g., basal cell carcinomas, which comprise the majority, and squamous cell carcinomas), which are common (from 400,000 to one million new cases/year) but relatively innocuous (±2700 deaths/year) and MALIGNANT MELANOMA, which is relatively rare (±34,000 new cases/year) but highly aggressive (±7000 deaths/year). The diagnosis of skin cancer requires a biopsy; if deep tissue invasion is a major issue, the biopsy should include a wide margin of normal tissue to eliminate or at least minimize the need for a second procedure.

skin window of Rebuck An uncommonly performed method for studying host response to antigenic stimuli, in which a sterile glass coverslip is placed over superficially abraded skin; after 3–4 hours, most of the cells picked up on the coverslip are neutrophils; at 12 hours, "round" cells (e.g., lymphocytes, plasma cells, and monocytes) are found, and at 24 hours, monocytes and macrophages are obtained.

skip lesion Any lesion in which normal tissue is interspersed with tissue affected by a pathologic condition. Skip lesions are described in metastatic cancer, polyarteritis nodosa, and Crohn's disease.

skip metastases The metastatic spread of a malignancy in which contiguous regions are skipped, while distant malignant tumors are present, a finding that has a poor prognosis. Skipping is typical of lymphatic permeation of a lymphoproliferative disease, such as Hodgkin's disease. It also occurs in rare osteosarcomas with multiple tumor nodules in the same bone but located at a distance from each other.

slant culture A bacterial culture grown on a solid (i.e., agar-based) growth medium that has been poured in a test tube and allowed to solidify at a slanted angle.

Southern blot A method used to detect the presence of specific segments of DNA that have been previously separated by gel electrophoresis.

Southwestern blot A technique that combines the principle of Southern hybridization, which identifies DNA fragments, with "Western" immunoblotting, which identifies proteins of interest.

special stain Any stain used in tissue pathology, other than the usual hematoxylin and eosin (H&E) stain which is the "workhorse" stain on which the vast majority of diagnoses in tissue pathology are based. Special stains used in diagnostic pathology include acid-fast stain for mycobacteria, Bodian stain for myelin, Congo red stain for amyloid, Fontana-Masson stain for melanin, Gomori-methenamine-silver (GMS) stain for fungi, gram stain for bacteria, Grimelius stain for tumors of neural crest origin, Masson's trichrome stain trichrome stain to differentiate between muscle and collagen, periodic acid Schiff stain for complex carbohydrate and mucosubstances, Prussian blue stain for iron, and reticulin stain for reticulin.

SPECT (single photon emission computed tomography) A noninvasive technique for reconstructing cross-sectional images of the distribution of radionuclide. It is used to evaluate changes in the central nervous system (e.g., acute ischemic episodes, seizure activity, vascular dementia, and Alzheimer's dementia), the heart (e.g., defects in myocardial perfusion), and to detect subtle changes in bone metabolism.

spectroscopy The use of a spectroscope to evaluate a fluid for the presence of a molecule of interest; it is based on the molecule's ability to absorb light at specific wavelengths. Spectroscopy is the most widely applied method in the clinical laboratory.

spike A sharp peak seen in a serum or urine protein electrophoresis, due to a marked increase in the production of a specific immunoglobulin produced by a clone of lymphocytes. "Clonal expansions" occur in malignancies of the lymphoid system, e.g., multiple myeloma and Waldenström's disease, as well as in a monoclonal gammopathy of undetermined significance. Spikes may not be seen if the immunoglobulin production is normally very low, because the spike may be obscured by the curves corresponding to more abundant immunoglobulin G, immunoglobulin A, or immunoglobulin M.

"spike-and-wave" pattern An electroencephalographic pattern seen in absences (formerly petit mal epilepsy), occurring as symmetric and synchronous, three or more discharges per second with an abrupt beginning and end.

spike potential A single, rapid voltage "transient" that occurs spontaneously in smooth muscle cells, as seen by electromyography, when the cells have resting membrane potentials above that of the spike potential threshold, as occurs in the lower esophageal sphincter. See *electromyography.*

spirochetes A general term for any spiral-shaped bacterium, which is usually understood to mean *Treponema pallidum*, the bacterial cause of syphilis. Other spirochetes of medical importance are *Borrelia burgdorferi*, which causes Lyme disease, and *Leptospira* species, which cause leptospirosis.

spur An arc seen on immunoelectrophoresis of the serum, often found in the presence of a monoclonal protein.

SQUID imaging (superconducting quantum interference device imaging) A highly sensitive low-noise amplifier currently used in research to measure the magnetic flux created when electrical energy flows through neurons. SQUIDs are currently expensive ($2–$3 million), but may prove useful in diagnosing epilepsy, strokes, migraines, language disorders, schizophrenia, motor and sensory defects, and cardiac arrhythmias.

stab culture A culture of bacteria that has been inoculated in an agar tube with a needle that reaches the deep portion of the tube. A stab culture allows the comparison of aerobic and anaerobic growth conditions. See *oxidative-fermentative test* in Glossary.

staging An evaluation or "work-up" of a patient to determine the severity and extent of a disease in order to guide therapy; this process is important in treating malignancies and other conditions because each stage has a relatively standard treatment. For most malignancies, there are four stages, ranging from the early and well-circumscribed stage I to the aggressive, metastatic, and preterminal stage IV.

stain A series of dyes used to selectively color tissues or cells for microscopic examination. The hematoxylin and eosin stain (H&E stain) colors the nuclei blue (basophilic) and the stromal or support tissue a light pink (acidophilic or eosinophilic) and is by far the most commonly used stain for examination of tissues removed during surgery. See *special stain* in Glossary.

standard deviation (square root of the variance) A statistical measure of the spread of a set of data about a mean, where a graph of the data points is described by a curve with Gaussian distribution, i.e., bell-shaped.

"stat" A specimen, often from the critical care unit or emergency room, that is given priority in the clinical laboratory in order to measure various analytes with immediate potential impact on patient management. "Stats" may include blood glucose levels, hematocrit, electronic leukocyte differential count, certain enzyme levels, prothrombin time, partial thromboplastin time, BUN, and creatinine.

statistical test A general term for any test that analyzes the degree to which results from a sample or specimen agree with those predicted. The statistical significance of the difference between that which is observed (e.g., the results of a laboratory test) and that which is predicted can be precisely expressed in terms of probability.

stem cell A primitive cell that is capable of dividing and giving rise to both primitive daughter cells like itself and cells capable of undergoing differentiation. In adults, the stem cell capability of the early embryo is lost except in the bone marrow where it is retained.

stimulated acid output (SAO) A stimulatory test used to evaluate the adequacy of vagal nerve resection in patients who required a vagotomy for gastric ulcer disease. See *maximum acid output.*

streak To inoculate a semisolid bacterial growth plate.

subfertility A term referring to a male condition in which semen parameters are below the lower limits of normal on two or more occasions. Criteria include volume, sperm density, sperm viability, motility, and abnormal forms. Subfertile semen may also demonstrate hyperviscosity, sperm agglutination, polyspermia, and/or hematospermia. See *antisperm antibodies, semen analysis.*

substance abuse An activity that is defined as the use of illicit, potentially addicting drugs (e.g., cocaine); the misuse of prescribed drugs with stimulatory or depressant activities on the nervous system (e.g., amphetamines or barbiturates); or the habitual use of readily available substances known to have deleterious effects (e.g., alcohol and tobacco).

surveillance The monitoring of diseases that have a certain prevalence in a population. Infectious disease surveillance methods include identifying contaminated food or other products, determining the current strains of influenza virus in the community, and monitoring the safety of the blood supply.

surveillance scanning A generic term for the use of various imaging modalities, such as CT and MRI to detect and follow patients with certain diseases, particularly brain tumors.

tanned red cell test A laboratory test in which the red blood cells are treated with highly diluted tannic acid. "Tanning" allows them to act as antigen carriers and enhances the visualization of certain antigen-antibody reactions.

TCBS agar (thiosulfate-citrate-bile salts-sucrose agar) A bacterial culture medium with a high salt concentration and alkaline pH that is the preferred "recovery" medium for vibrios, e.g., *Vibrio cholera* and *V. parahaemolyticus*. Other organisms that grow on TCBS agar are *Enterococcus faecalis, Escherichia coli, and Pseudomonas aeruginosa*.

T cell (T lymphocyte) The T (thymus-drived) cell is the most complex cell of the immune system, given the diversity of T cell types, such as T cells with activator, cytotoxic, delayed hypersensitivity, and suppressor activities; the wide range of cytokines, growth factors, and immune modulators produced by activated T cells; the complexity of T-cell interaction with exogenous and endogenous antigens; and the complexity of T-cell maturation in the thymus.

technician See *medical technician* in Glossary.

technologist See *medical technologist* in Glossary.

techoic acid antibody assay (TA-AB) A test that measures the titers of antibody to techoic acid, a component of the staphylococcal cell wall. 90% of patients with *S. aureus*-induced endocarditis have increased TA-AB levels, and the assay is used to diagnose such endocarditis, determine response to therapy, and detect possible relapse.

teleconsultation A general term for a medical consultation on an electronic network (usually the Internet).

telemedicine A general term for any form of medical practice in which the diagnostic information is transmitted to the physician for analysis via telecytometry, (cardiac) telemetry, telemicroscopy, telepathology, or teleradiology.

telepathology An evolving field that may eliminate the need for small rural hospitals to have an on-site surgical pathologist. It utilizes high-resolution video cameras and robotic microscopes to transmit images of tissue specimens over telephone lines or fiberoptic cables to a distant center with multiple, expert pathologists.

teleradiology A form of delivering expert radiology services by transmitting a digitalized image (obtained by angiography, CT, MRI, PET scanning, sonography, thermography, or other imaging devices) via satellite or telephone cabling to radiologists who may be located a great distance away.

tertiary care The most specialized level of health care, administered to patients who have complex diseases and/or who may require high-risk pharmacologic regimens or surgical procedures. Patients who receive tertiary care are usually referred by either a primary caregiver or by a specialist.

tertiary care center A hospital or medical center providing subspecialty expertise for patients referred from secondary care centers. Areas of expertise include surgery (organ transplantation, pediatric cardiovascular surgery, stereotactic neurosurgery); internal medicine (genetics, hepatology, adolescent psychiatry); diagnostic modalities (positron emission tomography, superconducting quantum interface device, color Doppler electrocardiography, electron microscopy, gene rearrangement, and molecular analysis); and therapies (experimental protocols for treating advanced and/or potentially fatal disease, including AIDS, cancer, and inborn errors of metabolism).

Thayer-Martin agar An enriched bacterial growth medium that incorporates antibiotics (colistin, nystatin, trimethoprim lactate, vancomycin).

therapeutic index The ratio of a drug's toxic level to its therapeutic level, calculated as the toxic concentration (TC) of a drug divided by the effective concentration, and expressed as TC_{50}/EC_{50}, a point at which 50% of patients have a toxic reaction to the drug being monitored. The lower the therapeutic index, the more difficult it is to adjust a drug's dose, and the more critical it is that the drug be monitored.

therapeutic range See *therapeutic index* in Glossary.

thermocycler A device used in polymerase chain reaction (PCR) that cycles between a low (72°C) temperature in which a round of DNA synthesis occurs, and a high (95°C) temperature during which the newly formed DNA duplexes are melted to prepare for another round of DNA synthesis.

thermography An obsolete method for diagnosing breast cancer which was based on the increased warmth of skin overlying malignancy. This relatively nonspecific finding also occurs in mastitis. See *mammography, xeroradiography* in Glossary.

thiamin deficiency A clinical condition that results in beri-beri; "wet" beri-beri results in congestive heart failure and dry beri-beri results in peripheral neuropathy.

Thörmahlen's test A sensitive and specific but rarely performed colorimetric method for detecting the presence of melanin in a fluid. Sodium nitroprusside, potassium hydroxide, and acetic acid are added to the fluid (e.g., urine) of interest, which in the presence of melanin is converted to a green-blue color; the intensity correlates with the quantity. A brown color is seen in absence of melanin.

three-glass test A crude clinical test in which the urinary stream is collected in succession in three different 3-ounce (±75 ml) glasses. The urine in the first contains cells from the anterior urethra; the second, from the urinary bladder; and the third, from the posterior urethra, seminal vesicles, and prostate.

thyroid suppression test A test once used to identify suspected thyrotoxicosis and subtle Graves' disease, which was based on the finding that adminstration of exogenous thyroid hormone suppresses endogenous thyroid hormone production. The test has fallen into disuse, as measurement of serum TSH levels and measurement of TSH response to thyroid-releasing hormone provide the same information at no risk to the patient.

timed collection The obtention of a laboratory specimen at either multiple specified intervals

(i.e., at one-half hour, 1 hour, 2 hours, and 3 hours) or at one specified time interval (e.g., a 24-hour urine).

tissue processor A laboratory instrument used to prepare formaldehyde-fixed tissues for embedding in paraffin, which are subsequently sectioned with a microtome and stained on a glass slide for examination by light microscopy.

titer The amount of a substance required to evoke a reaction to another substance. Determination of titers is of clinical use in determining a present infection or past exposure to an antigen or virus. Rising titers indicate a developing disease, while falling titers indicate a resolving condition.

TLC See *thin-layer chromatograhy.*

TNTC (too numerous to count) A colloquial abbreviation for a confluent "lawn" of bacteria on a culture plate that may be seen in urinary tract infections.

tolerance An increase in dosage of a drug required to achieve the same effect, which is a function of increased metabolism.

toluidine blue A metachromatic thiazin stain used for "thick" sections in ultrastructural studies.

toluidine method A technique in which O-toluidine, an aromatic amine, reacts with glucose in a hot acetic acid solution to produce colored derivatives, allowing the quantification of glucose; this method gives similar results to those generated by the enzymatic methodology used in multichannel analyzers.

toxicity testing A component of the risk assessment process, which is required by law in the United States for all new chemicals, for new purposes of old chemicals, or for combinations of new and old chemicals. Toxicity testing attempts to identify hazards (e.g., adverse effects, cancer, nephrotoxicity, and teratogenesis) and quantitate exposure-response relation (measured by LD_{50}, the chemical "dose" that is lethal in 50% of the test animals, and ED_{50}, the "effective dose" that causes a consistent change in 50% of tested animals). See *Ames test* in Glossary.

transfusion "trigger" The hematocrit and hemoglobin values at or below which packed red cells are usually ordered for transfusion by a clinician. In the current environment of potentially fatal transfusion-transmitted infections (e.g., HIV and hepatitis B), the most widely used current transfusion trigger is a hemoglobin of 7.0 g/dl, unless the hemoglobin level is falling rapidly.

transluminal angiography (balloon angioplasty) A general term for any procedure in which a device is introduced into an artery in order to dilate it and increase its internal diameter. Transluminal angiography is used both to establish the diagnosis of vascular occlusion (narrowing) and to treat it.

transmission electron microscope The most commonly used type of electron microscope, which has a resolution of up to 200,000 magnifications. In TEM, a beam of electrons passes through the specimen, providing a magnified image of an object on a fluorescent screen. TEM is used clinically to study glomerulonephritis and to classify tumors, e.g., cell junctions are found in poorly differentiated carcinoma, neurosecretory granules in tumors of neural crest origin, and premelanosomes in malignant melanoma. See *scanning electron microscopy.*

TRAP (tartrate-resistant acid phosphatase) A form of acid phosphatase that is used in hematology, because its presence is relatively specific for hairy cell leukemia. Weak TRAP staining occurs in infectious mononucleosis, chronic lymphocytic leukemia, lymphosarcoma, Sézary cells, osteoclastic bone tumors, and Gaucher cells.

Trendelenburg test A clinical maneuver used to determine the competency of the valves of the leg veins. The patient is lying down, and the leg being examined is raised to a 45° angle, allowing the veins to drain. An elastic band is place around the thigh to close off the superficial veins. The patient then stands up and the speed at which the veins refill is evaluated. In normal legs, venous refill is incomplete at 30 seconds; removal of the elastic band does not cause retrograde filling. Rapid venous refilling on release of the band suggests incompetent valves of saphenous veins. Filling of the superficial veins upon releasing the band indicates incompetent valves are also present in some perforating veins.

Treponema pallidum immobilization test (TPI test) A test that was developed in 1949 and served as the "gold standard" for the serologic diagnosis of syphilis. The TPI test is based on the immobilization of live, motile *Treponema pallidum* microorganisms by specific antibodies in serum from infected patients with syphilis. It is expensive to perform and no longer used in the United States. See *VDRL.*

trichrome stain A special stain used in pathology that colors collagen green, muscle red-purple, and myelin brown; it is used to detect the presence of muscle invasion in certain carcinomas (e.g., of the urinary bladder) and to diagnose collagenous colitis.

tricyclic antidepressants A family of drugs used to treat bipolar disorder (manic-depressive psychosis), by blocking the re-uptake of neurotransmitters, resulting in a prolonged action of neurotransmitters at the receptor site.

triple iron agar A bacterial growth medium that may be used to identify certain gram-negative bacteria, especially *Enterobacteriaceae.*

troponin A contractile protein composed of three subunits, troponin-I, troponin-T, and troponin-C. It is present in low concentrations in the thin filaments of striated muscle; it binds calcium and tropomyosin, inhibits actomyosin ATPase, and regulates muscle contraction. Troponins I and T are elevated after myocardial infarction and may be better than creatinine phosphokinase-MB for the early detection of heart attacks. See *creatine phosphokinase.*

trough The minimum serum concentration of a drug being administered for a prolonged period, the levels of which are measured immediately before administering the next dose. "Peaks" and "troughs" are measured for drugs that have a low therapeutic index and potentially serious side effects (e.g., aminoglycoside antibiotics, which have well-known ototoxic and nephrotoxic effects). Trough levels should be above the minimum inhibitory concentration of the infecting bacteria.

Trypanosoma detection The identification of *Trypanosoma cruzi*, a blood-borne pathogen endemic to the tropics of the Western hemisphere. *T. cruzi* is identified by direct examination of a smear of the peripheral blood, which is stained with a dye (Giemsa) and examined by high-power light microscopy.

tubeless test A general term for any pancreatic function test in which various substrate molecules for pancreatic enzymes are administered per os (i.e., without intubating the patient), followed by measurement of the digestion products. The most popular tubeless tests are the bentiromide and the pancreolauryl tests; others include fecal chymotrypsin, trypsin RIA, serum pancreatic polypeptide, dual-label Schilling, and quantitative stool fat tests.

turbidimetry A laboratory technique that semi-quantifies a substance in suspension, based on the decrease in forward light transmission by the suspension. See *nephelometry* in Glossary.

turnaround time   A parameter of a clinical laboratory's efficiency in performing and reporting test results, defined as the time between ordering a test and the reporting of results. See *turnover time* in Glossary.

turnover time   The time needed for a metabolite, nutrient, therapeutic agent, toxin, or other substance to be either completely removed from the system or replaced by more of the same substance, in the case of a therapeutic agent or metabolite. See *turnaround time* in Glossary.

ultrafast Papanicolaou stain   A recently developed stain for cytology specimens that improves the quality of preparation and facilitates the interpretation of specimens obtained by fine-needle aspiration. See *pap smear*.

ultrastructure   The sum total of organelles and structures (e.g., membranes, microtubules, microfilaments, and molecules) that are beyond the resolution of light microscopy; ultrastructural studies include scanning electron microscopy, used to study the surfaces of membranes and cells (magnifications of 2000x to 20,000x), transmission electron microscopy (resolution of structures from 2000x to 150,000x), and scanning tunnel electron microscopy, which has a magnification ceiling of up to 2 million-fold magnification. See *electron microscopy* in Glossary, *microscopy* in Glossary.

Ulysses syndrome   A complication of false-positive diagnostic tests or clinical observations that is responsible for a complete and aggressive diagnostic work-up to elucidate the nature of what is, in actual fact, a nondisease, before the patient is allowed to return to his original state of health.

undercall (underread)   A noun and a verb for an error in which a benign diagnosis is rendered on what later proves to be a malignant lesion; misinterpretation of this type may occur at any stage of patient evaluation, from the time of physical examination of a mass or complaint by a clinician to the endpoint of imaging analysis by the radiologist and microscopic examination by the pathologist.

universal precautions   A method of infection control in which all human blood, certain body fluids (e.g., amniotic, cerebrospinal, pericardial, peritoneal, pleural, and synovial fluids, saliva in dental procedures, maternal milk, semen, vaginal secretions, and any fluid grossly contaminated with blood), as well as unfixed organs or tissues of human origin, HIV-containing cell or tissue cultures, or HBV-containing culture medium or other solutions are treated as if known to be infected with HIV, HBV, and/or other blood-borne pathogens. Exposure to blood and body fluids is minimized by using isolation materials and removable and disposable barriers (latex and vinyl gloves, protective eyewear, masks and gowns and disposable sharps containers). Universal precautions serve to both protect the health care worker and prevent him from acting as a vector for these pathogens. See *biohazardous waste* in Glossary, *sharps* in Glossary.

Ureaplasma urealyticum (T strain mycoplasma)   A genus of small (0.3 μm) pleomorphic (coccal to coccobacillary), bacteria of the family *Mycoplasmataceae* that lack a cell wall and catabolize urea to ammonia. *U. urealyticum* reside in the genital tract and nasopharynx, are sexually transmitted, and cause nongonococcal urethritis, urethroprostatitis, and epididymitis in males, urinary tract infections, reproductive wastage and chorioamnionitis in females, and respiratory tract and central nervous system infection of neonates.

urinary tract infection   A condition that affects about seven million people per year in the United States alone; UTIs can be divided into those affecting young women with acute uncomplicated pyelonephritis or cystitis, or recurrent cystitis, and adults with asymptomatic bacteruria or with complicated urinary tract infections. Urinary tract infections are characterized by dysuria, burning, increased frequency, and urgency. The most common bacteria seen in urinary tract infections are *Escherichia coli* (±80%), *Staphylococcus saprophyticus, Proteus mirabilis,* and *Klebsiella pneumoniae.*

vaginal cornification test   An obsolete term for the evaluation of estrogenic activity, based on the finding of keratinized (cornified) squamous cells in cytologic smears of the vagina and uterine cervix.

vestibule (of ear)   The central cavity in the bony labyrinth of the inner ear that houses the utriculus and sacculus; it is posterior to the cochlea, anterior to the semicircular canals, and medial to the tympanic cavity, with which it is directly contiguous via the vestibular window.

video consultation   A facet of telemedicine in which video images are transmitted to an expert (consultant) located at a distance from the patient. See *teleconsultation* in Glossary, *telemedicine* in Glossary.

VIN (vulvar intraepithelial neoplasm) An umbrella term encompassing two clinically distinct, but histologically similar lesions: carcinoma in situ (Bowen's disease) and bowenoid papulosis (bowenoid dysplasia). See *carcinoma in situ* in Glossary, *cervical intraepithelial neoplasia, HPV, intraepithelial neoplasia* in Glossary.

viral neutralization assay A highly specific test of relatively low sensitivity, which is used to identify the presence of antibodies to a particular virus. These assays are complex, technically demanding, and only detect antibodies to specific sites on the virus, and are therefore not routinely performed.

viral profile A battery of immunoassays performed on the serum of patients suspected of being infected by, or having been recently exposed to, viruses. A viral profile from a commercial laboratory usually measures adenovirus and coxsackievirus (B1-B6) antibodies, IgG antibodies against CMV (cytomegalovirus), and IgG herpes simplex antibodies.

viral study A general term for any test or battery of tests used to detect or confirm past or present exposure to a particular virus. As with all microorganisms, viral studies can be either "indirect," where the effects of the virus on the host organism are measured by the formation of antibodies, or "direct," where the virus itself is cultured. The type of anti-viral antibodies produced reflect the temporal nature of exposure. They are, as a rule, either of the IgM class (produced after acute exposure to the virus), or IgGs, which indicates previous exposure to the virus, and often a status of adequate immunity to repeat exposure to the same virus. The vast number of viruses in a particular genus (e.g., arbovirus, coxsackievirus, echovirus, enterovirus, and others), each requiring a specific immune response, explains how one can get the "flu" on an annual basis, despite having mounted a previous, adequate, and "permanent" immune response.

vitamin Any of a number of organic accessory factors present in foods. Vitamins are necessary in minimal or trace amounts (daily requirements of individual vitamins are measured in milligram to microgram quantities), as the body either does not produce them or does so in minute quantities. Vitamins are the most commonly abused over-the-counter substances. Water-soluble vitamins (vitamins B_1, B_2, B_6, B_{12} and C) are reasonably well-tolerated because they are easily excreted by the kidneys; lipid-soluble vitamins (A, D, E and K) accumulate in fat, and in large doses, they can be toxic to the liver. Vitamin levels are not routinely measured in the serum in the absence of clinical suspicion of vitamin deficiency, given the relative rarity of such deficiencies in developed countries. See *pseudovitamin* in Glossary.

vocabulary test A general term for a component of intelligence tests in which an individual is asked to define words of varying level of difficulty, and use them in context, which provides the examiner with a measure of the person's intellectual achievement and aptitude.

Voges-Proskauer test A test used to differentiate among bacteria of the family *Enterobacteriaceae*, which is indicated by a red color, and based on the production of acetylmethylcarbonol from glucose by some genuses of bacteria.

Volhard's test A test of a person's renal function based on the ability to produce dilute urine after ingesting 1500 ml of water on an empty stomach. See *water deprivation test, water testing* in Glossary.

volume of distribution (V_d) A calculated value used to estimate the "pull" that a storage tissue has on drugs in the circulation. Lipotropic drugs have V_d of many liters, while high-molecular-weight substances stay within the blood vessels. The V_d is decreased with valproic acid, normal with lithium, phenobarbital, and chloramphenicol, and increased with lidocaine, procainamide, and thiopental. See *apparent volume of distribution* in Glossary, *therapeutic drug monitoring.*

waived test A test that is regarded as being of such simplicity that it would require a special talent *not* to perform it correctly. Waived tests include dipstick urinalysis (for bilirubin, glucose, hemoglobin, ketones, leukocytes, nitrite, pH, protein, specific gravity, and urobilirubinogen), visual color tests for ovulation and pregnancy, non-automated erythrocyte sedimentation rate, hemoglobin by copper sulfate method, fecal occult blood, spun microhematocrit, and glucose by FDA-approved home-monitoring devices.

warfarin An anticoagulant that inhibits the synthesis of liver-dependent coagulation factors (the prothrombin complex, factors II, VII, IX and X). Warfarin is used for long-term prevention of uncomplicated distal deep vein thrombosis, prophylaxis and prevention of thromboembolism of cardiac origin, in survivors of acute myocardial infarction, and to prevent cerebral infarction in older patients with atrial fibrillation. Warfarin levels are not routinely measured. Warfarin's activity is increased by phenylbutazone, clofibrate, and decreased by barbiturates.

warm antibody An antibody or agglutinin (usually IgG) that reacts optimally at 37°C and has an affinity for certain red blood cell antigens (e.g., Duffy, Kell, Kidd, MNSs, and Rh) and if produced by a blood cell recipient, may cause an immune hemolytic response.

warm nodule A relatively circumscribed increase in radioisotope concentration seen by radionuclide imaging of the thyroid ("thyroid scan") in which functional thyroid lesions suppress TSH synthesis, but do not cause hyperthyroidism, the latter of which evokes "hot" nodules. See *cold nodule* in Glossary.

washout test A crude method for estimating obstruction of the flow of urine, which is based on the time necessary for a radioactive substance to be completely cleared ("washed out") from the kidneys.

Waters' position A position used to visualize the maxillofacial bones and maxillary sinuses and determine the patency of the maxillary sinuses, in which the patient is placed at a 37° angle with the orbitomeatal line, perpendicular to the mid-sagittal plane.

water testing Any of a number of tests that can be performed on drinking water, usually intended to detect microorganisms, particularly those originating from improperly processed sewage. The most commonly perfomed test is the coliform count, in which the number of bacteria of colonic origin (by convention, *Escherichia coli*) is determined per volume of drinking water.

watery diarrhea-hypokalemia-achlorhydria syndrome (WDHA syndrome, Verner-Morrison syndrome, pancreatic cholera) A disease due to increased serum VIP (vasoactive intestinal polypeptide), caused by a VIPoma, a pancreatic islet cell tumor. WDHA syndrome is characterized by profuse watery diarrhea, dehydration, hypotension, shock, and episodic flushing. Laboratory findings in WDHA syndrome include achlorhydria, increased or decreased glucose, markedly decreased potassium, and increased calcium. In children, it is associated with ganglioneuromas.

waxy casts Cylindrical structures seen in the urine by light microscopy; they have a high refractile index and correspond to the degenerated cellular casts typical of long-term oliguria and renal tube obstruction, as seen in chronic renal failure, acute and chronic renal rejection, and amyloidosis. Very broad waxy casts or "renal failure" casts are typical of end-stage renal failure.

whiskey test A stimulation test of historic interest that was once used to determine calcitonin levels. Two ounces of whiskey was administered by mouth to patients with medullary thyroid carcinoma. Within 15 minutes, calcitonin increases to levels comparable to those produced by calcium infusions.

white blood cell (leukocyte) A general term for cells (WBCs) found in the peripheral blood, which include the granulated WBCs (basophils, eosinophils, and neutrophils) and the nongranulated WBCs (lymphocytes and monocytes).

white blood cell count (leukocyte count, WBC count) See *complete blood count.*

white coat hyperglycemia The false elevation of glucose levels related to the psychological stress of being examined by persons wearing "white coats" in a formal medical setting, e.g., a clinic or office practice.

white coat hypertension A transient increase in blood pressure that occurs in apprehensive patients faced with the "white coat" of the physician. White coat hypertension may result in inappropriate anti-hypertensive therapy. This form of pseudohypertension may be prevented by either having a nurse or technician measure the pressure or by measuring the pressure after a physical examination. See *pseudohypertension* in Glossary.

whole blood tonometry A technique in which fresh whole blood at a given temperature is equilibrated with known concentrations of O_2, CO_2, and nitrogen. Whole blood tonometry is useful for measuring the inaccuracy of blood gas analyzers. See *arterial blood gas.*

window period An interval between the time of inoculation or exposure to a microorganism, usually viral, and the ability to detect its presence by serological assays (i.e., by antigen-antibody reactions). Window periods are common in infections by hepatitis B virus and human immunodeficiency virus (HIV).

wood alcohol See *methanol.*

working diagnosis A diagnosis based on experience, clinical epidemiology, and confirmatory evidence provided by ancillary studies. Working diagnoses allow early treatment of a disease while awaiting special or more definitive studies.

work-up 1) The constellation of procedures, including obtaining the patient's medical history, performing a physical examination, and ordering and evaluating laboratory tests and imaging procedures, upon which diagnosis and therapy are based. 2) To evaluate a patient.

wristband An identifying label attached to a patient's wrist at the time of admission to a hospital or other health care institution.

xenodiagnosis A method for diagnosing an infection in one animal by inoculating the organism into a second animal of a different species; this allows detection of blood-borne parasites (*Trypanosoma cruzi* and *T. spiralis*) when the blood smears are negative. Insects are fed blood that is presumed to be positive for the hemoflagellate and "incubated" for 10–30 days, after which the insects' feces are examined for the parasites.

xeroradiography An obsolete radiologic imaging technique used to record an image, which is converted into a "positive" image by a dry photoelectric process. Xeromammography provides a relatively good image, since the entire breast is viewed at once and delineates variability in tissue density, blood vessels, calcification, and tumor masses.

XLD agar (Xylose-Lysine-Deoxycholate agar) A selective bacterial growth medium that contains substances that inhibit the growth of native coliform flora, allowing identification of *Enterobacteriaceae* (enteric gram-negative rods).

X ray A type of electromagnetic energy that is linked to the interactions of high-energy particles. These particles include electrons, which collide with targets and "bump" these targets to higher energy levels. As the targets fall back to lower energy levels, photons and X rays are released. Patient exposure levels to X rays are divided into those with an undesired side effect of a diagnostic procedure and those that are a necessary component of a therapeutic procedure. Diagnostic X rays expose patients to a relatively low (30 to 150 keV) level of energy. See *computed tomography, MRI, mammography.*

yeast culture A test in which clinical material is obtained from a patient and grown on a nutrient-enriched medium to identify the presence of a yeast.

yellow urine A yellow-tinged urine, which in acid pH urine may be due to excretion of picric acid, dinitrophenol, phenacetin, or chrysarobin; in alkaline pH urine, it may be due to increased secretion of anthocyanin or associated with ingestion of beets or blackberries. Pure yellow urine is associated with increased acriflavine and has a green fluorescence. Yellow-orange urine may be highly concentrated or contain increased bilirubin.

zero-order kinetics The dynamics related to the rate of drug elimination, which is linear with time and proportional to the concentration of the enzyme responsible for catabolism and independent of substrate concentration.

zonal centrifugation A method for separating molecules by size, as a function of the time of centrifugation and the mass of the molecule.

zone electrophoresis A general term for any electrophoretic technique in which components are separated into zones or bands in a buffer and stabilized in a solid, porous, or other support medium, including filter paper, agar gel, and polyacrylamide gel.

zone of equivalence A region in an antigen-antibody reacting system where the ratio of antigen to antibody is equivalent.

aa	Amino acid
ACE	Angiotensin-converting enzyme
AFB	Acid-fast bacillus
AIDS	Acquired immunodeficiency syndrome
aka	Also known as
ALL	Acute lymphocytic (lymphoid, lymphoblastic) leukemia
ALS	Amyotrophic lateral sclerosis
ALT	Alanine aminotransferase (formerly GPT)
AMA	American Medical Association
AML	Acute myelocytic (granulocytic, myeloid, myelogenous) leukemia
andr(o)–	male, man
ANLL	Acute nonlymphocytic leukemia
apo	Apolipoprotein
aPTT	Activated partial thromboplastin time
ARDS	Acute (or adult) respiratory distress syndrome
AST	Aspartate aminotransferase (formerly GPT)
AV	Atrioventricular
BCC	Basal cell carcinoma
BM	Bone marrow (or basement membrane)
BUN	Blood urea nitrogen
CAD	Coronary artery disease
cAMP	Cyclic adenosine monophosphate
CAP	College of American Pathologists
CBC	Complete blood count
CDC	Centers for Disease Control and Prevention
cDNA	Complementary DNA
CEA	Carcinoembryonic antigen

CHF	Congestive heart failure
Ci.e.	Counter-immunoelectrophoresis
CIN	Cervical intraepithelial neoplasia
CK	Creatinine phosphokinase
CLL	Chronic lymphocytic (lymphoblastic, lymphoid) leukemia
CML	Chronic myelocytic (granulocytic, myelogenous, myeloid) leukemia
CNS	Central nervous system
COD	Cause of death
COPD	Chronic obstructive pulmonary disease
CSF	Cerebrospinal fluid
CT	Computed tomography
CVA	Cerebrovascular accident
2-D	Two-dimensional
3-D	Three-dimensional
DAD	Diffuse alveolar damage
DDx	Differential diagnosis
DIC	Disseminated intravascular coagulation
DM	Diabetes mellitus
DNA	Deoxyribonucleic acid
DSM-IV	Diagnostic and Statistical Manual, fourth edition
E. coli	*Escherichia coli*
Ee.g.	Electroencephalogram
e.g.	*exempli gratia*, for example
EGF	Epidermal growth factor
EKG	Electrocardiography
ELISA	Enzyme-linked immunosorbent assay
EM	Electron microscopy, ultrastructure

EMG	Electromyography	**ICU**	Intensive care unit
ENT	Ears, nose, & throat, otorhino-laryngology	**IDDM**	Insulin-dependent diabetes mellitus
EPA	Environmental Protection Agency	**i.e.**	*id est*, that is (to say)
ER	Emergency room, emergency ward	**IFN**	Interferon
		Ig	Immunoglobulin
ERCP	Endoscopic retrograde cholangiography	**IL**	Interleukin
		IM	Intramuscular
ESR	Erythrocyte sedimentation rate	**ImPx**	Immunoperoxidase
ESRD	End-stage renal disease	**IQ**	Intelligence quotient
FDA	United States Food & Drug Administration	**IR**	Infrared
		ISH	In situ hybridization
FDP	Fibrinogen degradation product(s)	**ITP**	Idiopathic thrombocytopenic purpura
FISH	Fluorescence in situ hybridization	**IUD**	Intrauterine (contraceptive) device
FNA	Fine-needle aspiration (biopsy or cytology)	**IV**	Intravenous
FSH	Follicle-stimulating hormone	**JCAHO**	Joint Commission of Accredited Hospitals Organization
FUO	Fever of unknown origin	**K⁺**	Potassium
GABA	Gamma-aminobutyric acid	**kD**	Kilodalton
GC-MS	Gas chromatography-mass spectroscopy	**KS**	Kaposi sarcoma
		LDH	Lactate dehydrogenase
GFR	Glomerular filtration rate	**LDL**	Low-density lipoprotein
GGT	Gamma-glutamyl transferase	**LGV**	Lymphogranuloma venereum
GI	Gastrointestinal	**LH**	Luteinizing hormone
GM-CSF	Granulocyte-macrophage colony-stimulating factor	**LM**	Light microscopy
		LN	Lymph node
GMS	Gomori-methenamine-silver (a stain)	**MAOI**	Monoamine oxidase inhibitor
		MEN	Multiple endocrine neoplasia
GN	Glomerulonephritis	**MHC**	Major histocompatibility complex
GVHD	Graft-versus-host disease	**MI**	Myocardial infarction
HAV	Hepatitis A virus	**mo/ma**	Monocyte/macrophage (tissue histiocyte)
HBV	Hepatitis B virus		
hCG	Human chorionic gonadotropin	**min**	Minute (time)
HCV	Hepatitis C virus	**MPS**	Mucopolysaccharide(s), mucopolysaccharidosis
HDL	High-density lipoprotein		
H&E	Hematoxylin & eosin	**MRI**	Magnetic resonance imaging
HHV	Human herpesvirus (HHV-1, HHV-etc.)	**mRNA**	Messenger RNA (ribonucleic acid)
HIV	Human immunodeficiency virus	**MS**	Multiple sclerosis
HLA	Human leukocyte antigen (the major histocompatibility complex of humans)	**MVA**	Motor vehicle accident
		MW	Molecular weight
		Na⁺	Sodium
HMO	Health maintenance organization	**N/C ratio**	Nuclear/cytoplasmic ratio
HPLC	High-performance liquid chromatography	**N-CAM**	Neuronal-cell adhesion molecule
HPV	Human papillomavirus	**NGF**	Nerve growth factor
HSV	Herpes simplex virus	**NIH**	National Institutes of Health
HTLV-I	Human T cell leukemia/lymphoma virus, type 1	**NIDDM**	Non-insulin-dependent diabetes mellitus
HTLV-II	Human T cell leukemia/lymphoma virus, type 2	**NK cell**	Natural killer cell

NO	Nitric oxide
NSAID	Nonsteroidal anti-inflammatory drug
OR	Operating room, operating suite
OSHA	Occupational Safety and Health Administration
PAF	Platelet activating factor
PAS	Periodic acid-Schiff (a histologic stain)
PCP	*Pneumocystis carinii* pneumonia
PCR	Polymerase chain reaction
PDA	Patent ductus arteriosus
PG	Prostaglandin
PID	Pelvic inflammatory disease
PMN	Polymorphonuclear neutrophil or leukocyte, segmented neutrophil
ppb	Parts per billion
ppm	Parts per million
PT	Prothrombin time
PTE	Pulmonary thromboembolism
PTH	Parathyroid hormone
PTT	Partial thromboplastin time
QA	Quality assurance
QC	Quality control
RA	Rheumatoid arthritis
RBCs	Red blood cells, erythrocytes
RDS	Respiratory distress syndrome
REM sleep	Rapid eye movement sleep
RFLP	Restriction fragment length polymorphism
RIA	Radioimmunoassay
RR	Relative risk
rRNA	Ribosomal RNA (ribonucleic acid)
RSV	Respiratory syncytial virus
RT	Radiation therapy, reverse transcriptase
SD	Standard deviation
sec	Second (time)
SI	International System (of units)
SIDS	Sudden infant death syndrome
SLE	Systemic lupus erythematosus
STD	Sexually-transmitted disease
TAH-BSO	Total abdominal hysterectomy with bilateral salpingo-oophorectomy
TB	Tuberculosis
TDM	Therapeutic drug monitoring
TGF-β	Transforming growth factor-β
TIA	Transient ischemic attack
TIBC	Total iron-binding capacity
TLC	Thin-layer chromatography
TNF	Tumor necrosis factor
tRNA	Transfer RNA (ribonucleic acid)
T-S	Trimethoprim-sulfamethoxazole
TSH	Thyroid-stimulating hormone
TTP	Thrombotic thrombocytopenic purpura
TX	Thromboxane
U	1) Unit 2) University
UK	United Kingdom
URI	Upper respiratory tract infection
US	United States
UTI	Urinary tract infection
UV	Ultraviolet
VDRL	Venereal disease research laboratory (test) for syphilis
VIP	Vasoactive intestinal polypeptide
VLDL	Very low-density lipoprotein
V/Q	Ventilation/perfusion
vs	Versus, in contrast to, in comparison with
VSD	Ventricular septal defect
VZV	Varicella-zoster virus
WBCs	White blood cells, leukocytes
WHO	World Health Organization
X-R	X-linked recessive
<	Less than
<<<	Much less than
≤	Less than or equal to
>	More than
>>>	Much more than
≥	More than or equal to

INDEX

aspartate aminotransferase
41; gamma glutamyl
transferase 124; leucine
aminopeptidase 162
Liver function tests 362, 372
Liver panel 372
Liver-spleen scan 372
Load 373
Loading test 373
Locomotion index 373
Lombard (voice-reflex) test 373
Long-acting thyroid stimulator
373
Loop electrosurgical excision
procedure 161
Loop-o-gram 164
Lot 373
Low-density lipoprotein 161,
164
Low-grade squamous intraep-
ithelial lesion 347, 373
Lower GIseries 44
Lp(a) 372
LSIL 373
Lugol's solution 2, 78
Lumbar puncture 165
Lumpectomy 165
Lung
screening test 174
Lung cancer
small cell type 378
Lung panel 253
Lung profile 166
Lung testing
spirometry 287
Lung volumes 166
Lupus antibodies 32
Lupus anticoagulant 25, 31,
166
Lupus band test 373
Lupus erythematosus 31, 33,
80, 88, 161, 166, 208, 348,
366, 371
anti-double-stranded anti-
bodies 26; anti-histone
antibodies 28; anti-nuclear
antibodies 31; cardiolipin
antibodies 25; lupus antico-
agulants 166
Lupus inhibitor 166
Lupus test 373
Luteinizing hormone 167
Lyme disease 43, 167, 303
Lyme embryopathy 373
Lymphadenopathy 373
Lymphangiography 168
Lymphocyte 81–82, 373
Lymphocyte mitogen 383
Lymphocyte proliferation
test 182

Lymphocyte typing 169
Lymphocytotoxicity assay 169
Lymphokines 373
Lysozyme 169

- M -

M-mode display ultrasonogra-
phy 320
M-mode echocardiography
183
MAb 376
Macroglobulin 373
Macrophage 373
Macrophage migration
inhibition test 170
Magnesium 170
Magnetic resonance imaging
83, 184
Major crossmatch 171
Make-a-picture story 374
Malabsorption 101, 374
antigliadin antibodies 27
Malaria 172
Malignant 374
Malignant cell 374
Malignant melanoma 375,
389
Malnutrition 374
Malonate test 172
Mammography 147, 172
digital 355
Management test 374
Mandatory reporting 374
Manganese 173
Manic-depressive disease 163
Mantoux test 173
MAO 175
Marijuana 174
Mass spectrometry 374
Mass spectroscopy 374
Masson's trichrome stain 389
Match test 174
Maturation index 174
Maximum acid output 175
Maximum breathing capacity
175
Maximum expiratory flow rate
253
Maximum voluntary ventilation
175
MBP 189
MCH 81, 262
MCHC 176, 262
McMurray's test 374
MCV 81, 262
Mean cell (corpuscular) hemo-
globin 176
Mean cell hemoglobin concen-
tration 176

Mean cell volume 176
Mean corpuscular hemoglobin
262
Mean corpuscular volume 262
Measles 177
Mecholyl challenge 55
Meckel's diverticulum scan
374
Mediastinoscopy 177
Medical laboratory technician
374
Medical technologist 374
Medium 374
Medullary carcinoma of the
thyroid 60
Melanoma 375
Mercaptoethanol agglutination
inhibition test 178
Mercury 178
Messenger ribonucleic acid
375
Metabisulfite test 179
Metabolic acidosis 375
Metabolic alkalosis 375
Metabolic disease
amino acids 17
Metanephrines 179
Metastasis 375
Metastatic tumor cell 375
Methacholine provocation test
55
Methanol 179
Methemoglobin 38
Method of choice 375
Methotrexate 180
Methyl red test 375
Metyrapone test 180
MIC 375
Microbiology
diffusion test 23
Microbiology culture 43
Microhematuria 375
Microinvasive carcinoma 375
Microscopic hematuria 375
Microscopy 375
Migration inhibition assay 170
Milk intolerance 159
Millon clinical multiaxial inven-
tory (test) 375
Mills' test 375
Mini-mental test 181
Minimum bactericidal concen-
tration 375
Minimum inhibitory concentra-
tion 375
Minnesota Multiphasic
Personality Inventory 181
Mirror image biopsy 182
Mirror test 375
Miscall 375